Management of Lung Cancer in Older People

Cesare Gridelli • Riccardo A. Audisio
Editors

Riccardo A. Audisio
Series Editor

Management of Lung Cancer in Older People

Springer

SIOG
INTERNATIONAL SOCIETY
OF GERIATRIC ONCOLOGY

Editors
Cesare Gridelli, MD
Department of Oncology/Hematology
S.G. Moscati Hospital
Avellino
Italy

Riccardo A. Audisio, MD, FRCS
University of Liverpool
St Helens Teaching Hospital
St Helens
UK

Series Editor
Riccardo A. Audisio MD, FRCS
University of Liverpool
St Helens Teaching Hospital
St Helens
UK

ISBN 978-0-85729-792-1 ISBN 978-0-85729-793-8 (eBook)
DOI 10.1007/978-0-85729-793-8
Springer London Heidelberg New York Dordrecht

Library of Congress Control Number: 2013937329

Printed on acid-free paper

Springer is part of Springer Science+Business Media (www.springer.com)

Preface

Dramatic epidemiological changes are presently taking place in the western world as well as in rapidly developing countries such as China and India. These deep modifications in the distribution of malignant tumors impose a reassessment of our clinical practice. In the UK, 155,000 people aged >70 years are diagnosed with cancer every year. They represent 50% of all cancer diagnosis, and this number is expected to increase substantially over the next decades.

Cancer survival is poorer in senior patients than in the younger ones; numerous reasons have been taken into account to explain this phenomenon: delayed diagnosis, inaccurate staging, substandard treatment, and even patients' refusal. The common denominator is lack of knowledge: physicians are not entirely aware of how aggressive they can be in their treatment; patients are not adequately informed of the real risks of medical, surgical, and radiation management. This lack of knowledge is the result of the insufficient number of clinical investigations including older patients. When randomized clinical trials cannot be undertaken, good-quality epidemiological data should be made available to guide clinicians, patients, and their families.

The aim of this book is to provide a comprehensive collection of expert opinions on the important topic of lung cancer in older patients. An international panel of opinion leaders on this topic has generously contributed to this project. We would like to congratulate all contributors and acknowledge them for their time and efforts. The editors wish to acknowledge the enthusiastic editorial support of Margaret Burns and the Springer team.

Cesare Gridelli, MD
Riccardo A. Audisio, MD, FRCS

Contents

Contributors

Fiona H. Blackhall, PhD, FRCP Department of Medical Oncology, The Christie NHS Foundation Trust, Manchester, UK

Anna P. Britten, MRCP Department of Clinical Oncology, The Christie NHS Foundation Trust, Manchester, UK

Flavia Cantile, MD Department of Internal Medicine, Seconda Universita degli Studi di Napoli, Naples, Italy

Fortunato Ciardiello, MD, PhD Laboratory of Experimental Therapeutics, Division of Medical Oncology, Department of Clinical and Experimental Medicine, Second University of Naples, Naples, Italy

Rovel J. Colaco, FRCR Department of Clinical Oncology, The Christie NHS Foundation Trust, Manchester, UK

Dario Cova, MD Onco-Geriatric Unit, Department of Pharmacology, School of Clinical Pharmacology, University of Milan, Milan, Italy

Corinne Faivre-Finn, MD, PhD Department of Clinical Oncology, The Christie NHS Foundation Trust, Manchester, UK

Morena Fasano, MD Department of Internal Medicine, Seconda Universita degli Studi di Napoli, Naples, Italy

Enriqueta Felip, MD, PhD Oncology Department, Vall d'Hebron University Hospital, Barcelona, Spain

Domenico Galetta, MD, PhD Division of Thoracic Surgery, European Institute of Oncology, Milan, Italy

Nicolas Girard, MD, PhD Respiratory Medicine Department, Hôpital Louis Pradel, Lyon, France

Claude Bernard University, Lyon, France

Cesare Gridelli, MD Department of Oncology/Hematology, S.G. Moscati Hospital, Avellino, Italy

Michael P. W. Grocott, MD, FRCA, FRCP, FFICM Department of Anaesthesia and Critical Care, University of Southampton NHS Foundation Trust, Southampton, UK

Sandy Jack, MSc, PhD Department of Musculoskeletal Biology II, Institute of Ageing and Chronic Disease, University Hospital Aintree NHS Trust, Liverpool, UK

Michael T. Jaklitsch, MD Department of Surgery, Harvard Medical School, Boston, MA, USA

Maryska L.G. Janssen-Heijnen, PhD Department of Clinical Epidemiology, VieCuri Medical Centre, Venlo, The Netherlands

Siri Rostoft Kristjansson, MD, PhD Department of Internal Medicine, Diakonhjemmet Hospital, Oslo, Norway

Silvana Leo, MD Division of Medical Oncology, Department of Geriatric Oncology, Vito Fazzi Hospital, Lecce, Italy

Paolo Maione, MD Division of Medical Oncology, S.G. Moscati Hospital, Avellino, Italy

Floriana Morgillo, MD, PhD Department of Internal Medicine, Seconda Universita degli Studi di Napoli, Naples, Italy

Françoise Mornex, MD, PhD Radiation Oncology Department, Centre Hospitalier Lyon Sud, Lyon, France

Alejandro Navarro, MD Oncology Department, Vall d'Hebron University Hospital, Barcelona, Spain

Lazzaro Repetto, MD, PhD Oncology Unit, Istituto Nazionale Ricovero e Cura Anziani, INRCA-IRCCS, Rome, Italy

Antonio Rossi, MD Division of Medical Oncology, S.G. Moscati Hospital, Avellino, Italy

Weston Sacco, BS Tulane University, New Orleans, LA, USA

Steven E. Schild, MD Department of Radiation Oncology, Mayo Clinic, Scottsdale, AZ, USA

Suresh Senan, PhD, FRCR, MRCP Department of Radiation Oncology, VU University Medical Center, Amsterdam, The Netherlands

Frances A. Shepherd, MD, FRCPC Department of Medical Oncology and Hematology, Princess Margaret Hospital, Toronto, ON, Canada

Lorenzo Spaggiari, MD, PhD Division of Thoracic Surgery, European Institute of Oncology, Milan, Italy

University of Milan, School of Medicine, Milan, Italy

Naomi E. Verstegen, BSc Department of Radiation Oncology, VU University Medical Center, Amsterdam, The Netherlands

Paul P. Walker, BMedSci (Hons), MD, FRCP Department of Respiratory Medicine, University Hospital Aintree, Liverpool, UK

Malcolm West, MD, MRCS(Ed) Musculoskeletal Biology II, University Hospital Aintree NHS Foundation Trust, Liverpool, UK

Paul Wheatley-Price, BSc, MBChB, MRCP (UK), MD Division of Medical Oncology, Department of Medicine, Ottawa Hospital, Ottawa Hospital Cancer Centre, Ottawa, ON, Canada

Part I
Background and Epidemiology

Chapter 1
Basic Science of Lung Cancer in Older Patients

Morena Fasano, Flavia Cantile, Floriana Morgillo, and Fortunato Ciardiello

Abstract Lung cancer is the leading cause of cancer-related mortality in both men and women, with about 1.61 million new diagnoses and 1.38 million deaths worldwide in 2008. Non-small cell lung cancer (NSCLC), including squamous carcinoma, adenocarcinoma, and undifferentiated large cell carcinoma, accounts for more than 80 % of new lung cancer diagnoses. Unfortunately, at the time of diagnosis, the majority of patients have advanced disease, for which a systemic, palliative treatment is the primary therapeutic option. Considering that 47 % of all lung cancers are diagnosed in patients older than 70 years (14 % in patients older than 80 years), advanced NSCLC in elderly patients is an increasingly common problem, which the practitioner of oncology must face. The relationship between aging and cancer is not clear; considerable controversy surrounds the mechanisms that lead to increased incidence of cancer in the aged. It is worthy to note that frequencies of specific cancers are age-specific.

Keyword Lung cancer • Non-small cell lung cancer • Squamous carcinoma • Adenocarcinoma • Undifferentiated large cell carcinoma • Age-specific cancer • Elderly patients

M. Fasano, MD • F. Cantile, MD • F. Morgillo, MD, PhD
Department of Internal Medicine, Seconda Universita degli Studi di Napoli, Naples, Italy

F. Ciardiello, MD, PhD (✉)
Laboratory of Experimental Therapeutics, Division of Medical Oncology, Department of Clinical and Experimental Medicine, Second University of Naples, Naples, Italy
e-mail: fortunato.ciardiello@unina2.it

C. Gridelli, R.A. Audisio (eds.), *Management of Lung Cancer in Older People*, DOI 10.1007/978-0-85729-793-8_1, © Springer-Verlag London 2013

Lung cancer is the leading cause of cancer-related mortality in both men and women [1], with about 1.61 million new diagnoses and 1.38 million deaths worldwide in 2008 [2, 3]. Non-small cell lung cancer (NSCLC), including squamous carcinoma, adenocarcinoma, and undifferentiated large cell carcinoma, accounts for more than 80 % of new lung cancer diagnoses. Unfortunately, at the time of diagnosis, the majority of patients have advanced disease, for which a systemic, palliative treatment is the primary therapeutic option. Considering that 47 % of all lung cancers are diagnosed in patients older than 70 years (14 % in patients older than 80 years) [4], advanced NSCLC in elderly patients is an increasingly common problem, which the practitioner of oncology must face. Establishing the exact age, i.e., the biological age, is still difficult nowadays due to the lack of adequate laboratory tests and tools. Thus, the chronological age is the only indicator we have in defining the elderly, and 70 years may be the most appropriate boundary because the incidence of age-related changes starts to increase after this cutoff age [5]. Important concerns in evaluating the treatment of elderly patients are the presence of comorbidities and the progressive physiologic reduction of hepatic, renal, and bone marrow functions, which could have a negative impact on the degree of toxicity.

The relationship between aging and cancer is not clear; considerable controversy surrounds the mechanisms that lead to increased incidence of cancer in the aged. It is worthy to note that frequencies of specific cancers are age-specific [6, 7].

Cancer and Age

Three major hypotheses have been proposed to explain the association of cancer and age. The first hypothesis holds this association is a consequence of the duration of carcinogenesis. In other words, the sequential carcinogenic steps that are required for the neoplastic transformation of normal tissues develop over several years, and cancer is more likely to become manifest in older individuals by a process of natural selection [8, 9]. In an article entitled "There is no such thing as aging, and cancer is not related to it," Peto et al. [9] have proposed that the high prevalence of cancer in older individuals simply reflects a more prolonged exposure to carcinogens. In the estimate of these authors, the incidence of cancer is a power function of the duration of carcinogen exposure, rather than a power function of the tumor-host age.

The second hypothesis proposes that age-related progressive changes in the internal milieu of the organism may provide an increasingly favorable environment for the initiation of new neoplasms and for the growth of already existent, but latent, malignant cells [10–18]. These mechanisms may also include proliferate senescence, as the senescent cells lose the ability to undergo apoptosis [19–21] and, as it has been suggested, produce multiple factors, which act together, to stimulate epithelial cells with oncogenic mutations [22]. Specific potential soluble mediators of age-dependent changes in stromal-epithelial cell interaction are cytokine interleukin-1, transforming growth factor-b, keratinocyte growth factor, hepatocyte growth factor, and pigmented epithelium-derived factor/early population doubling clone-1 (PEDF/EPC-1), a member of the serine protease inhibitor family [23]. The third hypothesis proposes that the cancer-prone phenotype of older humans might reflect the combined effects of cumulative mutational load, increased epigenetic gene silencing, telomere dysfunction, and altered stromal milieu [16]. DePinho [16] stressed that telomere dysfunction might be leading among of several mechanisms driving epithelial carcinogenesis as humans advance in age. His telomeric instability model of epithelial carcinogenesis fits well with what is known about the timing of telomerase activation and evolving genomic changes during various stages of multistage process of carcinogenesis in humans, in particular those of the breast and colon. The elucidation of causes of an accelerated increase in cancer incidence may be the key to a strategy for primary cancer prevention.

Lung Cancer and Age

Lung carcinogenesis in older patients is a complex, multistep process that involves the acquisition of genetic mutations and epigenetic changes that alter cellular processes, such as proliferation, differentiation, invasion, and metastasis. For example, the concept of *field of cancerization* refers to areas of histologically normal-appearing tissue adjacent to neoplastic lesions that display molecular abnormalities, some of which are the same as those in the tumors [24, 25]. Several studies, using cytologic and molecular techniques, have established that cigarette smoking creates injury in all airway epithelial cells exposed to the cigarette smoke [25]. In addition, modulation of global gene expression in the normal bronchial epithelium in healthy smokers is similar in the large and small airways, and the smoking-induced alterations are mirrored in the epithelia of the main stem bronchus, buccal, and nasal cavities [26–30]. Auerbach and colleagues first described the observation of cellular atypia throughout the airways of smokers at autopsy [31], indicating that the cellular injury produced by smoking involves the whole respiratory tract. In the initial phase, injury leads to dysregulated repair by stem/progenitor cells, which form a clonal group of indefinitely self-renewing daughter cells. Additional genetic and epigenetic alterations result in proliferation of these cells and expansion of the field, gradually displacing the normal epithelium. Development of an expanding premalignant field appears to be a critical step in lung carcinogenesis that can persist even after smoking cessation. Also KRAS and epidermal growth factor receptor (EGFR) mutations have been described in nonmalignant histologically normal-appearing lung tissue adjacent to lung tumors [32–34]. More recently, global messenger RNA (mRNA) and microRNA (miRNA) expression profiles have been described in the normal-appearing bronchial epithelium of healthy smokers [35, 36]. It has also been shown that gene expression profiles in the cytologically normal bronchial airway epithelium can predict, with high sensitivity and specificity, the presence of lung cancer in current or former smokers being evaluated for clinical suspicion of lung cancer [37].

However, both carcinogenesis and aging are associated with genomic alterations, which may act synergistically in causing cancer [38–42]. In particular, three recently described age-related changes in DNA metabolism may favor lung cell transformation and cancer growth. These changes are genetic instability, DNA hypomethylation, and formation of DNA adducts. Genetic instability involves activation of genes that are normally suppressed, such as the cellular proto-oncogenes, and/or inactivation of some tumor suppression genes (p53, Rb, etc.) [38, 43]. DNA hypomethylation is characteristic of aging as well as of transformed cells. Hypomethylation, a potential mechanism of oncogene activation, may result in spontaneous deamination of cytosine and consequent base transition, i.e., substitution of the pair thymine to adenine. Accumulation of inappropriate base pairs may cause cell transformation by activation of cellular proto-oncogenes [38]. Age-related abnormalities of DNA metabolism may be, to some extent, tissue- and gene-specific. Within the same cell, different DNA segments express different degrees of age-related hypomethylation.

The uneven distribution of hypomethylation may underlie selective overexpression of proto-oncogenes by senescent cells. The different extent of DNA abnormalities among aging tissues may account in part for the different susceptibility of these tissues to carcinogens [39, 44].

There is evidence of an age-related accumulation of spontaneous mutations in somatic and germ cells [41]. Accumulation with age of some spontaneous mutations or mutations evoked by endogenous mutagens can induce genome instability and, hence, increase the sensitivity to carcinogens and/or tumor promoters. It has been shown that clonally expanded DNA mutations accumulate with age in normal human tissues as well as in human tumors [45–47].

In addition, miRNAs, i.e., small, noncoding RNA molecules, play important roles in the epigenetic control of diverse cellular processes by altering the translation of proteins from mRNAs. miRNAs are important transcriptional regulators of gene expression, involved in many physiological and pathological processes, such as proliferation, differentiation, death, and stress resistance, by altering levels of gene expression [48]. A single miRNA can target many different mRNAs, and an mRNA can be targeted by multiple miRNAs, thereby creating a complex network of molecular pathways in cells. Downregulation of miRNAs is commonly observed in human cancers and has been linked mechanistically to promotion of cellular transformation and tumorigenesis. More than 50 % of miRNA genes are located in cancer-associated genomic regions or in fragile sites, frequently amplified or deleted in human cancer, resulting in frequent copy number alterations, suggesting that differences in miRNA expression may be induced by genomic alterations. The multiple targets of each miRNA, in addition to the regulatory effects of many noncoding RNAs other than miRNAs, result in extremely complex regulatory networks present in normal and cancer cells.

Carcinogenesis is a multistage process: neoplastic transformation implies the engagement of a cell through sequential stages, and different agents may affect the transition between continuous stages [49–54]. Multistage carcinogenesis is accompanied by disturbances in tissue homeostasis and perturbations in nervous, hormonal, and metabolic factors which may affect antitumor resistance. The development of these changes depends on the susceptibility of various systems to a carcinogen and on the dose of the carcinogen. Changes in the microenvironment may condition key carcinogenic events and determine the duration of each carcinogenic stage, and sometimes they may even reverse the process of carcinogenesis. These microenvironmental changes influence the proliferation rate of transformed cells together, the total duration of carcinogenesis, and, consequently, the latent period of tumor development. Cross talk between mesenchyme and epithelium has been described as a known driver of differentiation and development [55, 56]. There is increasing evidence that age-related changes in tumor microenvironment might play a significant role. In some experiments, cells of rat rhabdomyosarcoma RA-2 selected for affinity to lung tissue were intravenously inoculated into rats of different ages [57]. It was observed that the number of lung tumor colonies was highest in 1- and 15-month-old animals and lowest in 3- and 12-month-old animals. A positive correlation was found between the number of tumor lung colonies and somatomedin (IGF-I) activity in the lung. In another experiment, RA-2 cells from a 3-month-old donor were inoculated into 2- or 21-month-old recipients and 3 weeks later were separately taken from young and old hosts and transplanted into 3-month-old recipients. The number of lung colonies was significantly decreased in 3-month-old recipients injected with RA-2 cell passed via old host [58]. The results obtained suggest the critical role of host and donor microenvironment in lung colony forming potential of RA-2 cells.

Free Radical Theory of Aging

One of the most advanced theories of aging is free radical theory proposed by in 1956 by Harman [59–61]. This theory postulated that various oxidative reactions occurring in the organism (mainly in mitochondria) generate free radicals as by-product which cause multiple lesions in macromolecules (nucleic acids, proteins, and lipids), leading to their damage and aging. This theory explains not only the mechanism of aging but also a wide variety of age-associated pathology, including cancer [60–65].

The damage caused by endogenous oxygen radicals has been proposed as a major contributor to both aging and cancer. Endogenous oxidative damage to lipids and proteins increases with age [66–68]. It was shown that oxygen free radicals may induce active mutations of the human c-H-ras proto-oncogene [69]. A variety of cellular defense systems are involved in protecting cellular macromolecules against devastating action of oxygen-based radicals. These systems include antioxidant enzymes (Cu, Zn- superoxide dismutase (SOD), manganese-containing SOD, catalase, glutathione peroxidase, glutathione reductase, glucose-6-phosphate dehydrogenase), some vitamins (atocopherol, ascorbic acid), uric acid, and the pineal indole hormone melatonin [59, 60, 70, 71].

The recent evidence suggests that key mechanisms of both aging and cancer are linked via endogenous stress-induced DNA damage caused by reactive oxygen species. They include oxidative nuclear and mitochondrial DNA damage and repair, the telomere shortening, and telomere-driven cellular senescence and have been intensively discussed in a number of comprehensive reviews [61–65, 72–74]. It is worthy to note that some other aspects of the relationships between aging and cancer, e.g., chemically and radiation-induced carcinogenesis, also are critically involved the free radical processes.

Inflammation and Immunosuppression

Two other conditions related to the increased risk of developing lung cancer in elderly patients are inflammation and immunosuppression. Chronic inflammation in numerous organ sites increases the risk for cancer development [75]. The link between inflammation and lung carcinogenesis is well established [76, 77]. Several changes in the airways are associated with chronic inflammation, in particular in older patients. Inflammation of the airway targets the epithelium for injury, which further drives an abnormal inflammatory response. In addition, immunosuppression may contribute to lung carcinogenesis by allowing lung cancer cells to escape immune surveillance. Tumor cells may contribute to immunosuppression by releasing suppressive cytokines, augmenting the trafficking of suppressor cells to the tumor site, and/or promoting differentiation of effector lymphocytes to a T-regulatory cell phenotype. One major impediment to effective therapy is our inadequate understanding of how lung cancer cells escape immune surveillance and inhibit antitumor immunity. In previous studies, an immune suppressive network in NSCLC that is due to overexpression of tumor COX-2 has been defined. COX-2 metabolites have been identified as mediators of immunosuppression. PGE2 promotes the CD4þCD25þT regulatory phenotype and increases the expression of the forkhead transcription factor FOXP3 that is known to program the development and function of T-regulatory cells [78, 79].

Conclusions

The relation between cancer and age is still not fully elucidated. Three major hypotheses and non-mutually exclusive hypotheses may explain the association of cancer and age:

- Carcinogenesis is a time-consuming process, whose final product, cancer, is more likely to occur in person of advanced age depending on accumulation of the dose to the environmental carcinogen(s).
- Aging tissues undergo molecular changes that parallel early carcinogenic changes and prime these tissues to the effects of carcinogens.
- Age-related changes in body microenvironment, including proliferative and immune senescence, may favor cancer development and growth.

Increased susceptibility to the effects of tumor promoters has been found both in aged animals and aged humans, as predicted by the multistage model of carcinogenesis. Old animals should be included in standard protocol for the long-term assay for carcinogenicity, in particular, of compounds with suggested tumor-promoting activity. Strategies for cancer prevention must include not only measures to minimize exposure to exogenous carcinogenic agents but also measures to normalize the age-related alterations in internal milieu.

References

1. Parkin DM, Bray F, Ferlay J, et al. Global cancer statistics. CA Cancer J Clin. 2005;55: 74–108.
2. Owonikoko TK, Ragin CC, Belani CP, et al. Lung cancer in elderly patients: an analysis of the surveillance, epidemiology, and end results database. J Clin Oncol. 2007;25:5570–7.
3. Wingo PA, Cardinez CJ, Landis SH, et al. Long term trends in cancer mortality in the United States. Cancer. 2003;97:3133–275.
4. Gridelli C, Perrone F, Monfardini S, et al. Lung cancer in the elderly. Eur J Cancer. 1997; 33(14):2313–4.
5. Havlik RJ, Yancik R, Long S, et al. The National Institute on Aging and the National Cancer Institute SEER collaborative study on comorbidity and early diagnosis of cancer in the elderly. Cancer. 1994;74(Suppl):2101–6.
6. Dix D, Cohen P. On the role of aging in carcinogenesis. Anticancer Res. 1999;19:723–6.
7. Parkin DM, Bray FI, Devesa S. Cancer burden in the year 2000. The global picture. Eur J Cancer. 2001;37:S4–66.
8. Peto R, Roe FJC, Lee PN, Levy L, Clack J. Cancer and ageing in mice and men. Br J Cancer. 1975;32:411–26.
9. Peto R, Parish SE, Gray RG. There is no such thing as ageing, and cancer is not related to it. In: Likhachev A, Anisimov V, Montesano R, editors. Age-related factors in carcinogenesis, vol. 58. Lyon: IARC; 1985. p. 43–53.
10. Anisimov VN. Carcinogenesis and aging. Adv Cancer Res. 1983;40:265–324.
11. Anisimov VN. Carcinogenesis and aging, vol. 1, 2. Boca Raton: CRC Press; 1987.
12. Anisimov VN. Age-related mechanisms of susceptibility to carcinogenesis. Semin Oncol. 1989;16:10–9.
13. Dilman VM. Development, aging, and disease. A new rationale for and intervention strategy. Chur: Harwood Acad Publ; 1994.
14. Simpson AJG. A natural somatic mutation frequency and human carcinogenesis. Adv Cancer Res. 1997;71:209–40.
15. Anisimov VN. Age as a factor of risk in multistage carcinogenesis. In: Balducci L, Lyman GH, Ershler WB, editors. Comprehensive geriatric oncology. Amsterdam: Harwood Academic Publishers; 1998. p. 157–78.
16. DePinho RA. The age of cancer. Nature. 2000;408:248–54.
17. Fernandez-Pol JA, Douglas MG. Molecular interactions of cancer and age. Hematol Oncol Clin North Am. 2000;14:25–44.
18. Rubin H. Selected cell and selective microenvironment in neoplastic development. Cancer Res. 2001;61:799–807.
19. Campisi J. Aging and cancer: the double-edged sword or replicative senescence. J Am Geriatr Soc. 1997;45:1–6.
20. Campisi J. Cancer, aging, and cellular senescence. In Vivo. 2000;14:183–8.

21. Campisi J, Kirn S, Lim CS, Rubio M. Cellular senescence, cancer and aging: the telomere connection. Exp Gerontol. 2001;36:1619–37.
22. Krtolica A, Parincllo S, Lockett S, Desprez P-Y, Campisi J. Senescent fibroblasts promote epithelial cell growth and tumorigenesis: a link between cancer and aging. Proc Natl Acad Sci USA. 2001;98:12072–7.
23. Rinehart CA, Torti VR. Aging and cancer: the role of stromal interactions with epithelial cells. Mol Carcinog. 1997;18:187–92.
24. Dakubo GD, Jakupciak JP, Birch-Machin MA, Parr RL. Clinical implications and utility of field cancerization. Cancer Cell Int. 2007;7:2.
25. Slaughter DP, Southwick HW, Smejkal W. Field cancerization in oral stratified squamous epithelium; clinical implications of multicentric origin. Cancer. 1953;6(5):963–8.
26. Steiling K, Ryan J, Brody JS, Spira A. The field of tissue injury in the lung and airway. Cancer Prev Res (Phila). 2008;1(6):396–403.
27. Wistuba II, Lam S, Behrens C, et al. Molecular damage in the bronchial epithelium of current and former smokers. J Natl Cancer Inst. 1997;89(18):1366–73.
28. Powell CA, Klares S, O'Connor G, Brody JS. Loss of heterozygosity in epithelial cells obtained by bronchial brushing: clinical utility in lung cancer. Clin Cancer Res. 1999;5(8):2025–34.
29. Bhutani M, Pathak AK, Fan YH, et al. Oral epithelium as a surrogate tissue for assessing smoking-induced molecular alterations in the lungs. Cancer Prev Res (Phila). 2008;1(1):39–44.
30. Sridhar S, Schembri F, Zeskind J, et al. Smoking-induced gene expression changes in the bronchial airway are reflected in nasal and buccal epithelium. BMC Genomics. 2008;9:259.
31. Auerbach O, Hammond EC, Kirman D, Garfinkel L. Effects of cigarette smoking on dogs, II: pulmonary neoplasms. Arch Environ Health. 1970;21(6):754–68.
32. Nelson MA, Wymer J, Clements Jr N. Detection of K-ras gene mutations in non-neoplastic lung tissue and lung cancers. Cancer Lett. 1996;103(1):115–21.
33. Tang X, Shigematsu H, Bekele BN, et al. EGFR tyrosine kinase domain mutations are detected in histologically normal respiratory epithelium in lung cancer patients. Cancer Res. 2005;65(17):7568–72.
34. Tang X, Varella-Garcia M, Xavier AC, et al. Epidermal growth factor receptor abnormalities in the pathogenesis and progression of lung adenocarcinomas. Cancer Prev Res (Phila). 2008;1(3):192–200.
35. Hackett NR, Heguy A, Harvey BG, et al. Variability of antioxidant-related gene expression in the airway epithelium of cigarette smokers. Am J Respir Cell Mol Biol. 2003;29(3 Pt 1):331–43.
36. Spira A, Beane J, Shah V, et al. Effects of cigarette smoke on the human airway epithelial cell transcriptome. Proc Natl Acad Sci USA. 2004;101(27):10143–8.
37. Spira A, Beane JE, Shah V, et al. Airway epithelial gene expression in the diagnostic evaluation of smokers with suspect lung cancer. Nat Med. 2007;13(3):361–6.
38. Hanahan D, Weinberg RA. The hallmarks of cancer. Cell. 2000;100:57–70.
39. Lindahl T. Instability and decay of the primary structure of DNA. Nature. 1993;362:709–15.
40. Pitot HC. The molecular biology of carcinogenesis. Cancer. 1993;72:962–70.
41. Vijg J. Somatic mutations and aging: a re-evaluation. Mutat Res. 2000;447:117–35.
42. Luzatto L. The mechanisms of neoplastic transformation. Eur J Cancer. 2001;37:S114–7.
43. Kinzler KW, Vogelstein B. Gatekeepers and caretakers. Nature. 1997;386:761–3.
44. Catania J, Fairweather DS. DNA methylation and cellular aging. Mutat Res. 1991;256:283–93.
45. Coller HA, Khrapko K, Bodyak ND, et al. High frequency of homoplasmic mitochondrial DNA mutations in human tumors can be explained without selection. Nat Genet. 2001;28:147–50.
46. Coller HA, Bodyak ND, Khrapko K. Frequent intracellular clonal expansions of somatic mtDNA mutations. Ann N Y Acad Sci. 2002;959:434–47.
47. Nekhaeva E, Bodyak ND, Kraytsberg Y, et al. Clonally expanded mtDNA point mutations are abundant in individual cells of human tissues. Proc Natl Acad Sci USA. 2002;99:5521–6.

48. Ambros V. MicroRNA pathways in flies and worms: growth, death, fat, stress, and timing. Cell. 2003;113(6):673–6.
49. Vanio H, Magee PN, McGregor D, McMichael AJ, editors. Mechanisms of carcinogenesis in risk identification. IARC science publication number 116. Lyon: IARC;1992. p. 9–56.
50. Moolgavkar S, Krewski D, Zeise L, et al., editors. Quantitative estimation and prediction of human cancer risk, IARC science publication number 131. Lyon: IARC; 1999.
51. Simons JW. Genetic, epigenetic, dysgenetic and non-genetic mechanisms in tumorigenesis. II. Further delineation of the rate limiting step. Anticancer Res. 1999;19:4781–9.
52. Ponten J. Cell biology of precancer. Eur J Cancer. 2001;37:S97–113.
53. Reya T, Morrison SJ, Clarke MF, Weissman IL. Stem cells, cancer, and cancer stem cells. Nature. 2001;414:105–11.
54. Schlessinger D, Van Zant G. Does functional depletion of stem cells drive aging. Mech Ageing Dev. 2001;122:1537–53.
55. Aboseif S, El-Sakka A, Young P, Cunha G. Mesenchymal reprogramming of adult human epithelial differentiation. Differentiation. 1999;65:113–8.
56. Liotta LA, Kohn EC. The microenvironment of the tumor-host interface. Nature. 2001;411:375–9.
57. Anisimov VN, Zhukovskaya NV, Loktionov AS, et al. Influence of host age on lung colony forming capacity of injected rat rhabdomyosarcoma cells. Cancer Lett. 1988;40:77–82.
58. Anisimov VN, Zhukovskaya NV, Loktionov AS, et al. Host and donor age dependency of colony forming capacity of lung-affine rat rhabdomyosarcoma RA-2 cells. In: Abstract of the international conference on tumor micro environment: progression, therapy and prevention. Israel: Tiberias; 1995. p. 6.
59. Harman D. Free-radical theory of aging: increasing the functional life span. Ann N Y Acad Sci. 1994;717:257–66.
60. Harman DH. Extending functional life span. Exp Gerontol. 1998;33:95–112.
61. Hamilton ML, Van Remmen H, Drake JA, et al. Does oxidative damage to DNA increase with age. Proc Natl Acad Sci USA. 2001;98:10469–74.
62. Skulachev VP. The programmed death phenomena, aging, and the Samurai law of biology. Exp Gerontol. 2001;36:995–1024.
63. Kawanishi S, Hiraki Y, Oikawa S. Mechanism of guanine-specific DNA damage by oxidative stress and its role in carcinogenesis and aging. Mutat Res. 2001;488:65–76.
64. Salvioli S, Bonafe M, Capri M, Monti D, Fransceschi C. Mitochondria, aging and longevity–a new perspective. FEBS Lett. 2001;492:9–13.
65. von Zglinicki T, Burkle A, Kirkwood TBL. Stress, DNA damage and aging-an integrative approach. Exp Gerontol. 2001;36:1049–62.
66. Yu BP, editor. Free radicals in aging. Boca Raton: CRC Press; 1993.
67. Shigenaga MK, Hagen TV, Ames BN. Oxidative damage and mitochondrial decay in aging. Proc Natl Acad Sci USA. 1994;91:10771–8.
68. Barja G. Endogenous oxidative stress: relation to aging, longevity and caloric restriction. Ageing Res Rev. 2002;1:397–411.
69. Du MQ, Carmichael PL, Phillips DH. Induction of activated mutations in the human c-Ha-ras proto-oncogene by oxygen free radicals. Mol Carcinog. 1994;11:170–5.
70. Ames BN, Shigenaga MB, Hagen TM. Oxidants, antioxidants, and the degenerative diseases of aging. Proc Natl Acad Sci USA. 1993;90:7915–22.
71. Reiter RJ. Reactive oxygen species, DNA damage, and carcinogenesis: intervention with melatonin. In: Bartsch C, Bartsch H, Blask DE, Cardinali DP, Hrushesky WJM, Mecke D, editors. The pineal gland and cancer neuroimmunoendocrine mechanisms in malignancy. Berlin: Springer; 2001. p. 442–55.
72. Saretzki G, Sitte N, Merkel U, Wurm RE. Telomere shortening triggers a p53-dependent cell cycle arrest via accumulation of Grich single stranded DNA fragments. Oncogene. 1999; 18:5148–58.
73. von Zglinicki T, Pilger R, Sitte N. Accumulation of single-strand breaks is the major cause of telomere shortening in human fibroblasts. Free Radic Biol Med. 2000;28:64–74.

74. Proctor CJ, Kikwood TBL. Modelling telomere shortening and the role of oxidative stress. Mech Ageing Dev. 2002;123:351–6.
75. Colotta F, Allavena P, Sica A, et al. Cancer-related inflammation, the seventh hallmark of cancer: links to genetic instability. Carcinogenesis. 2009;30(7):1073–81.
76. Brody JS, Spira A. State of the art: chronic obstructive pulmonary disease, inflammation, and lung cancer. Proc Am Thorac Soc. 2006;3(6):535–7.
77. Smith CJ, Perfetti TA, King JA. Perspectives on pulmonary inflammation and lung cancer risk in cigarette smokers. Inhal Toxicol. 2006;18(9):667–77.
78. Baratelli F, Lin Y, Zhu L, et al. Prostaglandin E2 induces FOXP3 gene expression and T regulatory cell function in human CD4þT cells. J Immunol. 2005;175(3):1483–90.
79. Gavin MA, Rasmussen JP, Fontenot JD, et al. Foxp3- dependent programme of regulatory T-cell differentiation. Nature. 2007;445(7129):771–5.

Chapter 2
Clinical Epidemiology and the Impact of Comorbidity on Treatment and Outcome

Maryska L.G. Janssen-Heijnen

Abstract In the beginning of the twentieth century lung cancer was a very rare disease, but rates have increased so dramatically that lung cancer can be considered one of the major epidemics of the twentieth century. Currently, lung cancer is still number one cause of death among cancer deaths. Over fifty percent of all newly diagnosed lung cancer patients are aged over 65 years at the time of lung cancer diagnosis, and about 30% are aged over 70. Since lung cancer is a disease that mainly occurs in elderly and smoking is the most important risk factor, many patients have (smoking-related) comorbidity at the time of lung cancer diagnosis. This may complicate the management of lung cancer in elderly patients. Elderly receive standard treatment less often, although standard treatment has a positive effect on prognosis of lung cancer, even after adjustment for differences in age and comorbidity. However, complications of treatment among elderly patients are very common, despite a strict selection of the fittest elderly for standard treatment. In elderly, the impact of toxicities on quality-of-life may be just as important as the prolongation of life expectancy. A proper selection of patients fit enough for surgery, chemotherapy and/or radiotherapy is therefore important and there is an urgent need for predictive models for treatment tolerance that can be easily used in everyday clinical practice.

Keywords Lung cancer • Comorbidity and lung cancer • Elderly lung cancer patients • Non-small cell lung cancer • Small cell lung cancer • Survival in elderly lung cancer patients

---

M.L.G. Janssen-Heijnen, PhD
Department of Clinical Epidemiology, VieCuri Medical Centre,
Tegelseweg 210, Venlo 5912 BL, The Netherlands
e-mail: mjanssenheijnen@viecuri.nl

C. Gridelli, R.A. Audisio (eds.), *Management of Lung Cancer in Older People*,
DOI 10.1007/978-0-85729-793-8_2, © Springer-Verlag London 2013

Trends in Incidence and Mortality of Lung Cancer

In the beginning of the twentieth century, lung cancer was a very rare disease, but rates have increased so dramatically that lung cancer can be considered one of the major epidemics of the twentieth century. Currently, lung cancer is still number one cause of death among cancer deaths (www.globocan.iarc.fr) [1].

Incidence and mortality rates for lung cancer have changed markedly over the past five decades [2]. In North America, Australia, New Zealand, and most countries of northwestern Europe, the age-standardized rate for men has increased markedly up to the 1970s or 1980s and then started to decline, first among middle-aged men and later in the older age groups [3–11]. In southern and eastern Europe, the incidence of lung cancer among men has increased up to the late 1980s or even up to the late 1990s [2, 12]. In Latin America, Africa, and Asia, lung cancer mortality has been increasing, except for Cuba, Argentina, Paraguay, and Peru [13–15]. Among women, the incidence of lung cancer (being much lower than that for men) started to increase later and is still on the rise in most countries. Dramatic increases have been seen in North America, Iceland, Ireland, the UK, and Denmark but also in the Netherlands and Hungary [3, 8, 11, 16]. Female lung cancer rates were also relatively high in Norway and Sweden, both countries with relatively low rates among males, and have been increasing over time [3]. In some countries (USA, Cuba, Argentina, Paraguay, Peru, Ireland, the United Kingdom, Hong Kong, Singapore, and Japan), the rates among women have already leveled off [3, 13, 17]. In the Netherlands and the USA, lung cancer incidence rates for females have started to decline among younger patients but are still increasing among the elderly (www.seer.cancer.gov and www.globocan.iarc.fr) [16].

Of all men aged 65–74 years and diagnosed with cancer, 15–20 % are diagnosed with lung cancer; among women this is 10–20 % (www.seer.cancer.gov). Among male cancer patients aged 75 or older, about 15 % have lung cancer; among women this is 10–15 %. Fifty percent of all newly diagnosed lung cancer patients in the USA were aged over 65 years at the time of lung cancer diagnosis, and 30 % were aged over 70 (www.seer.cancer.gov), and more than two thirds of patients dying of lung cancer in the USA were aged over 65 years [18].

Classification of Lung Cancer

Lung cancer is commonly classified as small cell carcinoma (SCLC, about 15 %) and non-small cell carcinoma (NSCLC, about 85 %). The latter includes squamous cell carcinoma, adenocarcinoma, large cell undifferentiated carcinoma, and some rare subtypes, such as adenosquamous cell carcinoma, mucoepidermoid carcinoma, and adenoid cystic carcinoma. Large cell undifferentiated carcinoma has frequently been called a "wastebasket" or nonentity, because the carcinomas are so poorly differentiated that squamous or glandular differentiation is no longer evident at the light microscopic level. Thus, the incidence of this histological subtype varies with the criteria used to classify the other forms of NSCLC. Squamous cell carcinoma used to be the most frequent type of lung cancer, but there has been a shift from squamous cell carcinoma to adenocarcinoma, first among younger age groups [10, 19–21]. This can probably be explained by a trend toward smoking filter cigarettes [21]. Among Dutch patients with SCLC, the proportion aged 75 or older has increased from 15 % in 2001–2003 to 18 % in 2007–2009; among those with NSCLC, the proportion aged 75+ has increased from 19 to 24 % (source: www.nkr.nl).

Risk Factors for Lung Cancer

Many studies have indicated that smoking tobacco is the main cause of lung cancer with a latency time between the start of smoking and lung cancer of 15–50 years [22, 23]. Also the number of pack years, the tar level of the cigarettes smoked, and the age at initiation of smoking are closely related to lung cancer risk [24, 25]. The relative risk of smoking is higher for squamous cell carcinoma and small cell carcinoma (RR between 10 and 200) than for adenocarcinoma (RR between 2 and 40) [23, 26–32]. The decline in risk after quitting smoking was also more consistent for squamous cell and small cell carcinoma than for adenocarcinoma [33]. However, the lower risk for adenocarcinoma could also be spurious, because the risk of adenocarcinoma in nonsmokers (= reference group) is also higher [23, 29, 30, 33, 34]. A meta-analysis in the IARC Monograph showed that the risk of lung cancer for involuntary smoking was 20–35 % higher than expected [25].

Other causes of lung cancer have been identified, such as air pollution and occupational exposure to arsenic, asbestos, radon, chloromethyl ethers, chromium, mustard gas, nickel refining, and polycyclic hydrocarbons (however, only a small proportion of the population was exposed). Vitamin A deficiency [35–39], indoor radon [40], possibly bird keeping [41–45], and previous chronic lung diseases [46] have also been identified as possible risk factors, but the effects of smoking are so predominant that other exposures seem unlikely to be largely responsible.

Comorbidity

Since lung cancer is a disease that mainly occurs in the elderly and smoking is the most important risk factor, many patients have (smoking-related) comorbidity at the time of lung cancer diagnosis. Figure 2.1 shows the prevalence of comorbidity among Dutch lung cancer patients by gender and age.

The prevalence of serious comorbid conditions among Dutch men who are diagnosed with lung cancer increases from 58 % in age group 50–64 to 80 % in age group 65–79 and 86 % in those aged 80 or older. Among Dutch women diagnosed with lung cancer, the prevalence of comorbidity increases from 58 % in age group 50–64 to 76 % in age group 65–79 and 79 % in those aged 80 or older. As expected, the most common comorbid conditions are smoking-related cardiovascular diseases (about 50 % in male lung cancer patients aged 65 or older and about 40 % in female patients) and chronic obstructive pulmonary diseases (COPD, about 30 % in male

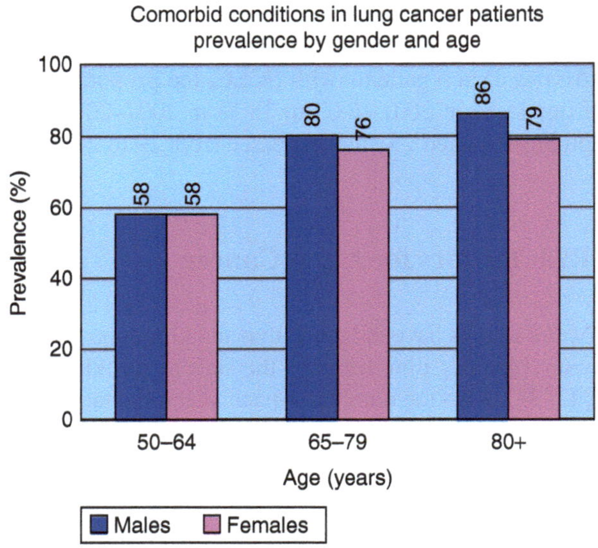

Fig. 2.1 Comorbid conditions in lung cancer patients (prevalence by gender and age) (Courtesy of the Eindhoven Cancer Registry)

patients aged 65+ and about 25 % in female patients). Since men have been smoking more than women in the past, the prevalence rates of these smoking-related comorbid conditions are higher among men [47, 48]. Several studies have also shown that the prevalence of comorbidity (especially smoking related) is higher among patients with lung cancer compared to those with other types of cancer [47, 49, 50].

Treatment of Elderly Lung Cancer Patients and Complications

Treatment of older cancer patients is challenging, since it is often complicated by comorbidity with subsequent postoperative complications, drug interactions, poor performance status, or social or psychological factors [51]. Complications/toxicity due to overtreatment on the one hand and undertreatment of elderly cancer patients on the other hand might lead to a poorer prognosis. The ultimate goal is not only to improve the duration of survival; maintaining an optimal quality of life (especially remaining independent) is probably even more important.

Nowadays, about 50 % of all lung cancer patients are 65 or older, and 30 % are 70 years or older. In contrast, only a small proportion of older patients is included in clinical trials [52–54]. Since elderly patients (especially those with serious comorbidity) are often excluded from clinical trials, it is not clear whether treatment guidelines can be generalized to these older patients. Population-based data can give insight into treatment and outcome in elderly cancer patients in everyday clinical practice. Both types of data (clinical trials and population based) are important. Population-based data can show adherence to treatment guidelines, whereas clinical trials can show the effect of treatment in randomized groups. The efficacy of treatment also depends on the life expectancy of the patients, given his/her comorbid conditions and functional status. Treatment for direct relief of symptoms is evident, whereas treatment for prevention of recurrences depends on the life expectancy of the patient. In addition, the elderly might have other preferences for treatment than younger patients. For example, the elderly seem to accept less toxicity for a given gain in survival time as compared to younger patients [55–57]. All these factors underscore the importance of studies of treatment and outcome in a graying population.

Non-small Cell Lung Cancer

Early Stages

Surgery

Surgery still remains the treatment of choice for early-stage non-small cell lung cancer (NSCLC). The proportion of Dutch patients with localized (stage I or II) NSCLC who underwent surgery was only 15 % of those aged 80 or older versus 88 and 66 % of age groups 50–64 and 65–79, respectively ($P<0.0001$, Fig. 2.2). Among patients up to 80 years, the resection rate was also significantly lower when COPD or cardiovascular diseases were present. Postoperative mortality was 2.5 % for patients younger than 75 years and 4 % for those aged 75 or older. An American study also showed the association between comorbidity and not undergoing surgery [58]. Postoperative death has been shown to be higher for elderly patients and is especially high for elderly patients undergoing pneumonectomy [48, 59–63]. Retrospective studies have shown that age alone is not a contraindication for thoracic surgery [64]. However, selection bias is present in retrospective studies. In case of pneumonectomy, high age should be considered because of the higher postoperative mortality rates among the elderly [59, 65]. Lung-sparing (segmentectomy and wedge resection) and video-assisted thoracic surgery (VATS) procedures could be particularly interesting to apply in elderly patients. These procedures have shown reduced postoperative mortality, complications, and lengths of hospital stay [66], but the long-term results are still controversial. A recent study has shown that the proportion of elderly patients (≥75 years) with stage I non-small cell lung cancer undergoing surgery has increased over time (1989–2009) from 35 to 49 % [67].

Radiotherapy

Nowadays, new nonsurgical treatment options as stereotactic radiotherapy are available for patients who are inoperable because of comorbidity, age, or functional status [68, 69]. Despite the high dose of radiation that is being used for this type of treatment, severe toxicity only occurs in 5 % of patients, and survival rates are almost equal to those for surgery [70–72]. However, results from randomized clinical trials comparing surgery and stereotactic radiotherapy among elderly lung cancer patients are not available yet.

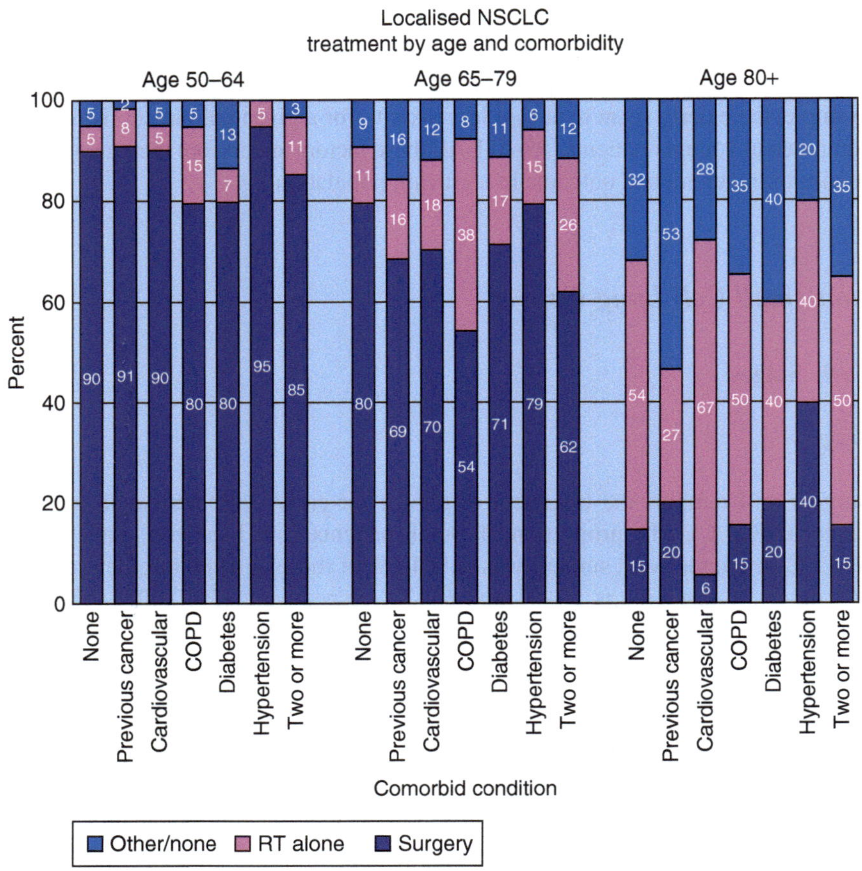

Fig. 2.2 Localized NSCLC treatment by age and comorbidity. *RT* radiotherapy (Courtesy of the Eindhoven Cancer Registry)

Adjuvant Therapy

Previous studies have shown that postoperative cisplatin-based chemotherapy improves survival in patients with stages II–IIIA NSCLC [73]. However, no prospective, elderly-specific data are available. In a recent population-based Dutch study, adjuvant chemotherapy for stage II increased from 0 to 24 % in younger patients but remained <5 % among those aged 75 years or older [67].

(Locally) Advanced Stages

Chemoradiation

Nowadays, preferred treatment for patients with locally advanced (stage IIIA and IIIB) NSCLC is concurrent chemoradiation. However, data are scarce for elderly

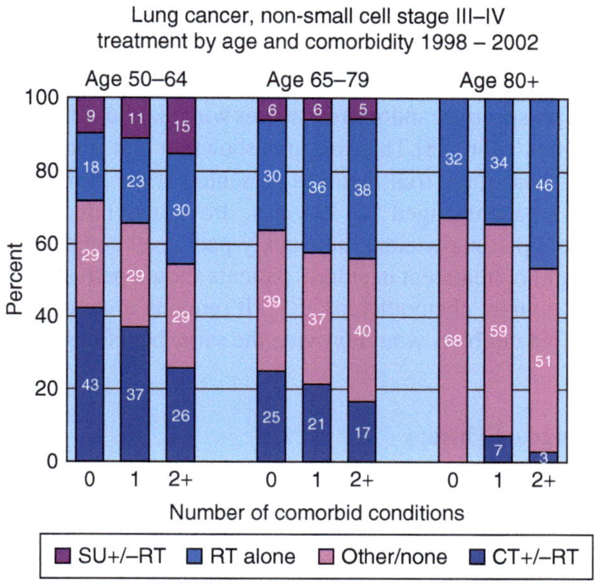

Fig. 2.3 Lung cancer, non-small cell stage III–IV treatment by age and comorbidity, 1998–2002. *SU* surgery, *RT* radiotherapy, *CT* chemotherapy (Courtesy of the Eindhoven Cancer Registry)

patients. Previous clinical trials have reported more hematological toxicity for elderly than for younger NSCLC patients receiving chemotherapy [74–76].

Among unselected Dutch patients with (locally) advanced (stage III or IV) NSCLC, the proportion receiving chemotherapy (whether or not in combination with radiotherapy) decreased with increasing age (Fig. 2.3). Within each age group, this proportion also decreased with an increasing number of comorbidities present at cancer diagnosis. The same was found in American population-based studies [74, 77]. Clinical studies have found that patients with comorbidity develop chemotherapy-related toxicity more often [75, 78, 79]. For this reason, the elderly more often receive only radiotherapy [61, 80]. Recent population-based studies have shown that the proportion of patients with stage III NSCLC receiving chemoradiation increased over time (1989–2009) from 8 to 43 % among patients younger than 75 years and from 1 to 13 % among the elderly [67]. No significant differences in comorbidity, age, or gender were observed between patients with stage III NSCLC treated with curative or palliative intent [81].

Palliative Chemotherapy

Unfortunately, about 50 % of all NSCLC patients have already metastasized at the time of diagnosis. Chemotherapy is the mainstay for treatment for advanced (stage IV) NSCLC. Chemotherapy can lead to a survival benefit of a few months, and quality of life can be improved. Although previous studies have shown that the benefit of chemotherapy for elderly patients is similar to younger patients [82], a minority of elderly patients receive chemotherapy. However, this proportion has increased over time (1989–2009): chemotherapy in younger patients increased from 10 to 54 % and in the elderly from 5 to 21 % [67]. Until now, single-agent chemotherapy should be considered a reasonable treatment of choice for elderly patients with advanced NSCLC [83–85]. Recently a favorable prognosis with acceptable toxicity was shown in prospective randomized studies with platinum-based chemotherapy among elderly patients [86–88].This was also shown in a recent publication with SEER data [77]. A phase three trial that was presented at the ASCO Meeting 2010 showed that PS 0–2 patients, aged 70–89 years, drove a significant benefit from a treatment with carboplatin associated to weekly paclitaxel compared to a monotherapy. The paradigm of treatment in elderly patients should perhaps be modified from a single-agent to doublet chemotherapy [88]. It remains to be evaluated whether other platinum-based doublets would provide the same benefit as the specific one studied.

Targeted Therapy

Although therapy for lung cancer has made progress in recent years, most patients will die of disease progression, and some current treatments are very toxic, in particular concomitant chemoradiotherapy for stage III disease. Therefore, the introduction of novel agents remains a high priority, especially for vulnerable elderly patients. Current interest is focused on molecular markers and biological therapies, such as targeting growth factors and growth factor receptors, suppressing angiogenesis and immunotherapy.

Small Cell Lung Cancer

Small cell lung cancer (SCLC) is an aggressive tumor which has frequently metastasized at the time of diagnosis. Because of its chemosensitivity, chemotherapy is the cornerstone of treatment. Several studies have reported an improvement in survival following the introduction of chemotherapy in the 1970s [89–93]. Preferred treatment for patients with limited disease (LD) SCLC who have a good performance score is concomitant chemoradiotherapy, while for those with extensive disease (ED), chemotherapy alone is recommended (and depending on locoregional symptoms also thoracic radiotherapy) [94, 95]. Due to the high probability of brain metastases, prophylactic cranial irradiation (PCI) for patients with LD is recommended since the early 2000s [96]. PCI substantially reduces the risk of brain recurrence, but the effect on survival has been debated [96, 97]. Since the study of Slotman and colleagues, PCI is also recommended for patients with ED [98]. New treatment modalities resulted in small improvements in survival in clinical trials with selected patients, mostly with good performance status and younger age.

In accordance with previous studies [99–104], elderly Dutch patients with LD SCLC received combined chemoradiation less often (27 % among age 75+ compared to 72 % among those aged 45–59, Fig. 2.4) [109]. Among elderly patients, the proportion receiving combined chemoradiation also decreased in the presence of

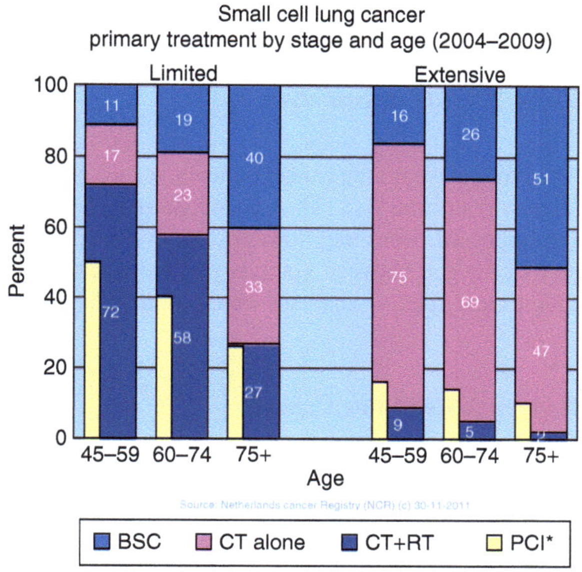

Fig. 2.4 Small cell lung cancer primary treatment by stage and age, 2004 to 2009. *BSC* best supportive care, *CT* chemotherapy, *RT* radiotherapy, *PCI* prophylactic cranial irradiation. *Percentage of patients who received chemotherapy (Courtesy of the Netherlands Cancer Registry)

comorbidity ($P=0.002$). The most common motives for withholding chemotherapy in elderly patients were refusal by patient or family, short life expectancy, or a combination of high age, comorbidity, and poor performance status. Two thirds of elderly (age 75+) SCLC patients receiving chemotherapy could not complete the full treatment, often due to hematological toxicity [105]. Sixty-five percent of patients aged 75+ receiving chemotherapy developed grade 3 or 4 toxicity, of which 43 % consisted of hematological toxicity [105]. Previous studies also report high toxicity rates for patients receiving chemotherapy for SCLC [100–102, 105–107]. A recent study has shown that the proportion of patients with LD receiving chemoradiation has increased over time: 36 % in 1997–2000 to 62 % in 2005–2007 among those aged 60–69, 28–49 % in age group 70–74, and 17–34 % in age group 75–79, but remaining less than 15 % among those aged 80 or older [109]. PCI was introduced in the Netherlands in 1999 and increased to 69 % in 2009 in patients aged 45–59 years who had received chemotherapy, 63 % in those aged 60–74, and 42 % of those aged 75 or older [109].

Among Dutch patients with ED, the proportion receiving chemotherapy clearly decreased with increasing age from 8 % of patients aged 45–59 to 49 % of those aged 75+ (Fig. 2.4), without significant changes in treatment modality over time [108]. Although PCI was not often applied to patients with extensive disease until 2006, 39 % of patients aged 45–59 who had received chemotherapy underwent PCI in 2009. This proportion was 32 % for those aged 60–74 and 25 % for those aged 75 or older [109]. A meta-analysis has shown that the effect of PCI on survival was not influenced by age [96]. However, clinical trials have shown that neuropsychological impairments were potentially related to PCI [110]. This means that preexisting neurocognitive problems in elderly patients should be carefully investigated, before PCI is advised [95].

Treatment Outcome

Time Trends in Survival

The prognosis for lung cancer patients, regardless of histological type, has improved slightly over time [1, 111]. A European study has shown that survival of all cancers has improved over time; however, survival increased at a slower rate in the elderly, so that the gap between younger and older patients widened [112]. Unfortunately, lung cancer-specific analyses were not included in this study.

Non-small Cell Lung Cancer

There was only a slight improvement in the prognosis of NSCLC during the last decades. Nowadays, the 5-year survival rate is 13–19 % [67, 113–116]. In Dutch patients, 5-year relative survival for females diagnosed with NSCLC improved significantly from 14 % in 1989–1993 to 18 % in 2004–2009 ($p < 0.001$), whereas 5-year relative survival for males remained stable at 15 % [67]. Although improvements in survival were observed among all age groups, survival remained significantly lower for the elderly (<75 years from 16 to 18 %, $p = 0.01$, and ≥75 years from 9 to 11 %, $p = 0.001$) [67].

Several studies indicate that survival differs according to histological subtype of NSCLC, being better for squamous cell carcinoma and adenocarcinoma (1-year survival rates of 40–50 %) than for large cell undifferentiated carcinoma (1-year survival rates of 25–30 %) [116–119]. Among Dutch patients, 5-year survival for patients with squamous cell carcinomas improved from 17 to 20 % between 1989 and 2009 and for those with non-squamous cell carcinomas from 11 to 14 % [67]. Since improvements in survival were especially seen among females, younger patients, and within each stage group, they probably could be partly explained by changes in treatment and better staging.

Small Cell Lung Cancer

SCLC can be distinguished from other forms of lung cancer. Its features are rapid progression, short doubling time, high growth fraction, and sensitivity to multiple chemotherapeutic agents and radiation therapy. Short-term survival has improved since the introduction of chemotherapy in the 1970s, but 5-year survival remains poor [89, 108, 120, 121]. Death from recurrent disease occurs within 2 years of diagnosis in 80–98 % of the cases [122–125]. A recent study has shown that improved staging resulted in improved survival for both limited and extensive SCLC, while survival of the total group has only significantly improved for patients younger than 60 years [109]. Although stage migration probably plays a role, the latter is possibly also related with improved treatment strategies.

Prognostic Factors for Survival in Elderly Lung Cancer Patients

Prognosis for elderly lung cancer patients is worse compared to younger patients, even after adjustment for higher mortality in the general population [48]. The poorer prognosis for the elderly might be explained by several factors: an increased risk of mortality due to comorbid conditions, death due to complications of treatment, or death from cancer due to less aggressive treatment.

Increased mortality due to comorbidity is probably of less importance in case of a lethal disease as lung cancer [48–50]. Most patients die of lung cancer before they are at risk of dying from the comorbid condition.

Comorbidity is of growing importance for the clinical management of elderly lung cancer patients. Elderly patients with localized NSCLC underwent less surgery than younger patients, and older patients with nonlocalized NSCLC received less chemotherapy [48, 126].

Treatment has been shown to be a strong prognostic factor for patients with localized NSCLC: those who only received radiotherapy (HR = 2.5) and those receiving only best supportive care (HR = 6.0) had a poorer prognosis compared to those who underwent surgery, even after adjustment for differences in age, gender, and comorbidity [127]. Comorbidity may increase the risk of preoperative and post-operative complications [128–131], especially those of the cardiorespiratory system [59, 132–134]. Previous studies have shown that pulmonary resection is justified, also for elderly lung cancer patients. However, a careful preoperative assessment ought to be performed, and standard resections should be preferred [133, 134]. Previous studies have shown that treatment is also an independent prognostic factor for patients with (locally) advanced NSCLC, even after adjustment for differences in age, gender, and comorbidity [48, 81]. Two recent publications have shown that with a proper patient selection, reasonable long-term survival rates can be achieved when treating elderly (75+) patients with stage III NSCLC with curative intent (15–20 % 5-year overall survival rate) [67, 81].

For patients with limited SCLC, treatment has been shown to be the strongest independent prognostic factor (hazard ratio up to 2 for those receiving chemotherapy alone and up to 3.5 for those receiving best supportive care compared to those receiving combined chemoradiation) [108]. This is not unexpected in studies in which generally only fit elderly were selected for aggressive treatment [135, 136]. Although thoracic radiation in combination with chemotherapy has been reported to improve survival moderately for younger patients with limited SCLC, the effect in the elderly is questionable [102, 104, 137, 138], because the evidence for a favorable prognosis after combined radiotherapy and chemotherapy is derived from studies in which only relatively fit elderly patients were selected for chemotherapy. Therefore, chemotherapy and the addition of radiotherapy to chemotherapy must be studied accurately in elderly patients, because relevant toxicity in the elderly has only been investigated in a few studies [105, 139, 140].

Smoking was also found to be a prognostic factor, even after adjustment for age, gender, illicit drug use, adverse symptoms, histology, stage, comorbidity, and treatment [141].

Some studies found higher survival rates for females than for males [142, 143]. Since survival rates are higher for younger persons than for older, some of the female–male survival differential may be due to a higher preponderance of younger-aged patients in the female group. The prognostic difference might also be due to a different histological distribution of the tumors or to the lower prevalence of comorbid conditions among women, such as chronic obstructive pulmonary diseases (COPD) or cardiovascular diseases [47].

Conclusions

Due to a growing proportion of elderly lung cancer patients, more patients present with serious comorbidity at diagnosis of cancer. This may complicate the management of lung cancer in elderly patients. This chapter has shown that receiving standard treatment has a positive effect on prognosis of lung cancer, even after adjustment for differences in age and comorbidity. However, (sometimes life-limiting) complications of treatment among elderly lung cancer patients are very common, despite a strict selection of the fittest elderly for standard treatment. In the elderly, the impact of toxicities on quality of life (especially maintaining independence) may be just as important as the prolongation of life expectancy. Previous studies have shown that elderly patients accept fewer complications for a given gain in life expectancy, compared to younger patients. A proper selection of patients fit enough for surgery, chemotherapy, and/or radiotherapy is therefore important, and there is an urgent need for predictive models for treatment tolerance that can be easily used in everyday clinical practice.

References

1. Levi F, Lucchini F, Negri E, et al. Cancer mortality in Europe, 1995–1999, and an overview of trends since 1960. Int J Cancer. 2004;110:155–69.
2. Janssen-Heijnen ML, Coebergh JW. The changing epidemiology of lung cancer in Europe. Lung Cancer. 2003;41:245–58.
3. Bray F, Tyczynski JE, Parkin DM. Going up or coming down? The changing phases of the lung cancer epidemic from 1967 to 1999 in the 15 European Union countries. Eur J Cancer. 2004;40:96–125.
4. Devesa SS, Silverman DT, Young JL, et al. Cancer incidence and mortality trends among whites in the United States, 1947–84. J Natl Cancer Inst. 1987;79:701–70.
5. Horm JW, Kessler LG. Falling rates of lung cancer in men in the United States. Lancet. 1986;1:425–6.
6. Janssen-Heijnen ML, Nab HW, van Reek J, et al. Striking changes in smoking behaviour and lung cancer incidence by histological type in south-east Netherlands, 1960–1991. Eur J Cancer. 1995;31A:949–52.
7. McCredie M, Coates MS, Ford JM. The changing incidence of cancer in adults in New South Wales. Int J Cancer. 1988;42:667–71.

8. O'Lorcain P, Comber H. Lung cancer mortality predictions for Ireland 2001–2015 and current trends in North Western Europe. Lung Cancer. 2004;46:157–63.
9. Skuladottir H, Olsen JH, Hirsch FR. Incidence of lung cancer in Denmark: historical and actual status. Lung Cancer. 2000;27:107–18.
10. Travis WD, Lubin J, Ries L, Devesa S. United States lung carcinoma incidence trends: declining for most histologic types among males, increasing among females. Cancer. 1996; 77:2464–70.
11. Tyczynski JE, Bray F, Aareleid T, et al. Lung cancer mortality patterns in selected Central, Eastern and Southern European countries. Int J Cancer. 2004;109:598–610.
12. Russo A, Crosignani P, Franceschi S, Berrino F. Changes in lung cancer histological types in Varese Cancer Registry, Italy 1976–1992. Eur J Cancer. 1997;33:1643–7.
13. Boffetta P, La Vecchia C, Levi F, Lucchini F. Mortality patterns and trends for lung cancer and other tobacco-related cancers in the Americas, 1955–1989. Int J Epidemiol. 1993;22:377–84.
14. La Vecchia C, Lucchini F, Negri E, et al. Trends in cancer mortality in the Americas, 1955–1989. Eur J Cancer. 1993;29A:431–70.
15. Morita T. A statistical study of lung cancer in the annual of pathological autopsy cases in Japan, from 1958 to 1997, with reference to time trends of lung cancer in the world. Jpn J Cancer Res. 2002;93:15–23.
16. Karim-Kos HE, Janssen-Heijnen ML, van Iersel CA, et al. The beginning of the end of the lung cancer epidemic in Dutch women? Int J Cancer. 2008;123:1472–5.
17. Chiu YL, Yu IT, Wong TW. Time trends of female lung cancer in Hong Kong: age, period and birth cohort analysis. Int J Cancer. 2004;111:424–30.
18. Havlik RJ, Yancik R, Long S, et al. The National Institute on Aging and the National Cancer Institute SEER collaborative study on comorbidity and early diagnosis of cancer in the elderly. Cancer. 1994;74:2101–6.
19. Janssen-Heijnen ML, Coebergh JW, Klinkhamer PJ, et al. Is there a common etiology for the rising incidence of and decreasing survival with adenocarcinoma of the lung? Epidemiology. 2001;12:256–8.
20. Levi F, Franceschi S, La Vecchia C, et al. Lung carcinoma trends by histologic type in Vaud and Neuchatel, Switzerland, 1974–1994. Cancer. 1997;79:906–14.
21. Thun MJ, Lally CA, Flannery JT, et al. Cigarette smoking and changes in the histopathology of lung cancer. J Natl Cancer Inst. 1997;89:1580–6.
22. Doll R, Peto R, Wheatley K, et al. Mortality in relation to smoking: 40 years' observations on male British doctors. BMJ. 1994;309:901–11.
23. Lubin JH, Blot WJ. Assessment of lung cancer risk factors by histologic category. J Natl Cancer Inst. 1984;73:383–9.
24. Harris JE, Thun MJ, Mondul AM, Calle EE. Cigarette tar yields in relation to mortality from lung cancer in the cancer prevention study II prospective cohort, 1982–8. BMJ. 2004;328:72.
25. Sasco AJ, Secretan MB, Straif K. Tobacco smoking and cancer: a brief review of recent epidemiological evidence. Lung Cancer. 2004;45 Suppl 2:S3–9.
26. de Waard F, Kemmeren JM, van Ginkel LA, Stolker AA. Urinary cotinine and lung cancer risk in a female cohort. Br J Cancer. 1995;72:784–7.
27. Denissenko MF, Pao A, Tang M, Pfeifer GP. Preferential formation of benzo[a]pyrene adducts at lung cancer mutational hotspots in P53. Science. 1996;274:430–2.
28. Engeland A, Haldorsen T, Andersen A, Tretli S. The impact of smoking habits on lung cancer risk: 28 years' observation of 26,000 Norwegian men and women. Cancer Causes Control. 1996;7:366–76.
29. Morabia A, Wynder EL. Cigarette smoking and lung cancer cell types. Cancer. 1991;68:2074–8.
30. Pezzotto SM, Mahuad R, Bay ML, et al. Variation in smoking-related lung cancer risk factors by cell type among men in Argentina: a case–control study. Cancer Causes Control. 1993;4:231–7.
31. Siemiatycki J, Krewski D, Franco E, Kaiserman M. Associations between cigarette smoking and each of 21 types of cancer: a multi-site case–control study. Int J Epidemiol. 1995; 24:504–14.

32. Simonato L, Agudo A, Ahrens W, et al. Lung cancer and cigarette smoking in Europe: an update of risk estimates and an assessment of inter-country heterogeneity. Int J Cancer. 2001;91:876–87.
33. Higgins IT, Wynder EL. Reduction in risk of lung cancer among ex-smokers with particular reference to histologic type. Cancer. 1988;62:2397–401.
34. Makitaro R, Paakko P, Huhti E, et al. An epidemiological study of lung cancer: history and histological types in a general population in northern Finland. Eur Respir J. 1999;13:436–40.
35. Dorant E, van den Brandt PA, Goldbohm RA. A prospective cohort study on Allium vegetable consumption, garlic supplement use, and the risk of lung carcinoma in The Netherlands. Cancer Res. 1994;54:6148–53.
36. Margetts BM, Jackson AA. Interactions between people's diet and their smoking habits: the dietary and nutritional survey of British adults. BMJ. 1993;307:1381–4.
37. Scali J, Astre C, Segala C, Gerber M. Relationship of serum cholesterol, dietary and plasma beta-carotene with lung cancer in male smokers. Eur J Cancer Prev. 1995;4:169–74.
38. Serdula MK, Byers T, Mokdad AH, et al. The association between fruit and vegetable intake and chronic disease risk factors. Epidemiology. 1996;7:161–5.
39. Ziegler RG, Colavito EA, Hartge P, et al. Importance of alpha-carotene, beta-carotene, and other phytochemicals in the etiology of lung cancer. J Natl Cancer Inst. 1996;88:612–5.
40. Lubin JH, Boice Jr JD. Lung cancer risk from residential radon: meta-analysis of eight epidemiologic studies. J Natl Cancer Inst. 1997;89:49–57.
41. Alavanja MC, Brownson RC, Berger E, et al. Avian exposure and risk of lung cancer in women in Missouri: population based case–control study. BMJ. 1996;313:1233–5.
42. Gardiner AJ, Forey BA, Lee PN. Avian exposure and bronchogenic carcinoma. BMJ. 1992;305:989–92.
43. Holst PA, Kromhout D, Brand R. For debate: pet birds as an independent risk factor for lung cancer. BMJ. 1988;297:1319–21.
44. Kohlmeier L, Arminger G, Bartolomeycik S, et al. Pet birds as an independent risk factor for lung cancer: case–control study. BMJ. 1992;305:986–9.
45. Modigh C, Axelsson G, Alavanja M, et al. Pet birds and risk of lung cancer in Sweden: a case–control study. BMJ. 1996;313:1236–8.
46. Littman AJ, Thornquist MD, White E, et al. Prior lung disease and risk of lung cancer in a large prospective study. Cancer Causes Control. 2004;15:819–27.
47. Janssen-Heijnen ML, Houterman S, Lemmens VE, et al. Prognostic impact of increasing age and co-morbidity in cancer patients: a population-based approach. Crit Rev Oncol Hematol. 2005;55:231–40.
48. Janssen-Heijnen ML, Smulders S, Lemmens VE, et al. Effect of comorbidity on the treatment and prognosis of elderly patients with non-small cell lung cancer. Thorax. 2004;59:602–7.
49. Piccirillo JF, Tierney RM, Costas I, et al. Prognostic importance of comorbidity in a hospital-based cancer registry. JAMA. 2004;291:2441–7.
50. Read WL, Tierney RM, Page NC, et al. Differential prognostic impact of comorbidity. J Clin Oncol. 2004;22:3099–103.
51. Extermann M, Overcash J, Lyman GH, et al. Comorbidity and functional status are independent in older cancer patients. J Clin Oncol. 1998;16:1582–7.
52. Aapro MS, Kohne CH, Cohen HJ, Extermann M. Never too old? Age should not be a barrier to enrollment in cancer clinical trials. Oncologist. 2005;10:198–204.
53. Talarico L, Chen G, Pazdur R. Enrollment of elderly patients in clinical trials for cancer drug registration: a 7-year experience by the US Food and Drug Administration. J Clin Oncol. 2004;22:4626–31.
54. Townsley CA, Selby R, Siu LL. Systematic review of barriers to the recruitment of older patients with cancer onto clinical trials. J Clin Oncol. 2005;23:3112–24.
55. Ayanian JZ, Zaslavsky AM, Fuchs CS, et al. Use of adjuvant chemotherapy and radiation therapy for colorectal cancer in a population-based cohort. J Clin Oncol. 2003;21:1293–300.
56. Bremnes RM, Andersen K, Wist EA. Cancer patients, doctors and nurses vary in their willingness to undertake cancer chemotherapy. Eur J Cancer. 1995;31A:1955–9.

57. Rose JH, O'Toole EE, Dawson NV, et al. Perspectives, preferences, care practices, and outcomes among older and middle-aged patients with late-stage cancer. J Clin Oncol. 2004;22:4907–17.
58. Cykert S, Dilworth-Anderson P, Monroe MH, et al. Factors associated with decisions to undergo surgery among patients with newly diagnosed early-stage lung cancer. JAMA. 2010;303:2368–76.
59. Damhuis RA, Schutte PR. Resection rates and postoperative mortality in 7,899 patients with lung cancer. Eur Respir J. 1996;9:7–10.
60. Finlayson EV, Birkmeyer JD. Operative mortality with elective surgery in older adults. Eff Clin Pract. 2001;4:172–7.
61. Janssen-Heijnen ML, Maas HA, Houterman S, et al. Comorbidity in older surgical cancer patients: influence on patient care and outcome. Eur J Cancer. 2007;43:2179–93.
62. Okami J, Higashiyama M, Asamura H, et al. Pulmonary resection in patients aged 80 years or over with clinical stage I non-small cell lung cancer: prognostic factors for overall survival and risk factors for postoperative complications. J Thorac Oncol. 2009;4:1247–53.
63. Veen EJ, Janssen-Heijnen ML, Ritchie ED, et al. Pneumonectomy for bronchogenic carcinoma: analysis of factors predicting short- and long-term outcome. Interact Cardiovasc Thorac Surg. 2009;9:260–4.
64. Dominguez-Ventura A, Allen MS, Cassivi SD, et al. Lung cancer in octogenarians: factors affecting morbidity and mortality after pulmonary resection. Ann Thorac Surg. 2006;82:1175–9.
65. Dyszkiewicz W, Pawlak K, Gasiorowski L. Early post-pneumonectomy complications in the elderly. Eur J Cardiothorac Surg. 2000;17:246–50.
66. Landreneau RJ, Sugarbaker DJ, Mack MJ, et al. Wedge resection versus lobectomy for stage I (T1 N0 M0) non-small-cell lung cancer. J Thorac Cardiovasc Surg. 1997;113:691–8; discussion 698–700.
67. Van der Drift MA, Karim-Kos HE, Siesling S, et al. Progress in standard of care therapy and modest survival benefits in the treatment of NSCLC patients in the Netherlands in the last 20 years. J Thorac Oncol. 2012;7:291–8.
68. Baumann P, Nyman J, Hoyer M, et al. Outcome in a prospective phase II trial of medically inoperable stage I non-small-cell lung cancer patients treated with stereotactic body radiotherapy. J Clin Oncol. 2009;27:3290–6.
69. Goldstraw P, Ball D, Jett JR, et al. Non-small-cell lung cancer. Lancet. 2011;378:1727–40.
70. Palma D, Visser O, Lagerwaard FJ, et al. Impact of introducing stereotactic lung radiotherapy for elderly patients with stage I non-small-cell lung cancer: a population-based time-trend analysis. J Clin Oncol. 2010;28:5153–9.
71. De Ruysscher D, Faivre-Finn C, Nestle U, et al. European Organisation for Research and Treatment of Cancer recommendations for planning and delivery of high-dose, high-precision radiotherapy for lung cancer. J Clin Oncol. 2011;28:5301–10.
72. Haasbeek CJ, Lagerwaard FJ, Antonisse ME, et al. Stage I nonsmall cell lung cancer in patients aged > or =75 years: outcomes after stereotactic radiotherapy. Cancer. 2011;116:406–14.
73. Pignon JP, Tribodet H, Scagliotti GV, et al. Lung adjuvant cisplatin evaluation: a pooled analysis by the LACE Collaborative Group. J Clin Oncol. 2008;26:3552–9.
74. Chrischilles EA, Pendergast JF, Kahn KL, et al. Adverse events among the elderly receiving chemotherapy for advanced non-small-cell lung cancer. J Clin Oncol. 2011;28:620–7.
75. Pallis AG, Karampeazis A, Vamvakas L, et al. Efficacy and treatment tolerance in older patients with NSCLC: a meta-analysis of five phase III randomized trials conducted by the Hellenic Oncology Research Group. Ann Oncol. 2011;22:2448–55.
76. Schild SE, Stella PJ, Geyer SM, et al. The outcome of combined-modality therapy for stage III non-small-cell lung cancer in the elderly. J Clin Oncol. 2003;21:3201–6.
77. Davidoff AJ, Tang M, Seal B, Edelman MJ. Chemotherapy and survival benefit in elderly patients with advanced non-small-cell lung cancer. J Clin Oncol. 2011;28:2191–7.
78. Gronberg BH, Sundstrom S, Kaasa S, et al. Influence of comorbidity on survival, toxicity and health-related quality of life in patients with advanced non-small-cell lung cancer receiving platinum-doublet chemotherapy. Eur J Cancer. 2011;46:2225–34.

79. Ngeow J, Leong SS, Gao F, et al. Impact of comorbidities on clinical outcomes in non-small cell lung cancer patients who are elderly and/or have poor performance status. Crit Rev Oncol Hematol. 2011;76:53–60.
80. de Rijke JM, Schouten LJ, ten Velde GP, et al. Influence of age, comorbidity and performance status on the choice of treatment for patients with non-small cell lung cancer; results of a population-based study. Lung Cancer. 2004;46:233–45.
81. Wanders R, Steevens J, Botterweck A, et al. Treatment with curative intent of stage III non-small cell lung cancer patients of 75years: a prospective population-based study. Eur J Cancer. 2011;47:2691–7.
82. Gridelli C, Perrone F, Gallo C, et al. Vinorelbine is well tolerated and active in the treatment of elderly patients with advanced non-small cell lung cancer. A two-stage phase II study. Eur J Cancer. 1997;33:392–7.
83. Gridelli C, Aapro M, Ardizzoni A, et al. Treatment of advanced non-small-cell lung cancer in the elderly: results of an international expert panel. J Clin Oncol. 2005;23:3125–37.
84. Pfister DG, Johnson DH, Azzoli CG, et al. American Society of Clinical Oncology treatment of unresectable non-small-cell lung cancer guideline: update 2003. J Clin Oncol. 2004;22: 330–53.
85. Gridelli C, Ardizzoni A, Douillard JY, et al. Recent issues in first-line treatment of advanced non-small-cell lung cancer: Results of an International Expert Panel Meeting of the Italian Association of Thoracic Oncology. Lung Cancer. 2010;68:319–31.
86. Biesma B, Wymenga AN, Vincent A, et al. Quality of life, geriatric assessment and survival in elderly patients with non-small-cell lung cancer treated with carboplatin-gemcitabine or carboplatin-paclitaxel: NVALT-3 a phase III study. Ann Oncol. 2011;22:1520–7.
87. Gridelli C, Maione P, Illiano A, et al. Cisplatin plus gemcitabine or vinorelbine for elderly patients with advanced non small-cell lung cancer: the MILES-2P studies. J Clin Oncol. 2007;25:4663–9.
88. Quoix E, Westeel V, Zalcman G, Milleron B. Chemotherapy in elderly patients with advanced non-small cell lung cancer. Lung Cancer. 2011;74:364–8.
89. Choi NC, Carey RW, Kaufman SD, et al. Small cell carcinoma of the lung. A progress report of 15 years' experience. Cancer. 1987;59:6–14.
90. Janssen-Heijnen ML, Schipper RM, Klinkhamer PJ, et al. Improvement and plateau in survival of small-cell lung cancer since 1975: a population-based study. Ann Oncol. 1998;9:543–7.
91. Lassen U, Osterlind K, Hansen M, et al. Long-term survival in small-cell lung cancer: post-treatment characteristics in patients surviving 5 to 18+ years–an analysis of 1,714 consecutive patients. J Clin Oncol. 1995;13:1215–20.
92. Skarin AT. Analysis of long-term survivors with small-cell lung cancer. Chest. 1993;103: 440S–4.
93. Souhami RL, Law K. Longevity in small cell lung cancer. A report to the Lung Cancer Subcommittee of the United Kingdom Coordinating Committee for Cancer Research. Br J Cancer. 1990;61:584–9.
94. Amarasena IU, Walters JA, Wood-Baker R, Fong K. Platinum versus non-platinum chemotherapy regimens for small cell lung cancer. Cochrane Database Syst Rev. 2008; (4): CD006849.
95. van Meerbeeck JP, Fennell DA, De Ruysscher DK. Small-cell lung cancer. Lancet. 2011;378: 1741–55.
96. Auperin A, Arriagada R, Pignon JP, et al. Prophylactic cranial irradiation for patients with small-cell lung cancer in complete remission. Prophylactic Cranial Irradiation Overview Collaborative Group. N Engl J Med. 1999;341:476–84.
97. Arriagada R, Le Chevalier T, Riviere A, et al. Patterns of failure after prophylactic cranial irradiation in small-cell lung cancer: analysis of 505 randomized patients. Ann Oncol. 2002;13:748–54.
98. Slotman B, Faivre-Finn C, Kramer G, et al. Prophylactic cranial irradiation in extensive small-cell lung cancer. N Engl J Med. 2007;357:664–72.

99. Deppermann KM. Influence of age and comorbidities on the chemotherapeutic management of lung cancer. Lung Cancer. 2001;33 Suppl 1:S115–20.
100. Janssen-Heijnen ML, Lemmens VE, van den Borne BE, et al. Negligible influence of comorbidity on prognosis of patients with small cell lung cancer: a population-based study in the Netherlands. Crit Rev Oncol Hematol. 2007;62:172–8.
101. Jara C, Gomez-Aldaravi JL, Tirado R, et al. Small-cell lung cancer in the elderly–is age of patient a relevant factor? Acta Oncol. 1999;38:781–6.
102. Ludbrook JJ, Truong PT, MacNeil MV, et al. Do age and comorbidity impact treatment allocation and outcomes in limited stage small-cell lung cancer? A community-based population analysis. Int J Radiat Oncol Biol Phys. 2003;55:1321–30.
103. Weinmann M, Jeremic B, Bamberg M, Bokemeyer C. Treatment of lung cancer in elderly part II: small cell lung cancer. Lung Cancer. 2003;40:1–16.
104. Lally BE, Geiger AM, Urbanic JJ, et al. Trends in the outcomes for patients with limited stage small cell lung cancer: an analysis of the Surveillance, Epidemiology, and End Results database. Lung Cancer. 2009;64:226–31.
105. Janssen-Heijnen ML, Maas HA, van de Schans SA, et al. Chemotherapy in elderly small-cell lung cancer patients: yes we can, but should we do it? Ann Oncol. 2010;22:821–6.
106. Kim HG, Lee GW, Kang JH, et al. Combination chemotherapy with irinotecan and cisplatin in elderly patients (>or = 65 years) with extensive-disease small-cell lung cancer. Lung Cancer. 2008;61:220–6.
107. Siu LL, Shepherd FA, Murray N, et al. Influence of age on the treatment of limited-stage small-cell lung cancer. J Clin Oncol. 1996;14:821–8.
108. Janssen-Heijnen ML, Maas HA, Siesling S, et al. Treatment and survival of patients with small-cell lung cancer: small steps forward, but not for patients >80. Ann Oncol. 2011;23: 954–60.
109. Janssen-Heijnen ML, Karim-Kos HE, van der Drift MA, et al. Modest improvements of survival for patients with small cell lung cancer aged 45 to 59 years only, diagnosed in the Netherlands, 1989 to 2008. J Thorac Oncol. 2011;7:227–32.
110. Crossen JR, Garwood D, Glatstein E, Neuwelt EA. Neurobehavioral sequelae of cranial irradiation in adults: a review of radiation-induced encephalopathy. J Clin Oncol. 1994; 12:627–42.
111. Capocaccia R, Negri E, La Vecchia C, Decarli A. Trends in lung cancer mortality in three broad Italian geographical areas between 1969 and 1987. Eur J Cancer. 1993;29A:1288–93.
112. Quaglia A, Tavilla A, Shack L, et al. The cancer survival gap between elderly and middle-aged patients in Europe is widening. Eur J Cancer. 2009;45:1006–16.
113. Foucher P, Coudert B, Arveux P, et al. Age and prognosis of non-small cell lung cancer. Usefulness of a relative survival model. Eur J Cancer. 1993;29A:1809–13.
114. Grosclaude P, Galat JP, Mace-Lesech J, et al. Differences in treatment and survival rates of non-small-cell lung cancer in three regions of France. Br J Cancer. 1995;72:1278–82.
115. Janssen-Heijnen ML, Gatta G, Forman D, et al. Variation in survival of patients with lung cancer in Europe, 1985–1989. EUROCARE Working Group. Eur J Cancer. 1998;34: 2191–6.
116. Pastorino U, Berrino F, Valente M, et al. Incident lung cancer survival. Long-term follow-up of a population-based study in Italy. Tumori. 1990;76:199–204.
117. Janssen-Heijnen ML, Schipper RM, Klinkhamer PJ, et al. Divergent changes in survival for histological types of non-small-cell lung cancer in the southeastern area of The Netherlands since 1975. Br J Cancer. 1998;77:2053–7.
118. Sant M, Gatta G, Capocaccia R, et al. Survival for lung cancer in northern Italy. Cancer Causes Control. 1992;3:223–30.
119. Travis WD, Travis LB, Devesa SS. Lung cancer. Cancer. 1995;75:191–202.
120. Connolly CK, Jones WG, Thorogood J, et al. Investigation, treatment and prognosis of bronchial carcinoma in the Yorkshire Region of England 1976–1983. Br J Cancer. 1990;61: 579–83.

121. Watkin SW, Hayhurst GK, Green JA. Time trends in the outcome of lung cancer management: a study of 9,090 cases diagnosed in the Mersey Region, 1974–86. Br J Cancer. 1990;61:590–6.
122. Davis S, Wright PW, Schulman SF, et al. Long-term survival in small-cell carcinoma of the lung: a population experience. J Clin Oncol. 1985;3:80–91.
123. Findlay MP, Griffin AM, Raghavan D, et al. Retrospective review of chemotherapy for small cell lung cancer in the elderly: does the end justify the means? Eur J Cancer. 1991;27: 1597–601.
124. Osterlind K, Andersen PK. Prognostic factors in small cell lung cancer: multivariate model based on 778 patients treated with chemotherapy with or without irradiation. Cancer Res. 1986;46:4189–94.
125. van der Gaast A, Postmus PE, Burghouts J, et al. Long term survival of small cell lung cancer patients after chemotherapy. Br J Cancer. 1993;67:822–4.
126. Potosky AL, Saxman S, Wallace RB, Lynch CF. Population variations in the initial treatment of non-small-cell lung cancer. J Clin Oncol. 2004;22:3261–8.
127. Janssen-Heijnen ML, Van de Schans SA. Epidemiology of geriatric oncology. In: Pérez-Manga G, Repetto L, editors. Geriatric oncology. 3rd ed. Madrid: Grupo Aula Médica, S.L; 2011. p. 1–18.
128. Guadagnoli E, Weitberg A, Mor V, et al. The influence of patient age on the diagnosis and treatment of lung and colorectal cancer. Arch Intern Med. 1990;150:1485–90.
129. Monfardini S, Yancik R. Cancer in the elderly: meeting the challenge of an aging population. J Natl Cancer Inst. 1993;85:532–8.
130. Satariano WA. Comorbidities and cancer. Cancer in the elderly. In: Hunter CP, Johnson KA, Muss HB, editors. New York: Dekker; 2000. 48: p. 505–12.
131. Wei JY. Cardiovascular comorbidity in the older cancer patient. Semin Oncol. 1995; 22:9–10.
132. Ginsberg RJ, Hill LD, Eagan RT, et al. Modern thirty-day operative mortality for surgical resections in lung cancer. J Thorac Cardiovasc Surg. 1983;86:654–8.
133. Osaki T, Shirakusa T, Kodate M, et al. Surgical treatment of lung cancer in the octogenarian. Ann Thorac Surg. 1994;57:188–92; discussion 192–183.
134. Thomas P, Sielezneff I, Ragni J, et al. Is lung cancer resection justified in patients aged over 70 years? Eur J Cardiothorac Surg. 1993;7:246–50; discussion 250–241.
135. Chen J, Jiang R, Garces YI, et al. Prognostic factors for limited-stage small cell lung cancer: a study of 284 patients. Lung Cancer. 2010;67:221–6.
136. Shepherd FA, Amdemichael E, Evans WK, et al. Treatment of small cell lung cancer in the elderly. J Am Geriatr Soc. 1994;42:64–70.
137. Pignon JP, Arriagada R, Ihde DC, et al. A meta-analysis of thoracic radiotherapy for small-cell lung cancer. N Engl J Med. 1992;327:1618–24.
138. Schild SE, Stella PJ, Brooks BJ, et al. Results of combined-modality therapy for limited-stage small cell lung carcinoma in the elderly. Cancer. 2005;103:2349–54.
139. Gridelli C, De Vivo R, Monfardini S. Management of small-cell lung cancer in the elderly. Crit Rev Oncol Hematol. 2002;41:79–88.
140. Quon H, Shepherd FA, Payne DG, et al. The influence of age on the delivery, tolerance, and efficacy of thoracic irradiation in the combined modality treatment of limited stage small cell lung cancer. Int J Radiat Oncol Biol Phys. 1999;43:39–45.
141. Tammemagi CM, Neslund-Dudas C, Simoff M, Kvale P. Smoking and lung cancer survival: the role of comorbidity and treatment. Chest. 2004;125:27–37.
142. Batevik R, Grong K, Segadal L, Stangeland L. The female gender has a positive effect on survival independent of background life expectancy following surgical resection of primary non-small cell lung cancer: a study of absolute and relative survival over 15 years. Lung Cancer. 2005;47:173–81.
143. Xie L, Ugnat AM, Morriss J, et al. Histology-related variation in the treatment and survival of patients with lung carcinoma in Canada. Lung Cancer. 2003;42:127–39.

Part II
Special Considerations in the Management of Older Patients

Chapter 3
Physiological Assessment and Cardiopulmonary Exercise Testing

Paul P. Walker, Malcolm West, Michael P.W. Grocott, and Sandy Jack

Abstract There have been significant advances in the management and treatment of lung cancer over the last 10–20 years, but surgical resection remains the primary treatment that results in cure and long-term survival. However, factors that predispose to the development of lung cancer also increase the incidence of chronic obstructive pulmonary disease. Physiological testing before lung cancer surgery is important, and every patient should undergo detailed lung function testing including measurement of the transfer factor for carbon dioxide (TL_{CO}). Patients with a predicted postoperative FEV_1 and TL_{CO} of <40 % predicted should undergo cardiopulmonary exercise testing to further detail their risk status. Only in this way can a fully informed decision take place between the patient and surgeon as to the best treatment which not only attempts "cure" but also minimizes postoperative mortality while delivering acceptable postoperative breathlessness and quality of life. Age alone should never be used to deny surgery and function should be formally assessed as we have detailed.

P.P. Walker, BMedSci (Hons), MD, FRCP
Department of Respiratory Medicine, University Hospital Aintree,
Liverpool, UK

M. West, MD, MRCS(Ed) (✉)
Department of Musculoskeletal Biology II, Faculty of Health and Life Sciences,
University of Liverpool, Liverpool, UK
e-mail: malcolmwest@nhs.net

M.P.W. Grocott, MD, FRCA, FRCP, FFICM
Integrative Physiology and Critical Illness Group, Clinical and Experimental Sciences,
Faculty of Medicine, University of Southampton, Southampton, UK

S. Jack, MSc, PhD
Critical Care Research Area, NIHR Respiratory Biomedical Research Unit,
University Hospital Southampton NHS Foundation Trust, Southampton, UK

C. Gridelli, R.A. Audisio (eds.), *Management of Lung Cancer in Older People*,
DOI 10.1007/978-0-85729-793-8_3,

Keywords Cardiopulmonary exercise testing in the elderly with lung cancer • Lung cancer and exercise testing in the elderly • Physiological testing before lung cancer surgery • Lung function assessment in the elderly with cancer • Chemotherapy effects on lung function in elderly cancer patients

There have been significant advances in the management and treatment of lung cancer over the last 10–20 years, but surgical resection remains the primary treatment that results in cure and long-term survival. However, factors that predispose to the development of lung cancer also increase the incidence of chronic obstructive pulmonary disease. This is not related to cigarette smoking alone as the incidence of lung cancer in patients with COPD exceeds that expected due to cigarette smoking. Common genetic links have recently been identified [1–3]. In addition, the risk of lung cancer is increased multifold in patients with pulmonary fibrosis [4], and the presence of either pulmonary fibrosis or significant COPD increases the risk from surgery and potentially renders some patients inoperable.

Ultimately, the aim of surgery is to completely resect the tumor while leaving the patient with an acceptable quality of life and level of breathlessness. Without effective treatment, survival with lung cancer is poor, with 5-year survival in Europe of less than 15 % [5], but this has to be balanced against postoperative symptoms and function. Ultimately, these decisions have to be made at patient level as, while multidisciplinary team (MDT) discussion is important to outcomes [6], it results in recommendations and only the individual can ultimately decide what is and is not an acceptable function. In most cases, resection involves a pneumonectomy or lobectomy though alternatives, such as sleeve, sub-lobar, or wedge resection, may be both acceptable and lung preserving in patients with poorer preoperative function. In addition, the advent of stereotactic radiotherapy [7, 8] means that some patients with early-stage tumors considered unresectable can benefit from potentially curative treatment where previously they would have been managed palliatively because they could not receive external beam radiotherapy due to the damage it caused to the surrounding lung. In addition, stereotactic radiotherapy has shown good results in elderly patients (>75 years) in whom surgical resection is considered high risk [9].

There are a variety of methods with which suitability for radical treatment of lung cancer is assessed. The main body of evidence relates to surgical resection, and specific recommendations about fitness for radical therapy have been published by the European Respiratory Society/European Society for Thoracic Surgeons [10, 11] and the British Thoracic Society/the Society for Cardiothoracic Surgery in Great Britain/Ireland Lung Cancer Guideline Group [12]. The effects of external beam radiotherapy and chemotherapy have been studied previously though the studies have often been of modest size with a variety of different treatments and doses administered and a variety of different effects seen on physiological parameters. This will be discussed in more detail later in the chapter. This chapter will not cover cardiological assessment but will focus entirely on lung function and exercise testing.

Despite lung cancer being a disease of the elderly, there is little specific evidence base for an older population, in particular in relation to trials using standard, first-line platinum-based chemotherapy [13]. This limits the evidence base for physiological assessment though means it should be utilized irrespective of age.

Lung Function Assessment

The role of preoperative physiological assessment is twofold – assessment of the risk of operative mortality in patients considered for surgery and assessment of the risk of posttreatment breathlessness. Lung function relates relatively poorly to postoperative quality of life [14] though this is impacted by the surgical technique employed [15]. The two main measurements used are the forced expiratory volume in 1 s (FEV_1), measured using spirometry, and a measure of the oxygen diffusing capacity of the lung – usually the transfer factor for carbon monoxide (TL_{CO}). There is ample evidence that the two measures are relatively poorly related [16], indicating that they measure different aspects of lung function. Measurement of FEV_1 can be performed with a simple handheld spirometer, but measurement of lung diffusing capacity using the single breath-hold technique requires more complex equipment.

Spirometry and Forced Expiratory Volume in 1 Second (FEV_1)

The basis on which spirometry, more specifically FEV_1, is used to assess suitability for surgery is based on an estimation of predicted postoperative FEV_1 ($ppoFEV_1$) [17, 18]; this measure is being used as a surrogate for perioperative complications, postoperative dyspnea, and consequently health status. However, FEV_1 is predominantly used to determine where more detailed assessment is required using measurement of lung diffusion and exercise testing. In this situation, FEV_1 is best expressed as a percentage of predicted value rather than absolute value [19].

In a number of case series, a $ppoFEV_1$ of less than 40 % predicted has been associated with poor outcome, in particular high perioperative mortality [20, 21]. Where $ppoFEV_1$ is less than 30 % predicted, the risks are even higher [22, 23]. However, this evidence is based on data collected more than 20 years ago, and more recent series have indicated that mortality can be modest even in patients with a $ppoFEV_1$ of 30–40 % predicted likely due to better perioperative management and use of different surgical techniques allowing lung parenchymal sparing [24]. As a result, current guidelines suggest that a $ppoFEV_1$ of 30 % predicted should be the current lower limit for surgery [10–12].

The surgeon should consider two important additional aspects when recommending surgery. This first is the potential lung volume reduction effect in patients with extensive emphysema. This is discussed in detail later in the chapter, but in some patients this may extend the lower limit of $ppoFEV_1$. However, this has to be balanced against the immediate postoperative FEV_1 which is often significantly lower than the $ppoFEV_1$, in particular on postoperative day 1 [25], with $ppoFEV_1$ being a better estimate of FEV_1 3–6 months after the operation. However, in patients with COPD, lung function is often little changed or improved after 3–6 months [26, 27], with improvement in lung function being more common in patients with static hyperinflation likely secondary to emphysema [28].

Diffusion Capacity for Carbon Monoxide

The diffusing capacity for carbon monoxide, TL_{CO} (or more accurately transfer factor for carbon monoxide), is an accurate measure of alveolar oxygen exchange and is an independent predictor of perioperative complications and mortality in patients with and without COPD [29–31]. Reduction in the transfer factor is seen in patients with COPD (usually those with predominant emphysema) and pulmonary fibrosis and patients with pulmonary hypertension. The latter condition is often seen in patients with COPD or fibrosis secondary to the underlying lung disease and can further reduce transfer factor in these patients.

In clinical practice, diffusing capacity has often not been measured in patients with a reduced FEV_1 (less than 80 % of predicted value). However, data showing that TL_{CO} is useful in predicting postoperative complications even in patients with a normal FEV_1 [31] as well as the recognition that some patients with a normal FEV_1 may have a significant reduction in lung diffusion has led to the recommendation that all patients being assessed for lung resection should have DLCO measured. Traditionally, a $ppoTL_{CO}$ of 40 % has been used to determine high-risk patients [18] though more recent guidelines [10–12] have suggested that a $ppoTL_{CO}$ of 30 % is used to define high-risk threshold.

Split Lung Function Testing

Where radiological assessment suggests that a ventilation or perfusion mismatch may be present, ventilation scintigraphy and perfusion scintigraphy can be used to more accurately determine ppo lung function [32–35]. Although there are concerns about the accuracy of the measurement [32, 33], the technique allows a more detailed assessment of the contribution to ventilation by individual lung lobes. This technique is best reserved for patients where it has been assessed that any further loss of lung function would present an unacceptable perioperative risk or that postoperative dyspnea would be unacceptably great. One example is where predominantly destroyed emphysematous lung, which is contributing little to ventilation, would be removed. A similar situation could occur where the tumor is obstructing the arterial supply to an area targeted for resection and is again contributing little to ventilation.

Calculation of Estimated Postoperative Lung Function

Postoperative lung function is assessed by segment counting. The lung has 19 segments – ten on the right and nine on the left. The right upper lobe has three, middle lobe two, and the right lower lobe five segments. The left upper lobe division has three segments with an additional two in the lingular segment of the upper lobe. The left lower lobe has four segments. If there are no obstructed segments, then

$$\text{ppo value} = \text{pre-operative value} \times \frac{(19 - \text{number of segments resected})}{19}$$

However, if there are obstructed segments, measured by imaging, then these segments must be included in the equation. In this case,

$$\text{ppo value} = \text{pre-op value} \times \frac{(19 - \text{obstructed segments} - \text{number of segments resected})}{19 - \text{obstructed segments}}$$

If the ppo value falls below that recommended, surgery may still be possible utilizing "lung-sparing" surgical techniques in place of a pneumonectomy or lobectomy.

If $ppoFEV_1$ and/or TL_{CO} are <40 % predicted, the patient would be considered high risk for surgery, and functional assessment with exercise testing is recommended as shown in Fig. 3.1 taken from the UK guidelines [12]. This is discussed in more detail later in the chapter.

Change in Lung Function with Aging and the Impact on Reference Ranges

The effect of aging on the human lung results in dilatation of the alveoli, a reduction in the surface area available for gas exchange, and loss of tissue that supports the small airways resulting in a similar situation to that seen in patients with emphysema. This leads to reduced lung elastic recoil and an increase in functional residual capacity. Under conditions of forced spirometry, seen when FEV_1 is measured, there is a reduction in flow consistent with small airway collapse and closure. Respiratory muscle strength also decreases with aging as does the transfer factor for carbon monoxide, reflecting mainly this loss of surface area [36].

Significant challenges to accurate use of pulmonary function in the elderly include the underrepresentation of subjects over 65 years in populations used to derive reference ranges. When an individual is both elderly and from an

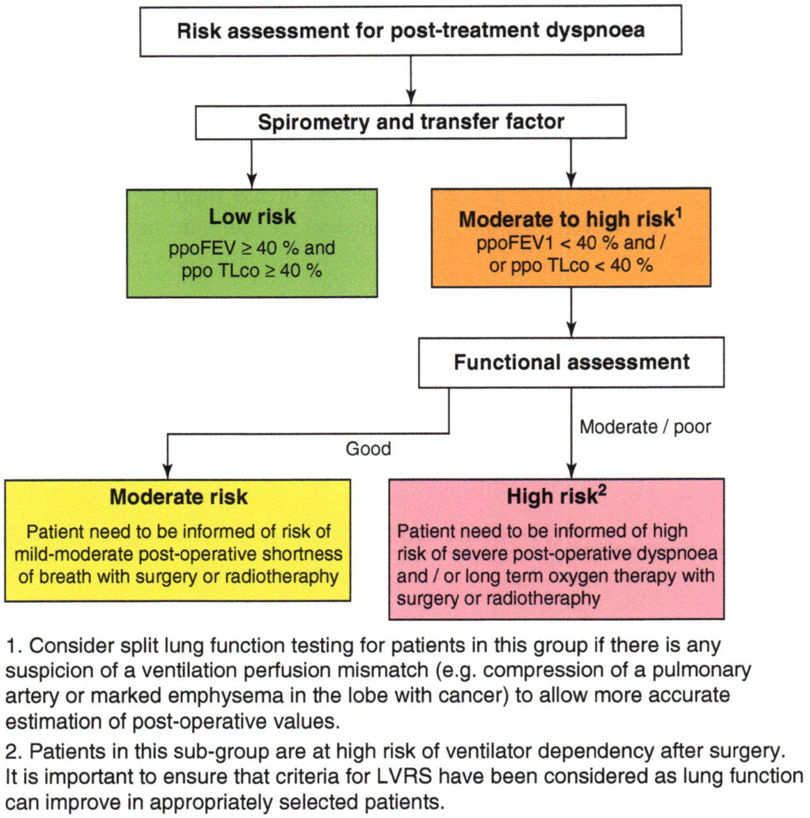

Fig. 3.1 Risk assessment for patients considered for surgery for lung cancer [12]. All patients should have FEV_1 and TL_{CO} measured. Patients at moderate to high risk should undergo CPET testing

ethnic minority population, finding accurate reference ranges can be even more challenging. Traditional datasets include the European Community for Coal and Steel [37] and the National Health and Nutrition Examination Survey (NHANES). The latter has involved three data collections with the latter (NHANES III) collected between 1988 and 1994 [38].

Considerable worldwide effort has been invested to improve accuracy of reference ranges using spirometry datasets collected over a number of decades [39]. Interpretative strategies for lung function have been reviewed previously and recommendations made [40]. It has previously been recommended that reference ranges used should be assessed against the local population, but it is now accepted that this is impractical; for spirometry alone, every center would need to perform in excess of 100 measurements to obtain representative values. Hence, use of ranges derived from larger populations is currently recommended. However, where the measuring device provides reference ranges, it is imperative that the physiologist ensures the range quoted is derived from the most applicable population.

Effects of Neoadjuvant Chemotherapy on Pulmonary Function

In specific patients with more advanced lung cancer, there is a role for neoadjuvant radiotherapy, chemoradiotherapy, or chemotherapy alone or to downstage a tumor prior to surgery. The effect of radical radiotherapy regimes on lung function has been long recognized [41, 42] and is caused by radiation pneumonitis followed by fibrosis, thickening of the alveolar walls, and damage to the microvasculature [43]. External beam radiotherapy results in a reduction in FEV_1, lung volumes including TLC, and lung diffusing capacity [44, 45], and the effect on lung diffusion is accentuated by the addition of sequential and in particular concurrent radiotherapy. Borst et al. also showed that in long-term survivors after radical radiotherapy, there was no “late” recovery in lung function.

Induction treatment with chemotherapy alone has been examined in a number of studies, and there is usually little effect or improvement in spirometry and lung volumes, probably as a result of tumor shrinkage and recruitment of previously nonfunctioning airways. Conversely, a considerable proportion of patients suffered reduction in lung diffusion – in some cases greater than 20 % of baseline value [46, 47]. In some studies, the fall in diffusion appeared to relate to perioperative complications [48]. In another study, pulmonary function was measured at baseline, post-chemotherapy, and postoperatively for 1 year after surgery, and this demonstrated the cumulative impact of chemotherapy and surgery on lung diffusion [49]. This study also suggested that while lung diffusion improved postoperatively in younger patients (<65 years), the same did not occur in older patients though the small number of subjects limits any applicability of this finding.

As a result, patients with reduced baseline lung diffusion who undergo induction chemotherapy, radiotherapy, or a combination should have pulmonary function reassessed after neoadjuvant treatment but before surgery as there may have been a significant impact upon ppoTLco. The effect of neoadjuvant therapy should be carefully considered in patients with borderline lung diffusion at baseline.

Although the overall effect of radiotherapy and chemotherapy on lung function has been established, pulmonary physiology cannot accurately predict the effect of treatment on lung function or the risks associated with treatment for an individual patient. Specific treatment algorithms based on the effects of either radiotherapy, chemotherapy, or a combination do not exist, and safe lower limits of lung function have not been defined. Currently, a decision to treat is primarily based on a combination of symptoms, FEV_1, and performance status.

Lung Volume Reduction Surgery

In one situation, surgery could be considered in patients with poorer lung function than usual – where the patient may benefit from lung volume reduction surgery (LVRS). This particular operation has been shown to benefit a subgroup of patients with COPD and a FEV_1 of <45 % predicted and works by removing grossly emphysematous lung (usually the upper lobes bilaterally) allowing the remaining less damaged lung to function better. The National Emphysema Treatment Trial (NETT) showed improved exercise capacity and a survival advantage in patients with homogenous emphysema and poor function (as formally assessed on a walking test) who were taking maximal bronchodilator therapy and who had completed pulmonary rehabilitation [50]. There was no upper age limit for inclusion though the mean age of participants was 67 (±6) years and mean FEV_1 was 27 % of predicted. An earlier publication from the same trial indicated an unacceptably high early mortality in patients with a FEV_1 <20 % predicted, a TL_{CO} <20 % predicted, and homogeneous emphysema [51]. Despite this a number of patients with poorer lung function than would normally be considered for surgery (FEV_1 20–40 % of predicted) could be considered for curative resection of their tumor as long as the tumor lies within the area of emphysema that would be removed by LVRS.

Cardiopulmonary Exercise Testing

Almost two decades ago, Older and colleagues identified an association between low functional capacity (low fitness level), as determined by cardiopulmonary exercise testing (CPET), and poor patient outcome following major non-cardiopulmonary surgery [52]. Based on this, and subsequent published literature, CPET-derived variables have been increasingly adopted as objective measures of fitness prior to surgery, particularly within the National Health Service (NHS) in the UK [53]. This information is used to inform operative decisions and choice of perioperative management and to discuss risk with patients [54]. CPET is not routinely used in all, or even a majority of, patients undergoing lung cancer resection; however, along with lung function testing, it has an important role in higher-risk patients as shown in Fig. 3.1 (patients with a ppoFEV_1 and/or TL_{CO} <40 % of predicted value).

Understanding the Basics of Cardiopulmonary Exercise Testing

Cardiopulmonary exercise testing (CPET) involves the measurement of physiological variables during incremental exercise, in order to assess a patient's functional capacity representing an index of their physiological reserve. CPET provides a global assessment of the integrated response to increasing work by the coordinated action of the cardiovascular, respiratory, skeletal muscle, and metabolic systems, all of which are activated during the stress response to surgery [54]. CPET allows evaluation of the integrated function of the oxygen transport system under conditions of physiological stress when the demand for oxygen is high and the system is required to function near to its maximum capacity. Despite requiring a moderate to high level of exertion, CPET is well tolerated by patients [55, 56] and is safe to conduct on most patient cohorts [57].

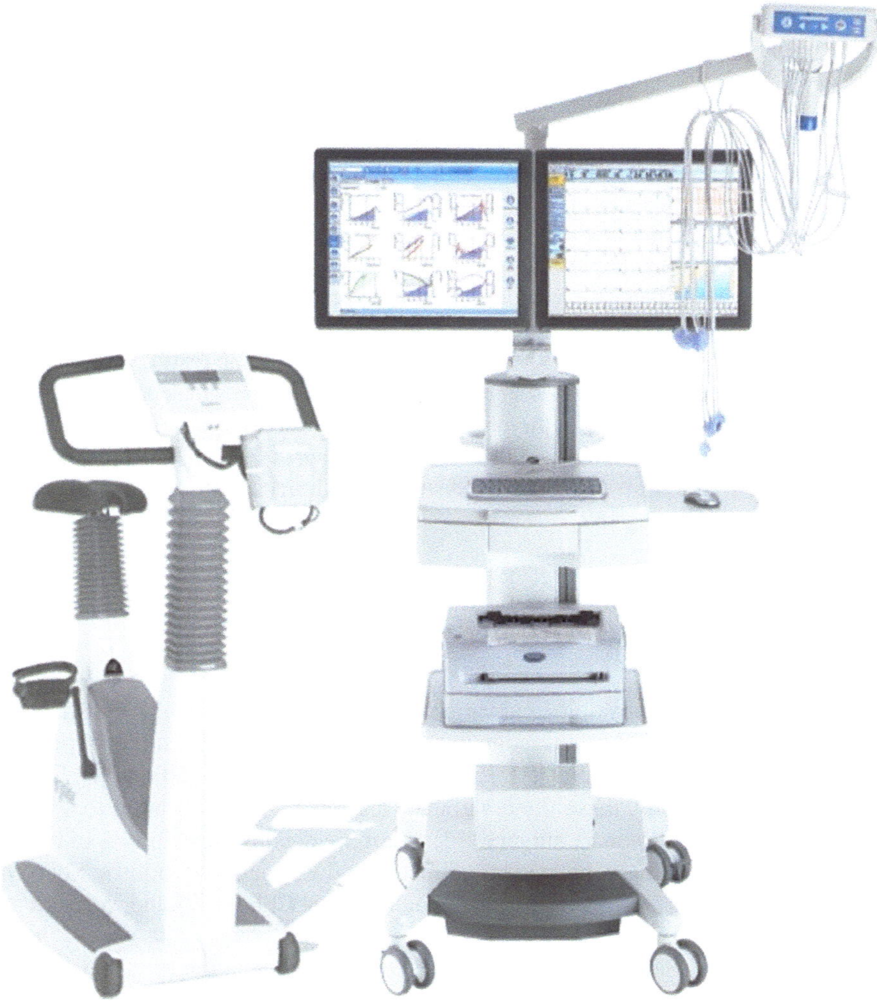

Fig. 3.2 CPET setup including metabolic cart, bike, and ECG (Courtesy of Ergostik, Geratherm Respiratory, Bad Kissingen, Germany)

In the assessment of preoperative risk, CPET is usually conducted on an electromagnetically braked cycle ergometer with the patient breathing through a mouthpiece through which gas exchange is measured. ECG and oxygen saturation monitoring with periodic measurement of blood pressure are continuously assessed. A typical CPET setup is shown in Fig. 3.2, and the common CPET variables are detailed in Table 3.1. The test protocol normally includes four phases. Typically, an initial rest phase (approximately 3 min) is employed to establish baseline values, followed by an unloaded cycling phase (3 min freewheel pedalling) to allow the patient to become familiar with the cycling motion [58]. Following this, the incremental exercise phase begins. A ramp protocol is commonly used, during which the set work rate is increased linearly with time, with a corresponding increase in the intensity of exercise. There are a variety of ways to determine the increment which will vary based on patient factors [58]. The criteria for test termination differ between laboratories; in some, the test is terminated by the patient at volitional exhaustion, while others perform a submaximal test and stop exercise when a particular criterion is met, such as a respiratory exchange ratio (RER) above 1 [57]. Following test completion, a recovery period of low-intensity exercise should be performed to maintain venous return, thereby reducing the risk of pooling of blood in the leg veins which can be associated with symptomatic hypotension (e.g., light-headedness, fainting). The patient should be observed throughout recovery until physiological variables including heart rate, blood pressure, ventilation, and oxygen saturation have returned close to baseline levels and any exercise-induced ECG changes have resolved.

Each laboratory will have specific exclusion criteria for testing. The test is stopped if the patient experiences any adverse symptoms (e.g., chest pain, dizziness, or severe breathlessness) or if the physiological data indicates a potential adverse event (e.g., ECG abnormalities, a fall in systolic pressure >20 mmHg from the highest value during the test, and a rise in systolic blood pressure to >250 mmHg and diastolic to >120 mmHg [57]).

Cardiopulmonary Exercise Testing Variables

A number of different physiological variables are recorded (Table 3.1), of which the following have been used by investigators to identify patients at high risk of perioperative morbidity and mortality: AT [52, 55, 56, 59], $VO_{2\ peak/max}$ [60], and V_E/VCO_2 [56, 61]. Consequently, these three variables are most commonly used to stratify risk for non-cardiopulmonary surgery [53]. For more detailed descriptions of CPET protocols and physiology, the reader is directed to the American Thoracic Society/American College of Chest Physicians' statement on CPET [57] and Wasserman et al. [58].

During exercise when the net increase in lactate accumulation produces an acidosis, the buffering of lactic acid causes an obligatory increase in carbon dioxide output (VCO_2) relative to oxygen uptake (VO_2) from the CO_2 produced when HCO_3^- buffers lactic acid. When these variables (VCO_2 and VO_2) are plotted against each other, the relationship is composed of two apparently linear components, the lower of which has a slope of slightly less than 1.0. The intercept of these two slopes is the anaerobic threshold (sometimes called the lactate threshold) as measured by gas exchange. This technique is referred to as the V-slope method [58] because it relates the increase in volume of CO_2 output to volume of O_2 uptake and is represented in Fig. 3.3, though the physiological basis for this variable remains controversial [62]. A potential limitation in the accurate determination of AT is that it is a noninvasive estimation which depends on CO_2 stores; therefore, alteration in these stores may introduce inaccuracy relevant to the context of risk stratification. Alteration in CO_2 stores may occur due to anticipatory anxiety causing acute hyperventilation [58, 62]. Ozcelik and colleagues demonstrated that the early dynamics of the CO_2 wash-in to

Table 3.1 Cardiopulmonary exercise testing variable definitions

Anaerobic threshold (AT)	The exercise VO_2 above which anaerobic high-energy phosphate production supplements aerobic high-energy phosphate production, with consequential lowering of the cellular redox state, increase in lactate/pyruvate (L/P) ratio, and net increase in lactate production at the site of anaerobiosis. Exercise above the AT is reflected in the muscle effluent and central blood by an increase in lactate concentration, L/P ratio, and metabolic acidosis
Heart rate reserve (HRR)	The difference between the predicted highest heart rate attainable during maximum exercise and the actual highest heart rate
Maximal oxygen uptake ($VO_{2\,max}$)	Describes the VO_2 when it reaches a plateau value during a single maximum work rate test. Repeated measurements necessary to obtain the VO_2 that cannot be exceeded by the subject
Oxygen pulse (O_2 pulse)	The oxygen uptake divided by the heart rate. Hence, this represents the amount of oxygen extracted by the tissue of the body from the O_2 carried in each stroke volume
Oxygen uptake (VO_2)	The amount of oxygen extracted from the inspired gas in a given period of time, expressed in ml or L per minute
Peak oxygen uptake ($VO_{2\,peak}$)	The highest oxygen uptake achieved during a maximum work rate test
Work rate	The rate at which work is preformed in Watts
Ventilatory equivalents for CO_2 and O_2 (V_E/VCO_2 and V_E/VO_2)	The ventilatory equivalents for CO_2 and O_2 are measurements of the ventilatory requirement for a given metabolic rate
Minute ventilation (V_E)	The volume of gas exhaled divided by the time of collection in minutes
Respiratory exchange ratio (RER)	The ratio between the molecules of O_2 breathed in and the molecules of CO_2 breathed out

From Onishi et al. [7]. With permission of Wolters Kluwer

the previously depleted body stores could result in a pseudo-AT, which arises significantly before the onset of the true lactic acidosis. They advocate using precautions to avoid hyperventilation prior to noninvasive estimation of the lactate threshold [63].

Peak oxygen uptake is another useful measure of functional reserve and VO_2 is related to age, sex, weight, and type of work performed. A formula for estimating VO_2 reported by Wasserman and Whipp is as follows [64]:

$$\text{Predicted } VO_2 \text{ during unloaded pedalling (ml / min)} = (5.8 \times \text{weight in kg}) + 151$$

$$\text{Peak } VO_2 \text{(ml / min)} = \text{Height (cm)} - \text{age (years)} \times 20 \text{ (sedentary males) or } \times 14 \text{ (sedentary females)}$$

$VO_{2\,Peak}$ is the highest VO_2 achieved during CPET and generally occurs at or near peak exercise. Moreover, if the VO_2 trace demonstrates a plateau, such that the VO_2

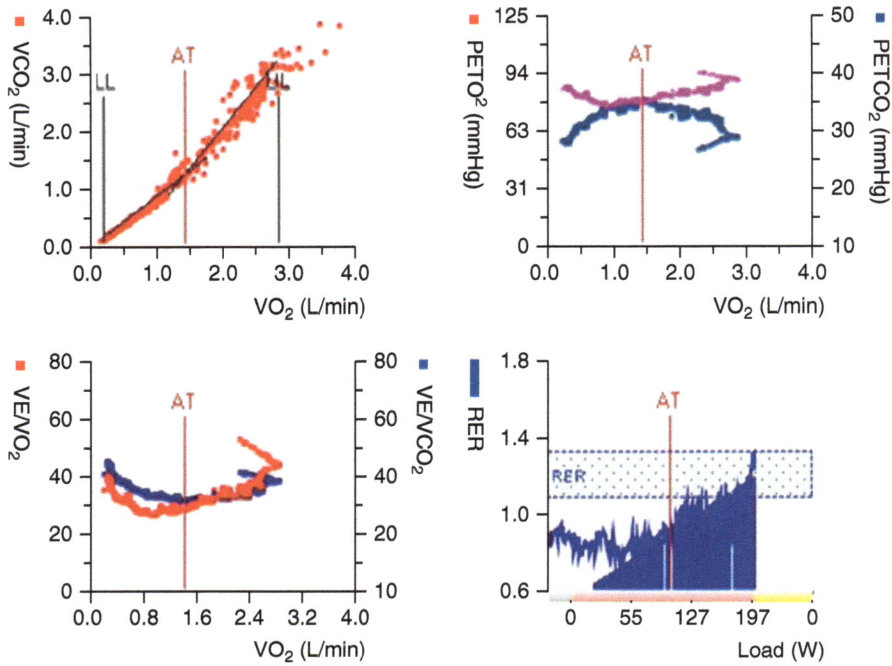

Fig. 3.3 An example trace showing AT and how it is determined

no longer increases despite progressive increments in workload, then the $VO_{2\,Peak}$ can also be labelled as the $VO_{2\,Max.}$ The two measures are often used interchangeably though can differ. $VO_{2\,Max}$ is the best and most reproducible index of cardiopulmonary fitness or disability [58].

The major link between the circulatory and ventilatory responses to exercise is carbon dioxide production. Ventilatory efficiency describes the relationship between minute ventilation and CO_2 production and is in part affected by matching of ventilation to perfusion. V_E/VCO_2 is a respiratory control function that reflects chemoreceptor sensitivity, acid–base balance, and diffusion efficiency at the alveolar-capillary interface [58].

Effect of Age on Fitness and Preoperative Risk

An age-related decline in peak oxygen consumption ($VO_{2\,Peak}$) and AT has been observed in both longitudinal [65, 66] and cross-sectional studies [67, 68]. The decline in $VO_{2\,Peak}$ and AT with age is multifactorial and associated with alterations in both central and peripheral factors. Changes in body composition and physical activity can also contribute to this decline. The reduction in $VO_{2\,Peak}$ in older patients has been associated with a greater risk of mortality primarily because of an increased cardiovascular risk [69]. $VO_{2\ Peak}$ has been shown to decline more with age in males (decline of 0.034 L/min each year) than in females (decline of 0.028 L/min each year). This decline is greater still in males if fat-free mass and fat mass are controlled for [70]. AT also decreases with age, but slower than $VO_{2\ Peak}$, at a rate of 0.0049 L/min each year. The mechanisms accounting for the differing rates of decline in AT and $VO_{2\ Peak}$ are unknown [71]. Older and colleagues [59] discuss how this reduction is believed to be more dependent on the presence of comorbidity, the prevalence of which increases with age, rather than with age per se. They have also shown that the variation in AT across all age groups is such that it lies within one standard deviation. Consequently, age is a poor guide to fitness and should not be used as a criterion on which to base judgements about perioperative risk.

Current Applications of Cardiopulmonary Exercise Testing in Major Surgery

Early publications in the 1990s showed a clear relationship between presurgical CPET variables and postoperative outcomes. It should be noted that because mortality is usually low, few of the studies are powered to look at differences in mortality but provide insight into the impact on postoperative complications. Older et al. [52] recorded the AT of 187 elderly patients undergoing major intra-abdominal surgery. They found that an AT <11 ml/kg/min was associated with increased cardiovascular mortality and patients with a low AT and preoperative myocardial ischemia mortality rose from 4 to 42 %. This supported the idea of preoperative risk stratification and use of targeted enhanced postoperative care. In a later study [59], the authors investigated the impact of triaging patients on the basis of the above data. In the study, 28 % patients with an AT <11 ml/min/kg were assigned to ICU preoperatively, while the other patients with an AT >11 ml/min/kg were assigned to HDU care if they had preoperative myocardial ischemia or a VE/VO_2 >35 (21 % patients) or ward care (51 %) if they had none of these factors. Of the nine patients who died postoperatively from cardiopulmonary complications, seven had an AT <11 ml/min/kg with the other two in the HDU category, while no deaths were recorded in the ward population.

Since these publications in the 1990s, several studies have addressed the association between CPET-derived variables and perioperative outcome in a variety of clinical contexts [72–74], and some of these studies have also evaluated the predictive utility of CPET-derived variables as a means of describing perioperative risk in clinical practice [72–74]. However, cardiopulmonary risk may differ in patients undergoing resection for lung cancer compared with major surgery for other reasons, making lung cancer-specific studies important.

Thoracic and Lung Cancer Surgery in the Elderly

The incidence of postoperative pulmonary complications after thoracotomy and lung resection is about 30 % and is related not only to the removal of lung tissue and alterations in chest wall mechanics [75] but also to patient comorbidities and physiological reserve. Hence, pulmonary function testing alone fails to fully assess the entire cardiovascular response to exercise and reserve.

In the mid-1980s, Smith et al. [76] assessed patients undergoing thoracotomy and concluded that those patients without complications had a significantly higher $VO_{2\,Max}$ than did patients who experienced complications (22.4 ± 1.4 vs. 14.9 ± 0.9 ml/kg/min; $p < 0.001$). However, after this study, a series of other studies were published showing no or inconsistent correlations between $VO_{2\ Peak}$ and postoperative complications [21, 77, 78]. Later the same decade, Bechard and Wetstein [79] correlated preoperative static pulmonary function, FEV_1, and $VO_{2\,Max}$ with postoperative morbidity and mortality in 50 consecutive patients in one of the first attempts to risk stratify lung cancer patients according to an objectively measured oxygen consumption. The authors concluded that exercise testing was an important criterion in the preoperative evaluation of patients for pulmonary surgery and that a $VO_{2\,Max}$ of less than 10 ml/kg/min was associated with significant morbidity and mortality. Finally, Gerson et al. [80] performed supine exercise ergometry in 177 patients, aged 65 and over, undergoing elective major noncardiac thoracic surgery. Patients who were unable to perform 2 min of supine bicycle exercise raising the heart rate above 99 beats/min had higher perioperative pulmonary and cardiac complications with five deaths and a 42 % rate of complications in 69 patients who were unable to exercise satisfactorily.

These studies stimulated interest in patients undergoing resections specifically for lung cancer rather than just patients undergoing a thoracotomy, in part because of the potentially greater cardiovascular stress associated with cancer surgery. Epstein and colleagues [81] were the first group in the 1990s that analyzed the findings in 42 patients who had CPET prior to lung cancer resections. They found that patients with a peak VO_2 of less than 500 ml/min/m^2 were six times more likely to experience a cardiopulmonary complication ($p < 0.05$). Larsen et al. [82] prospectively recruited 97 patients who had CPET prior to lung cancer resection. They found that maximal oxygen uptake and forced expiratory volume were predictive of postoperative complications. They also found that a maximal oxygen uptake <50 % of predicted value was associated with higher risk of death from cardiopulmonary causes. Kaplan-Meier survival curves showed that maximal oxygen uptake was correlated to long-term survival, while spirometric variables were not. Brutsche et al. [83] found similar results when they also conducted a prospective trial, to identify predictors of postoperative complications and death after lung resection, in 125 non-small cell lung cancer patients amenable to resection. All underwent functional assessment including spirometry and cardiopulmonary exercise tests and lung resection via thoracotomy. Complications occurred in 31 of 125 (25 %) patients including two (1.6 %) deaths. On logistic regression analysis, only maximal oxygen uptake ($VO_{2\,Max}$) per kg body weight expressed as a percentage of the predicted value ($p<0.0001$) and the estimated extent of lung tissue resection ($p=0.02$) were independent predictors of postoperative complications. The authors concluded that these simple parameters should be integrated into the preoperative decision analysis for operability in patients undergoing lung resection for lung cancer.

In the early part of the twenty-first century, Villani and Busia [84] set out to evaluate which parameters of preoperative spirometry, arterial blood gas, radionuclide lung scanning, and cardiopulmonary exercise test are the best predictor of postoperative morbidity and mortality in 150 relatively young patients specifically undergoing pneumonectomy for lung cancer. These subjects were undergoing resection of a large volume of lung tissue previously shown to be associated with a greater risk of complications and death [83]. Forty-four patients (29.3 %) had postoperative complications, of which four patients (2.7 %) died within 1 month of surgery. Patients with complications had significantly lower postoperative predicted (ppo) FEV_1 and lower $VO_{2\,Max}$, and those who died also had a significant decrease in PaO_2 during exercise. They also considered the ppoFEV_1 expressed as percentage and found significant differences between patients who suffered and did not suffer complications (55 ± 3 vs. 46 ± 1.9; $p<0.05$). They concluded that these data support the use of exercise testing as a useful adjunct in the evaluation of postoperative risk for pneumonectomy, especially in patients with obstructive pulmonary disease. In particular, they concluded that patients with a $VO_{2\,Max}$ <50 % of predicted should be considered at high risk of morbidity from cardiopulmonary causes.

Nagamatsu et al. [85] also studied 211 patients undergoing lung resection for cancer. The results of expired gas analysis during exercise testing showed that $VO_{2\,Max}$ ($P<0.0005$), anaerobic threshold ($P<0.01$), and vital capacity ($P<0.005$) were lower in patients with cardiopulmonary complications. In the same period, Win et al. [86] studied 130 patients with operable lung cancer. Mean $VO_{2\,Peak}$ was 18.3 ml/kg/ml and mean percentage predicted $VO_{2\,Peak}$ was 84.4 %. Poor surgical outcome was significantly related to $VO_{2\,Peak}$ percentage of predicted ($p<0.01$) but not to the actual oxygen uptake value; hence, this would be a better indicator of surgical outcome as it corrects for normal physiologic ranges. They concluded that the threshold of $VO_{2\,Peak}$ for surgical intervention could be set between 50 and 60 % predicted without excess surgical mortality. In another study, Bolliger et al. [87] set this threshold at 75 % of predicted $VO_{2\,Max}$, leading to uneventful operations in nine out of ten patients (mean age 61 years). Patients with a value of <50 % are regarded as being high risk for postoperative pulmonary complications. These and other works are now the basis of the current guidelines for preoperative exercise testing for patients amenable for lung cancer resection [10–12].

In an attempt to summarize the evidence from a significant number of smaller primary studies, all of which had methodological differences, Benzo et al. [88] performed a meta-analysis looking at whether $VO_{2\,Max}$ differed between patients who develop postoperative cardiopulmonary complications. Fourteen studies representing a total of 955 men and women were included. They concluded that exercise capacity expressed as $VO_{2\,Max}$ is lower in patients that develop clinically relevant complications after curative lung resection. Interestingly, subjects without postoperative cardiopulmonary complications were 4 years younger (mean age 61 years) than subjects who developed complications (mean age 65.4 years) which likely reflects increasing comorbidity with increasing age. This supports the usefulness of measuring preoperative exercise capacity as a tool for decision making for lung resection.

CPET is considered of value in patients who after lung resection are expected to have a forced expiratory volume in 1 s (FEV_1) or transfer factor (TL_{CO}) of less than 40 % predicted (Fig. 3.1). Patients who have a $VO_{2\ Peak}$ of less than 15 ml/kg/min are considered to be high risk. A recent literature review by Tilburg et al. [89] also confirms that CPET is a better predictor of postoperative complications than the resting assessment of cardiac and pulmonary function in an elderly lung cancer population (patients included in the review were mostly aged >65 years). It also concluded that $VO_{2\,Max}$ is the best indicator of aerobic capacity and cardiorespiratory fitness and that if $VO_{2\ Max}$ was >20 ml/kg/min, postoperative morbidity would be <10 % and mortality close to zero. Patients having curative lung cancer surgery with a $VO_{2\ Peak}$ of less than 15 ml/kg/min and/or a $VO_{2\,Max}$ of less than 20 ml/kg/min are at high risk of developing clinically relevant postoperative complications. As discussed previously, establishing that a patient is "high risk" does not necessarily rule out surgery; however, it represents important information for both patient and surgeon when making a decision about best treatment in light of other therapeutic options.

Conclusions

Physiological testing before lung cancer surgery is important, and every patient should undergo detailed lung function testing including measurement of TL_{CO}. Patients with a predicted postoperative FEV_1 and TL_{CO} of <40 % predicted should undergo CPET testing to further detail their risk status. Only in this way can a fully informed decision take place between the patient and surgeon as to the best treatment which not only attempts "cure" but also minimizes postoperative mortality while delivering acceptable postoperative breathlessness and quality of life. Age alone should never be used to deny surgery, and function should be formally assessed as we have detailed.

References

1. Young RP, Hopkins RJ. How the genetics of lung cancer may overlap with COPD. Respirology. 2011;16:1047–55.
2. Adcock IM, Caramori G, Barnes PJ. Chronic obstructive pulmonary disease and lung cancer: new molecular insights. Respiration. 2011;81:265–84.
3. Rooney C, Sethi T. The epithelial cell and lung cancer: the link between chronic obstructive pulmonary disease and lung cancer. Respiration. 2011;81:89–104.

4. Harris JM, Johnston ID, Rudd R, et al. Cryptogenic fibrosing alveolitis and lung cancer: the BTS study. Thorax. 2010;65:70–6.
5. Berrino F, De Angelis R, Sant M, et al. Survival for eight major cancers and all cancers combined for European adults diagnosed in 1995-99: results of the EUROCARE-4 study. Lancet Oncol. 2007;8:773–83.
6. Forrest LM, McMillan DC, McArdle CS, et al. An evaluation of the impact of a multidisciplinary team, in a single centre, on treatment and survival in patients with inoperable non-small-cell lung cancer. Br J Cancer. 2005;93(9):977–8.
7. Onishi H, Shirato H, Nagata Y, et al. Hypofractionated stereotactic radiotherapy (HypoFXSRT) for stage I non-small cell lung cancer: updated results of 257 patients in a Japanese multi-institutional study. J Thorac Oncol. 2007;2:S94–100.
8. Lagerwaard FJ, Haasbeek CJ, Smit EF, et al. Outcomes of risk-adapted fractionated stereotactic radiotherapy for stage I non-small-cell lung cancer. Int J Radiat Oncol Biol Phys. 2008;70:685–92.
9. Palma D, Visser O, Lagerwaard FJ, et al. Treatment of stage I NSCLC in elderly patients: a population-based matched-pair comparison of stereotactic radiotherapy versus surgery. Radiother Oncol. 2011;101:240–4.
10. Brunelli A, Charloux A, Bolliger CT, et al. European Sespiratory Society and European Society of Thoracic Surgeons joint task force on fitness for radical therapy. ERS/ESTS clinical guidelines on fitness for radical therapy in lung cancer patients (surgery and chemo-radiotherapy). Eur Respir J. 2009;34:17–41.
11. Brunelli A, Charloux A, Bolliger CT, European Respiratory Society, European Society of Thoracic Surgeons Joint Task Force on Fitness For Radical Therapy, et al. The European Respiratory Society and European Society of Thoracic Surgeons clinical guidelines for evaluating fitness for radical treatment (surgery and chemoradiotherapy) in patients with lung cancer. Eur J Cardiothorac Surg. 2009;36:181–4.
12. Lim E, Baldwin D, Beckles M, British Thoracic Society, Society for Cardiothoracic Surgery in Great Britain and Ireland, et al. Guidelines on the radical management of patients with lung cancer. Thorax. 2010;65 Suppl 3:iii1–27.
13. Goffin J, Lacchetti C, Ellis PM, Lung Cancer Disease Site Group of Cancer Care Ontario's Program in Evidence-Based Care, et al. First-line systemic chemotherapy in the treatment of advanced non-small cell lung cancer: a systematic review. J Thorac Oncol. 2010;5:260–74.
14. Greillier L, Thomas P, Loundou A, et al. Pulmonary function tests as a predictor of quantitative and qualitative outcomes after thoracic surgery for lung cancer. Clin Lung Cancer. 2007;8:554–61.
15. Balduyck B, Hendriks J, Lauwers P, et al. Quality of life evolution after lung cancer surgery: a prospective study in 100 patients. Lung Cancer. 2007;56:423–31.
16. Cerveri I, Dore R, Corsico A, et al. Assessment of emphysema in COPD: a functional and radiologic study. Chest. 2004;125:1714–8.
17. Kearney DJ, Lee TH, Reilly JJ, et al. Assessment of operative risk in patients undergoing lung resection. Importance of predicted pulmonary function. Chest. 1994;105:753–9.
18. Colice GL, Shafazand S, Griffin JP, et al. Physiologic evaluation of the patient with lung cancer being considered for resectional surgery: ACCP evidence-based clinical practice guidelines (2nd edition). Chest. 2007;132(3 Suppl):161S–77.
19. Win T, Jackson A, Sharples L, et al. Relationship between pulmonary function and lung cancer surgical outcome. Eur Respir J. 2005;25:594–9.
20. Pierce RJ, Copland JM, Sharpe K, et al. Preoperative risk evaluation for lung cancer resection: predicted postoperative product as a predictor of surgical mortality. Am J Respir Crit Care Med. 1994;150:947–55.
21. Markos J, Mullan BP, Hillman DR, et al. Preoperative assessment as a predictor of mortality and morbidity after lung resection. Am Rev Respir Dis. 1989;139:902–10.
22. Nakahara K, Monden Y, Ohno K, et al. A method for predicting postoperative lung function and its relation to postoperative complications in patients with lung cancer. Ann Thorac Surg. 1985;39:260–5.

23. Nakahara K, Ohno K, Hashimoto J, et al. Prediction of postoperative respiratory failure in patients undergoing lung resection for lung cancer. Ann Thorac Surg. 1988;46:549–52.
24. Brunelli A, Al Refai M, Monteverde M, et al. Predictors of early morbidity after major lung resection in patients with and without airflow limitation. Ann Thorac Surg. 2002;74: 999–1003.
25. Varela G, Brunelli A, Rocco G, et al. Predicted versus observed FEV1 in the immediate postoperative period after pulmonary lobectomy. Eur J Cardiothorac Surg. 2006;30:644–8.
26. Zeiher BG, Gross TJ, Kern JA, et al. Predicting postoperative pulmonary function in patients undergoing lung resection. Chest. 1995;108:68–72.
27. Schattenberg T, Muley T, Dienemann H, et al. Impact on pulmonary function after lobectomy in patients with chronic obstructive pulmonary disease. Thorac Cardiovasc Surg. 2007;55: 500–4.
28. Baldi S, Ruffini E, Harari S, et al. Does lobectomy for lung cancer in patients with chronic obstructive pulmonary disease affect lung function? A multicenter national study. J Thorac Cardiovasc Surg. 2005;130:1616–22.
29. Ferguson MK, Little L, Rizzo L, et al. Diffusing capacity predicts morbidity and mortality after pulmonary resection. J Thorac Cardiovasc Surg. 1988;96:894–900.
30. Wang J, Olak J, Ferguson MK. Diffusing capacity predicts operative mortality but not long-term survival after resection for lung cancer. J Thorac Cardiovasc Surg. 1999;117:581–7.
31. Ferguson MK, Vigneswaran WT. Diffusing capacity predicts morbidity after lung resection in patients without obstructive lung disease. Ann Thorac Surg. 2008;85:1158–65.
32. Williams AJ, Cayton RM, Harding LK, et al. Quantitative lung scintigrams and lung function in the selection of patients for pneumonectomy. Br J Dis Chest. 1984;78:105–12.
33. Olsen GN, Block AJ, Tobias JA. Prediction of postpneumonectomy pulmonary function using quantitative macroaggregate lung scanning. Chest. 1974;66:13–6.
34. Cordiner A, De Carlo F, De Gennaro R, et al. Prediction of postoperative pulmonary function following thoracic surgery for bronchial carcinoma. Angiology. 1991;42:985–9.
35. Bria WF, Kanarek DJ, Kazemi H. Prediction of postoperative pulmonary function following thoracic operations. Value of ventilation-perfusion scanning. J Thorac Cardiovasc Surg. 1983;86:186–92.
36. Janssens JP, Pache JC, Nicod LP. Physiological changes in respiratory function associated with ageing. Eur Respir J. 1999;13:197–205.
37. Quanjer PH, Tammeling GJ, Cotes JE, et al. Lung volumes and forced ventilatory flows. Report Working Party Standardization of Lung Function Tests, European Community for Steel and Coal. Official Statement of the European Respiratory Society. Eur Respir J. 1993;6:5–40.
38. Hankinson JL, Odencrantz JR, Fedan KB. Spirometric reference values from a sample of the general U.S. population. Am J Respir Crit Care Med. 1999;159:179–87.
39. Quanjer PH, Stocks J, Cole TJ, et al. Global lungs initiative. Influence of secular trends and sample size on reference equations for lung function tests. Eur Respir J. 2011;37:658–64.
40. Pellegrino R, Viegi G, Brusasco V, et al. Interpretative strategies for lung function tests. Eur Respir J. 2005;26:948–68.
41. Brady LW, Germon PA, Cander L. The effects of radiation therapy on pulmonary function in carcinoma of the lung. Radiology. 1965;85:130–4.
42. Germon PA, Brady LW. Physiologic changes before and after radiation treatment for carcinoma of the lung. JAMA. 1968;206:809–14.
43. Gross NJ. Pulmonary effects of radiation therapy. Ann Intern Med. 1977;86:81–92.
44. Borst GR, De Jaeger K, Belderbos JS, et al. Pulmonary function changes after radiotherapy in non-small-cell lung cancer patients with long-term disease-free survival. Int J Radiat Oncol Biol Phys. 2005;2:639–44.
45. Gopal R, Starkschall G, Tucker SL, et al. Effects of radiotherapy and chemotherapy on lung function in patients with non-small-cell lung cancer. Int J Radiat Oncol Biol Phys. 2003;56:114–20.
46. Leo F, Solli P, Spaggiari L, et al. Respiratory function changes after chemotherapy: an additional risk for postoperative respiratory complications? Ann Thorac Surg. 2004;77:260–5.

47. Takeda S, Funakoshi Y, Kadota Y, et al. Fall in diffusing capacity associated with induction therapy for lung cancer: a predictor of postoperative complication? Ann Thorac Surg. 2006; 82:232–6.
48. Cerfolio RJ, Talati A, Bryant AS. Changes in pulmonary function tests after neoadjuvant therapy predict postoperative complications. Ann Thorac Surg. 2009;88:930–6.
49. Margaritora S, Cesario A, Cusumano G, et al. Is pulmonary function damaged by neoadjuvant lung cancer therapy? A comprehensive serial time-trend analysis of pulmonary function after induction radiochemotherapy plus surgery. J Thorac Cardiovasc Surg. 2010;139: 1457–63.
50. Fishman A, Martinez F, Naunheim K, National Emphysema Treatment Trial Research Group, et al. A randomized trial comparing lung-volume-reduction surgery with medical therapy for severe emphysema. N Engl J Med. 2003;348:2059–73.
51. National Emphysema Treatment Trial Research Group. Patients at high risk of death after lung-volume-reduction surgery. N Engl J Med. 2001;345:1075–83.
52. Older P, Smith R, Courtney P, et al. Preoperative evaluation of cardiac-failure and ischemia in elderly patients by cardiopulmonary exercise testing. Chest. 1993;104:701–4.
53. Simpson JC, Sutton H, Grocott MPW. Cardiopulmonary exercise testing - a survey of current use in England. J Intensive Care Soc. 2009;10:275–8.
54. Ridgway ZA, Howell SJ. Cardiopulmonary exercise testing: a review of methods and applications in surgical patients. Eur J Anaesthesiol. 2010;27:858–65.
55. Snowden CP, Prentis JM, Anderson HL, et al. Submaximal cardiopulmonary exercise testing predicts complications and hospital length of stay in patients undergoing major elective surgery. Ann Surg. 2010;251:535–41.
56. Wilson RJ, Davies S, Yates D, et al. Impaired functional capacity is associated with all-cause mortality after major elective intra-abdominal surgery. Br J Anaesth. 2010;105:297–303.
57. American Thoracic Society, American College of Chest Physicians. ATS/ACCP statement on cardiopulmonary exercise testing. Am J Respir Crit Care Med. 2003;167:211–77.
58. Wasserman K, Hansen JE, Sue DY, et al. Principles of exercise testing and interpretation. 4th ed. Baltimore: Lippincott Williams & Wilkins; 2005.
59. Older P, Hall A, Hader R. Cardiopulmonary exercise testing as a screening test for perioperative management of major surgery in the elderly. Chest. 1999;116:355–62.
60. McCullough PA, Gallagher MJ, Dejong AT, et al. Cardiorespiratory fitness and short-term complications after bariatric surgery. Chest. 2006;130:517–25.
61. Carlisle J, Swart M. Mid-term survival after abdominal aortic aneurysm surgery predicted by cardiopulmonary exercise testing. Br J Surg. 2007;94:966–9.
62. Hopker JG, Jobson SA, Pandit JJ. Controversies in the physiological basis of the "anaerobic threshold" and their implications for clinical cardiopulmonary exercise testing. Anaesthesia. 2011;66:111–23.
63. Ozcelik O, Ward SA, Whipp BJ. Effect of altered body CO_2 stores on pulmonary gas exchange dynamics during incremental exercise in humans. Exp Physiol. 1999;84:999–1011.
64. Wasserman K, Whipp BJ. Exercise physiology in health and disease. Am Rev Respir Dis. 1975;112:219–59.
65. Pollock ML, Foster C, Knapp D, et al. Effect of age and training on aerobic capacity and body composition of master athletes. J Appl Physiol. 1987;62:725–31.
66. Rogers MA, Hagberg JM, Martin WH, et al. Decline in $VO_{2\,Max}$ with aging in master athletes and sedentary men. J Appl Physiol. 1990;68:2195–9.
67. Hossack KF, Bruce RA. Maximal cardiac function in sedentary normal men and women: comparison of age-related changes. J Appl Physiol. 1982;53:799–804.
68. Ogawa TR, Spina RJ, Martin WH, et al. Effects of aging, sex and physical training on cardiovascular responses to exercise. Circulation. 1992;86:494–503.
69. Sandvik L, Erikssen J, Thaulow E, et al. Physical fitness as a predictor of mortality among healthy, middle-aged Norwegian men. N Engl J Med. 1993;328:533–7.
70. Toth MJ, Gardner AW, Ades PA, et al. Contribution of body composition and physical activity to age-related decline in peak VO_2 in men and women. J Appl Physiol. 1994;77:647–52.

71. Posner JD, Gorman KM, Klein HS, et al. Ventilatory threshold: measurement and variation with age. J Appl Physiol. 1987;63:1519–25.
72. Smith TB, Stonell C, Purkayastha S, et al. Cardiopulmonary exercise testing as a risk assessment method in non cardio-pulmonary surgery: a systematic review. Anaesthesia. 2009;64: 883–9.
73. West M, Jack S, Grocott MP. Perioperative cardiopulmonary exercise testing in the elderly. Best Pract Res Clin Anaesthesiol. 2011;25:427–37.
74. Hennis PJ, Meale PM, Grocott MPW. Cardiopulmonary exercise testing for the evaluation of perioperative risk in non-cardio-pulmonary surgery. Postgrad Med J. 2011;87:550–7.
75. Epstein SK, Faling J, Daly BDT, et al. Inability to perform bicycle ergometry predicts increased morbidity and mortality after lung resection. Chest. 1995;107:311–6.
76. Smith TP, Kinasewitz GT, Tucker WY, et al. Exercise capacity as a predictor of post-thoracotomy morbidity. Am Rev Respir Dis. 1984;129:730–4.
77. Colman NC, Schraufnagel DE, Rivington RN, et al. Exercise testing in evaluation of patients for lung resection. Am Rev Respir Dis. 1982;125:604–6.
78. Ussetti P, Roca J, Agusti AGN, et al. Failure of exercise tolerance and hemodynamic studies t predict early post-thoracotomy morbidity and mortality. Am Rev Respir Dis. 1988; A94.
79. Bechard D, Wetstein L. Assessment of exercise oxygen consumption as preoperative criterion for lung resection. Ann Thorac Surg. 1987;44:344–9.
80. Gerson MC, Hurst JM, Hertzberg VS, et al. Prediction of cardiac and pulmonary complications related to elective abdomen and non-cardiac thoracic surgery in geriatric patients. Am J Med. 1990;88:101–7.
81. Epstein SK, Faling LJ, Daly BD, et al. Predicting complications after pulmonary resection. Preoperative exercise testing vs. a multifactorial cardiopulmonary risk index. Chest. 1993;104: 694–700.
82. Richter Larsen K, Svendsen UG, et al. Exercise testing in the preoperative evaluation of patients with bronchogenic carcinoma. Eur Respir J. 1997;10:1559–65.
83. Brutsche MH, Spiliopoulos A, Bolliger CT, et al. Exercise capacity and extent of resection as predictors of surgical risk in lung cancer. Eur Respir J. 2000;15:828–32.
84. Villani F, Busia A. Preoperative evaluation of patients submitted to pneumonectomy for lung carcinoma: role of exercise testing. Tumori. 2004;90:405–9.
85. Nagamatsu Y, Shima I, Hayashi A, et al. Preoperative spirometry versus expired gas analysis during exercise testing as predictors of cardiopulmonary complications after lung resection. Surg Today. 2004;34:107–10.
86. Win T, Jackson A, Sharples L, et al. Cardiopulmonary exercise tests and lung cancer surgical outcome. Chest. 2005;127:1159–65.
87. Bolliger CT, Jordan P, Soler M, et al. Exercise capacity as a predictor of post-operative complications in lung resection candidates. Am J Respir Crit Care Med. 1995;151:1472–80.
88. Benzo R, Kelley GA, Recchi L, et al. Complications of lung resection and exercise capacity: a meta-analysis. Respir Med. 2007;101:1790–7.
89. Tilburg PMB, Stam H, Hoogsteden HC. Pre-operative pulmonary evaluation of lung cancer patients: a review of the literature. Eur Respir J. 2009;33:1206–15.

Chapter 4
A Practical Mini-Guide to Geriatric Assessment

Siri Rostoft Kristjansson

Abstract The heterogeneity of the aging process has practical consequences for the assessment of older cancer patients: Patients need individualized assessments to approximately determine their physiological age. There is no simple way to assess physiological age, but an approach frequently used by geriatricians involves a comprehensive geriatric assessment (CGA). Unfortunately, there is no such thing as an internationally standardized CGA. Oncologists often ask for a copy of "the CGA" scoring sheet, which does not exist. However, there is general agreement within the literature of the components that comprise a CGA: Areas where older adults often present with problems are systematically assessed. The general composition of a CGA involves functional status, comorbidity, polypharmacy, nutritional status, cognitive function, emotional status, and social support. It is important to know that in clinical geriatric medicine, the CGA is carried out in the presence of a multidisciplinary team and involves the process of developing an intervention plan for the patient. The multidisciplinary team usually includes some or all of the following specialists: a geriatrician, a geriatric nurse, a physiotherapist, an occupational therapist, a dietician, a social worker, and a pharmacist. Thus, it is more correct to speak about a geriatric assessment (GA) than a CGA in this context where isolated scoring tools are presented. We will present some of the tools that are most frequently used in the field of geriatric oncology.

Keywords Geriatric assessment • Functional measurements • Objective physical performance assessment • Comorbidity assessment • Nutritional status assessment • Screening tools for the elderly

S.R. Kristjansson, MD, PhD (✉)
Department of Internal Medicine, Diakonhjemmet Hospital,
Diakonveien 12, Oslo 0319, Norway
e-mail: sirikristjansson@gmail.com

C. Gridelli, R.A. Audisio (eds.), *Management of Lung Cancer in Older People*,
DOI 10.1007/978-0-85729-793-8_4,

Table 4.1 Eastern cooperative oncology group performance status

Grade	ECOG
0	Fully active, able to carry on all pre-disease performance without restriction
1	Restricted in physically strenuous activity but ambulatory and able to carry out work of a light or sedentary nature, e.g., light housework, office work
2	Ambulatory and capable of all self-care but unable to carry out any work activities. Up and about more than 50 % of waking hours
3	Capable of only limited self-care, confined to bed or chair more than 50 % of waking hours
4	Completely disabled. Cannot carry on any self-care. Totally confined to bed or chair
5	Dead

From Oken et al. [1]. The ECOG Performance Status is in the public domain and therefore available for public use. The Eastern Cooperative Oncology Group, Robert Comis M.D., Group Chair

The heterogeneity of the aging process has practical consequences for the assessment of older cancer patients: Patients need individualized assessments to approximately determine their physiological age. There is no simple way to assess physiological age, but an approach frequently used by geriatricians involves a comprehensive geriatric assessment (CGA). Unfortunately, there is no such thing as an internationally standardized CGA. Oncologists often ask for a copy of "the CGA" scoring sheet, which does not exist. However, there is general agreement within the literature of the components that comprise a CGA: Areas where older adults often present with problems are systematically assessed. The general composition of a CGA involves functional status, comorbidity, polypharmacy, nutritional status, cognitive function, emotional status, and social support. It is important to know that in clinical geriatric medicine, the CGA is carried out in the presence of a multidisciplinary team and involves the process of developing an intervention plan for the patient. The multidisciplinary team usually includes some or all of the following specialists: a geriatrician, a geriatric nurse, a physiotherapist, an occupational therapist, a dietician, a social worker, and a pharmacist. Thus, it is more correct to speak about a geriatric assessment (GA) than a CGA in this context where isolated scoring tools are presented. We will present some of the tools that are most frequently used in the field of geriatric oncology.

Functional Measurements

These measurement tools help define a patient's functional capabilities.

Eastern Cooperative Oncology Group Performance Status

The Eastern Cooperative Oncology Group Performance Status (ECOG) scale (Table 4.1) is well known to oncologists, but not to doctors outside the oncology setting such as internal medicine specialists and surgeons.

Table 4.2 Katz index of independence in activities of daily living

Activities	Independence	Dependence
Points (1 or 0)	(1 point) No supervision, direction, or personal assistance	(0 point) With supervision, direction, personal assistance, or total care
Bathing Points: ______	(1 point) Bathes self completely or needs help in bathing only a single part of the body such as the back, genital area, or disabled extremity	(0 point) Need help with bathing more than one part of the body, getting in or out of the tub or shower. Requires total bathing
Dressing Points: ______	(1 point) Get clothes from closets and drawers and puts on clothes and outer garments complete with fasteners. May have help tying shoes	(0 point) Needs help with dressing self or needs to be completely dressed
Toileting Points: ______	(1 point) Goes to toilet, gets on and off, arranges clothes, cleans genital area without help	(0 point) Needs help in transferring to the toilet and cleaning self or uses bedpan or commode
Transferring Points: ______	(1 point) Moves in and out of bed or chair unassisted. Mechanical transfer aids are acceptable	(0 point) Needs help in moving from bed to chair or requires a complete transfer
Continence Points: ______	(1 point) Exercises complete self-control over urination and defecation	(0 point) Is partially or totally incontinent of bowel or bladder
Feeding Points: ______	(1 point) Gets food from plate into mouth without help. Preparation of food may be done by another person	(0 point) Needs partial or total help with feeding or requires parenteral feeding
Total points: ________		

From Katz et al. [2]. With permission of the Gerontological Society of America
Score of 6 high, patient is independent, *Score of 0* low, patient is very dependent

Katz Index of Independence in Basic Activities of Daily Living

This index measures basic activities of daily living including toileting, feeding, transferring, grooming, continence, and bathing (Table 4.2). Dependency in any of these activities will usually require help from a caregiver on a daily basis.

The Lawton Instrumental Activities of Daily Living Scale

Instrumental activities of daily living include more specialized activities such as abilities to manage money, to shop, to use transportation, housekeeping, and food preparation (Table 4.3).

Table 4.3 Instrumental activities of daily living scale (IADL)

A. Ability to use telephone	
1. Operates telephone on own initiative, looks up and dials numbers, etc.	1
2. Dials a few well-known numbers	1
3. Answers telephone but does not dial	1
4. Does not use telephone at all	0
B. Shopping	
1. Takes care of all shopping needs independently	1
2. Shops independently for small purchases	0
3. Needs to be accompanied on any shopping trip	0
4. Completely unable to shop	0
C. Food preparation	
1. Plans, prepares, and serves adequate meals independently	1
2. Prepares adequate meals if supplied with ingredients	0
3. Heats, serves, and prepares meals or prepares meals but does not maintain adequate diet	0
4. Needs to have meals prepared and served	0
D. Housekeeping	
1. Maintains house alone or with occasional assistance (e.g., "heavy work domestic help")	1
2. Performs light daily tasks such as dishwashing and bed making	1
3. Performs light daily tasks but cannot maintain acceptable level of cleanliness	1
4. Needs help with all home maintenance tasks	1
5. Does not participate in any housekeeping tasks	0
E. Laundry	
1. Does personal laundry completely	1
2. Launders small items, rinses stockings, etc.	1
3. All laundry must be done by others	0
F. Mode of transportation	
1. Travels independently on public transportation or drives own car	1
2. Arranges own travel via taxi, but does not otherwise use public transportation	1
3. Travels on public transportation when assisted or accompanied by another	1
4. Travel limited to taxi or automobile with assistance of another	0
5. Does not travel at all	0
G. Responsibility for own medications	
1. Is responsible for taking medication in correct dosages at correct time	1
2. Takes responsibility if medication is prepared in advance in separate dosages	0
3. Is not capable of dispensing own medication	0
H. Ability to handle finances	
1. Manages financial matters independently (budgets, writes checks, pays rent, bills goes to bank), collects and keeps track of income	1
2. Manages day-to-day purchases, but needs help with banking, major purchases, etc.	1
3. Incapable of handling money	0

From Lawton and Brody [3]. With permission and copyright The Gerontological Society of America

Objective Physical Performance Assessments

The ability to perform certain physical tests can predict mortality and physical dependence, and objective physical measurements are included in the definition of the phenotypic frailty syndrome [4].

A widely used example of a physical test is the timed "Up & Go" (TUG): A person sits on an armchair and is asked to walk 3 m, turn around, then walk back, and sit down on the chair [5]. The time used to complete this task is recorded. A cutoff of 19 s approximately identifies the slowest quintile in a sample of noninstitutionalized elderly individuals [6].

Afilalo and colleagues recently showed that *gait speed* might identify a subgroup of patients with increased risk of mortality and major morbidity after cardiac surgery [7]. Slow walkers were identified when the time taken to walk 5 m was 6 s or more.

Comorbidity

Comorbidity can be assessed using a numbered scale, such as Cumulative Illness Rating Scale (CIRS) or Charlson Comorbidity Index (CCI). The manual for scoring the CIRS is published as an appendix to the paper "A Manual of Guidelines to Score the Modified Cumulative Illness Rating Scale and Its Validation in Acute Hospitalized Elderly Patients" [8]. The Charlson Comorbidity Index was published in 1987 [9]. An example of the scoring sheet is shown in Table 4.4.

Nutritional Status

A well-validated tool in the geriatric population is the Mini Nutritional Assessment (MNA) (Fig. 4.1).

Cognitive Function

The mini-mental state examination (MMSE) is a 30-point cognitive test that comprises 11 items and takes approximately 8 min to complete. It is widely used and well validated. People with high education often score in the "normal" range of 25–30 points even when mild cognitive impairment is present. A score of less than 24 is indicative of cognitive impairment. MMSE is widely used, but copyright protection is now enforced, and the MMSE must be purchased from the publishers (www.parinc.com/). A shorter test for cognitive impairment is the abbreviated

Table 4.4 Charlson comorbidity index

Comorbidity	Present	Points
Myocardial infarct		1
Congestive heart failure		1
Peripheral vascular disease		1
Cerebrovascular disease (except hemiplegia)		1
Dementia		1
Chronic pulmonary disease		1
Connective tissue disease		1
Ulcer disease		1
Mild liver disease		1
Diabetes (without complications)		1
Diabetes with end-organ damage		2
Hemiplegia		2
Moderate or severe renal disease		2
2nd solid tumor (nonmetastatic)		2
Leukemia		2
Lymphoma, MM, etc.		2
Moderate or severe liver disease		3
2nd metastatic solid tumor		6
AIDS		6
	Total points:	_______

From Charlson et al. [9]. With permission

mental test score (AMTS) [14]. It includes ten questions, and a score of 7 or less suggests cognitive impairment.

Score 1 for each correct answer. A score of ≤7 out of a possible ten suggests cognitive impairment.

1. How old are you?
2. What is the time (to the nearest hour)?
3. Give the patient an address (such as “42 West Street”) for recall at the end of the test.
4. What year is it?
5. What is the name of this place?
6. Can the patient recognize two relevant people (such as a nurse and a doctor)?
7. What was the date of your birth?
8. When was the Second World War?
9. Who is the present prime minister?
10. Count down from 20 to 1. (Allow no errors and give no cues.)

It has also been shown that only four items from AMTS perform well as a screening for cognitive impairment in the emergency room with a cutoff of three points (How old are you, what is your date of birth, what place is this, what year is it?) [15].

Nestlé Nutrition Institute

Mini Nutritional Assessment MNA®

Last name: Firs name:

Sex: Age: Weight, kg: Height, cm: Date:

Complete the screen by filling in the boxes with the appropriate numbers. Total numbers for the final screening score.

Screening

A Has food intake declined over the past 3 months due to loss of appetite, digestive problems, chewing or swallowing difficulties?
0 = severe decrease in food intake
1 = moderate decrease in food intake
2 = no decrease in food intake ☐

B Weight loss during the last 3 months
0 = weight loss greater the 3 kg (6.6 lbs)
1 = does not know
2 = weight loss between 1 and 3 kg (2.2 and 6.6 lbs)
3 = no weight loss ☐

C Mobility
0 = bed or chair bound
1 = able to get out of bed / chair but does not go out
2 = goes out ☐

D Has suffered psychological stress or acute disease in the past 3 months?
0 = yes 2 = no ☐

E Neuropsychological problems
0 = severe dementia or depression
1 = mild dementia
2 = no psychological problems ☐

F1 Body Mass Indux (BMI) (weight in kg) / (height in m^2)
0 = BMI less than 19
1 = BMI 19 to less than 21
2 = BMI 21 to less than 23
3 = BMI 23 or greater ☐

IF BMI IS NOT AVAILABLE, REPLACE QUESTION F1 WITH QUESTION F2.
DO NOT ANSWER QUESTION F2 IF QUESTION F1 IS ALREADY COMPLETED.

F2 Calf circumference (CC) in cm
0 = CC less than 31
3 = CC 31 or greater ☐

Screening score
(max. 14 points) ☐☐

12–14 points:	Normal nutritional status
8–11 points:	At risk of malnutrition
0–7 points:	Malnourished

Fig. 4.1 Mini Nutritional Assessment (© Nestlé, 1994, Revision 2009. N67200 12/99 10 M 5. ®Société des Produits Nestlé S.A., Vevey, Switzerland, Trademark Owners. Sources: Vellas et al. [10], Rubenstein et al. [11], Guigoz [12], Kaiser et al. [13])

Table 4.5 Geriatric depression scale: (short form – GDS-15)

Choose the best answer for how you have felt over the past week:

1. Are you basically satisfied with your life? YES/**NO**
2. Have you dropped many of your activities and interests? **YES**/NO
3. Do you feel that your life is empty? **YES**/NO
4. Do you often get bored? **YES**/NO
5. Are you in good spirits most of the time? YES/**NO**
6. Are you afraid that something bad is going to happen to you? **YES**/NO
7. Do you feel happy most of the time? YES/**NO**
8. Do you often feel helpless? **YES**/NO
9. Do you prefer to stay at home, rather than going out and doing new things? **YES**/NO
10. Do you feel you have more problems with memory than most? **YES**/NO
11. Do you think it is wonderful to be alive now? YES/**NO**
12. Do you feel pretty worthless the way you are now? **YES**/NO
13. Do you feel full of energy? YES/**NO**
14. Do you feel that your situation is hopeless? **YES**/NO
15. Do you think that most people are better off than you are? **YES**/NO

Yesavage et al. [16]
Answers in **bold** indicate depression. Although differing sensitivities and specificities have been obtained across studies, for clinical purposes a score >5 points is suggestive of depression and should warrant a follow-up interview. Scores >10 are almost always depression

Depression

Depression is common among elderly patients, and a screening instrument for depression is often included in a GA. The Geriatric Depression Scale (GDS) is validated in an elderly population (Table 4.5). GDS-15 can also be found as a free application for iPhone (by Yesavage).

Screening Tools

The need for shorter screening tools to identify patients who need a complete GA has been advocated. The Vulnerable Elders Survey (VES-13) (Box 4.1) is an example of such a tool [17]. The G8 questionnaire is a very simple screening tool, which includes seven Mini Nutritional Assessment items and age (<80, 80–85, >85), for a total score ranging from 0 (poor score) to 17 (good score). In an exploratory study of 364 cancer patients older than 70, with a cutoff score of 14, G8 had 90 % sensitivity and 60 % specificity [18].

Predictive Models for Chemotherapy Toxicity

Hurria and colleagues recently published a predictive model for chemotherapy toxicity (grades 3–5) in older adults (65 years and older) where geriatric assessment variables were included [19]. Twenty-nine percent of the patients had stage I to IV

Box 4.1. Vulnerable Elders Survey (VES-13)

1. Age_____ (one point for age 75–84, three points for age 85 or greater)
2. In general, compared to other people at your age, would you say that your health is:
   (a) Poor, * (1 point)
   (b) Fair, * (1 point)
   (c) Good
   (d) Very good
   (e) Excellent
3. How much difficulty, on average, do you have with the following physical activities: (score 1 point for each* response, maximum of two points)

	No difficulty	A little difficulty	Some difficulty*	A lot of difficulty*	Unable to do*
Stooping, crouching, or kneeling					
Lifting or carrying objects as heavy as 10 lb					
Reaching or extending arms above shoulder level					
Writing, or handling and grasping small objects					
Walking a quarter of a mile					
Heavy housework such as scrubbing floors or washing windows					

4. Because of your health or a physical condition, do you have any difficulty: (score 4 points for one or more* YES responses in this section)
   (a) Shopping for personal items (like toilet items or medicine)?
   - YES>>Do you get help with shopping? YES* NO
   - NO
   - DON'T DO>>Is that because of your health? YES* NO

   (b) Managing money (like keeping track of expenses or paying bills)?
   - YES>>Do you get help with managing money? YES* NO
   - NO
   - DON'T DO>>Is it because of your health? YES* NO

   (c) Walking across the room? Use of cane or walker is okay.
   - YES>>Do you get help with walking? YES* NO
   - NO
   - DON'T DO>>Is that because of your health? YES* NO

   (d) Doing light housework (like washing dishes, straightening up, or light cleaning?)
   - YES>>Do you get help with light housework? YES* NO
   - NO
   - DON'T DO>>Is that because of your health? YES* NO

(e) Bathing or showering?
- YES>>Do you get help with bathing or showering? YES* NO
- NO
- DON'T DO>>Is that because of your health? YES* NO

Scoring 3 or greater identifies an individual that has 4.2 times the risk of death or functional decline over the next 2 years.
From Saliba et al. [17], with permission of The Rand Corporation http://www.rand.org/health/projects/acove/ve_survey.html - Accessed 18 Jan 2006

lung cancer. The following factors were included in the predictive model (score in parenthesis):

- Age >71 years (2)
- Cancer type, genitourinary or gastrointestinal (2)
- Chemotherapy dosing, standard dose (2)
- Number of chemotherapy drugs, polychemotherapy (2)
- Hemoglobin <11 g/dL (male), <10 g/dL (female) (3)
- Creatinine clearance <34 mL/min (3)
- Hearing, fair or worse (2)
- No. of falls in the last 6 months, one or more (3)
- IADL: taking medications with some help/unable (1)
- Walking 1 block, somewhat limited/limited a lot (2)
- Decreased social activity because of physical/emotional health, limited at least sometimes (1)

Patients with a risk score of 12–19 points had an 89 % risk of grade 3–5 toxicity, while patients scoring zero to three points had a risk of 25 %.

References

1. Oken MM, Creech RH, Tormey DC, Horton J, Davis TE, McFadden ET, et al. Toxicity and response criteria of the Eastern Cooperative Oncology Group. Am J Clin Oncol. 1982;5:649–55.
2. Katz S, Downs TD, Cash HR, et al. Progress in the development of the index of ADL. Gerontologist. 1970;10:8–12.
3. Lawton MP, Brody EM. Assessment living. Gerontologist. 1969;9:179–86.
4. Fried LP, Tangen CM, Walston J, Newman AB, Hirsch C, Gottdiener J, et al. Frailty in older adults: evidence for a phenotype. J Gerontol A Biol Sci Med Sci. 2001;56(3):M146–56.
5. Podsiadlo D, Richardson S. The timed "Up & Go": a test of basic functional mobility for frail elderly persons. J Am Geriatr Soc. 1991;39(2):142–8.
6. Rockwood K, Andrew M, Mitnitski A. A comparison of two approaches to measuring frailty in elderly people. J Gerontol A Biol Sci Med Sci. 2007;62(7):738–43.
7. Afilalo J, Eisenberg MJ, Morin JF, Bergman H, Monette J, Noiseux N, et al. Gait speed as an incremental predictor of mortality and major morbidity in elderly patients undergoing cardiac surgery. J Am Coll Cardiol. 2010;56(20):1668–76.

8. Salvi F, Miller MD, Grilli A, Giorgi R, Towers AL, Morichi V, et al. A manual of guidelines to score the modified cumulative illness rating scale and its validation in acute hospitalized elderly patients. J Am Geriatr Soc. 2008;56(10):1926–31.
9. Charlson ME, Pompei P, Ales KL, MacKenzie CR. A new method of classifying prognostic comorbidity in longitudinal studies: development and validation. J Chronic Dis. 1987;40(5): 373–83.
10. Vellas B, Villars H, Abellan G, et al. Overview of the MNA - Its history and challenges. J Nutr Health Aging. 2006;10:456–65.
11. Rubenstein LZ, Harker JO, Salva A, Guigoz Y, Vellas B. Screening for undernutrition in geriatric practice: developing the short-form Mini Nutritional Assessment (MNA-SF). J Gerontol. 2001;56A:M366–77.
12. Guigoz Y. The Mini-Nutritional Assessment (MNA) review of the literature - What does it tell us? J Nutr Health Aging. 2006;10:466–87.
13. Kaiser MJ, Bauer JM, Ramsch C, et al. Validation of the Mini Nutritional Assessment short-form (MNA-SF): a practical tool for identification of nutritional status. J Nutr Health Aging. 2009;13:782–8.
14. Hodkinson HM. Evaluation of a mental test score for assessment of mental impairment in the elderly. Age Ageing. 1972;1(4):233–8.
15. Schofield I, Stott DJ, Tolson D, McFadyen A, Monaghan J, Nelson D. Screening for cognitive impairment in older people attending accident and emergency using the 4-item Abbreviated Mental Test. Eur J Emergency Med. 2010;17(6):340–2.
16. Yesavage JA, Brink TL, Rose TL, Lum O, Huang V, Adey MB, et al. Development and validation of a geriatric depression scale: a preliminary report. J Psychiatr Res. 1983;17:37–49.
17. Saliba D, Elliott M, Rubenstein LZ, Solomon DH, Young RT, Kamberg CJ, et al. The vulnerable elders survey: a tool for identifying vulnerable older people in the community. J Am Geriatr Soc. 2001;49(12):1691–9.
18. Pallis AG, Wedding U, Lacombe D, Soubeyran P, Wildiers H. Questionnaires and instruments for a multidimensional assessment of the older cancer patient: what clinicians need to know? Eur J Cancer. 2010;46(6):1019–25.
19. Hurria A, Togawa K, Mohile SG, Owusu C, Klepin HD, Gross CP, et al. Predicting chemotherapy toxicity in older adults with cancer: a prospective multicenter study. J Clin Oncol. 2011;29(25):3457–65.

Chapter 5
Impact of the Physiological Effects of Aging on the Pharmacokinetics and Pharmacodynamics of Systemic Lung Cancer Treatment

Antonio Rossi, Dario Cova, Silvana Leo, and Lazzaro Repetto

Abstract Pharmacokinetics includes the study of the mechanisms of absorption and distribution of an administered drug, the rate at which a drug action begins and the duration of the effect, the chemical changes of the substance in the body, and the effects and routes of excretion of the metabolites of the drug. Pharmacodynamics is the study of the biochemical and physiological effects of drugs on the body and the relationship between drug concentration and effect. Overall, pharmacokinetics is the study of what the body does to a drug, whereas pharmacodynamics is often summarized as the study of what a drug does to the body. Pharmacokinetic interactions involve one drug or substance altering the absorption, distribution, metabolism, or elimination of another drug or substance. A common example of a pharmacokinetic interaction occurs when two drugs compete for the same metabolic pathway. When the pathway becomes saturated neither drug can be metabolized fully, which results in higher serum concentrations of the agents and can lead to clinically unfavorable consequences. Pharmacodynamic interactions occur when two drugs or substances have similar molecular targets, but do not affect the pharmacokinetic parameters of

A. Rossi, MD
Division of Medical Oncology,
S.G. Moscati Hospital, Avellino, Italy

D. Cova, MD
Emeritus Head of Oncogeriatrics, Department of Pharmacology,
School of Clinical Pharmacology,
University of Milan, Milan, Italy

S. Leo, MD
Onco-Geriatric Unit, Division of Medical Oncology,
Vito Fazzi Hospital, Lecce, Italy

L. Repetto, MD, PhD (✉)
Department of Oncology,
Sanremo Hospital - ASL 1 Imperiese,
Via G. Borea 56 -18038, Sanremo (IM), Italy
e-mail: l.repetto@asl1.liguria.it

C. Gridelli, R.A. Audisio (eds.), *Management of Lung Cancer in Older People*,
DOI 10.1007/978-0-85729-793-8_5, © Springer-Verlag London 2013

each other. Pharmacodynamics is related to the pharmacological activity of the interacting drugs, e.g., synergism, antagonism, altered cellular transport, and effect on the receptor site. When two or more drugs that have similar pharmacodynamic activity are coadministered, the additive effects might result in an excessive response or toxicity. Pharmacodynamic interactions occur when two or more drugs have mechanisms of action that result in the same physiological outcome.

Keywords Pharmacokinetics in the elderly with lung cancer • Lung cancer treatment and pharmacokinetics in the elderly • Drug interactions in the elderly with lung cancer • Chemotherapy and drug interactions • Aging effects in pharmacokinetics

Pharmacokinetics includes the study of the mechanisms of absorption and distribution of an administered drug, the rate at which a drug action begins and the duration of the effect, the chemical changes of the substance in the body, and the effects and routes of excretion of the metabolites of the drug. Pharmacodynamics is the study of the biochemical and physiological effects of drugs on the body and the relationship between drug concentration and effect. Overall, pharmacokinetics is the study of what the body does to a drug, whereas pharmacodynamics is often summarized as the study of what a drug does to the body [1]. Pharmacokinetic interactions involve one drug or substance altering the absorption, distribution, metabolism, or elimination of another drug or substance. A common example of a pharmacokinetic interaction occurs when two drugs compete for the same metabolic pathway. When the pathway becomes saturated neither drug can be metabolized fully, which results in higher serum concentrations of the agents and can lead to clinically unfavorable consequences. Pharmacodynamic interactions occur when two drugs or substances have similar molecular targets, but do not affect the pharmacokinetic parameters of each other. Pharmacodynamics are related to the pharmacological activity of the interacting drugs, e.g., synergism, antagonism, altered cellular transport, and effect on the receptor site. When two or more drugs that have similar pharmacodynamic activity are coadministered, the additive effects might result in an excessive response or toxicity. Pharmacodynamic interactions occur when two or more drugs have mechanisms of action that result in the same physiological outcome. Pharmacodynamic interactions can be categorized broadly as synergistic (when the effect of two drugs is greater than the sum of their individual effects), antagonistic (when the effect of two drugs is less than the sum of their individual effects), additive (when the effect of two drugs is merely the sum of the effects of each), and sequence-dependent (when the order in which two drugs are given governs their effects). Although pharmacodynamic interactions are relatively common in clinical practice, adverse effects can usually be minimized if the interactions are anticipated and appropriate countermeasures are taken. Pharmacodynamic interactions between drugs with opposing effects can reduce the response to one or both drugs [2].

There are few studies in the literature reporting the pharmacokinetics in elderly patients suffering from cancer, especially regarding the potential risk of drug interactions and proposing optimal dosing for individual elderly patient in order to achieve targeted drug exposure. Usually pharmacokinetics can help answer the fundamental questions in delivery of drugs: what route of administration? how often (schedule)? how much (dose)? Knowing the pharmacokinetics of a given agent, specifically its route of elimination, adjustments in dose can be made for altered renal or hepatic function to accommodate abnormalities in individual patient. In general, these adjustments would be expected to be less precise than adjustments based on drug level measurements [3, 4].

Of special interest is a study by Borkowski et al. [5], who investigated the pharmacokinetics of nine cytotoxic drugs in patients aged <65 and ≥65 years. A total of 51 % of patients over 65 and 53 % of those under 65 received a dose of chemotherapy equal to or higher than the maximum tolerated dose (MTD); 25.9 % of the older patients and 31.7 % of the younger experienced dose-limiting toxicity (DLT) equal or higher than grade 3. This study is very important for several reasons: it was the first study to include older individuals in phase I trials and demonstrated that the pharmacokinetics of many drugs does not change with the age of the patient; in this study, the possibility of compensatory changes in drug clearance for agents with mixed excretion has been suggested. The main flaw of the study was the limited representation of patients aged ≥75 years.

Another important aspect, but relatively unexplored, is the clinical pharmacokinetics monitoring of drug interactions. Polypharmacy is quite frequent in older cancer patient. In fact, in about 90 % of elderly, the average of administered drugs, due to comorbidities, is four per patient. Moreover, all treatment protocols include combinations of drugs, encompassing two or more anticancer drugs as well as various other drugs related to general symptomatic and supportive therapy of the patient. This large number of drugs leads to a high possibility of drug interactions, particularly with the cytochrome P450 (CYP450) system, and mainly CYP3A4 enzyme, and for drug excreted by renal route [6–8].

The fundamental obstacle to greater success in application of pharmacokinetics and clinical monitoring to anticancer therapy is our limited knowledge of pharmacodynamics. We need to develop pharmacologic goals, based upon measurements of drugs in body.

Special considerations are related to the use of new cytotoxic agents that have been developed over the last decade and present distinctive characteristic of special interest to older patients. These include a favorable toxicity profile and improved dose flexibility due to oral or weekly intravenous administration. Oral therapy [9] can eliminate charges for items such as administration and nursing, central intravenous catheter, and infusion pump costs, and costs related to adverse effects of intravenous administration such as line sepsis. Patient preferences and quality of life issues are important factors for the development of oral chemotherapy. More than 90 % of patients prefer an oral agent, if efficacy was maintained. Patient noncompliance is a potential major obstacle in oral therapy and may influence survival. Factors associated with noncompliance include lower socioeconomic status, treatment in a community-based setting, and number of doses per day.

Important Considerations When Prescribing Chemotherapy in the Elderly

Aging is associated with multidimensional changes, such as alterations of physiological functions, comorbidities, and polypharmacy. The main physiological changes of aging that are strictly related to pharmacological management of cancer in the elderly [9, 10] are related to:

- Decreased brain weight and cerebral blood flow affect the patient's ability to tolerate some drug's neurotoxicity and may result in interaction with special senses, such as taste, smell, and salivary flow, and skin changes that decrease wound healing; these alterations have implications for the patient's nutritional status.
- Cardiopulmonary changes must be considered in the use of surgery and drugs with cardiopulmonary toxicity.
- The hematopoietic system diminishes the response under stress of chemoradiation therapy; the decreased immune response leads to a greater rate of infection.
- Changes in body composition from less leanness to greater fat may influence drugs distribution, decreases in liver mass/flow and oxidative metabolism affect hepatic drug metabolism, and reduced kidney functioning alters renal drug excretion.

Changes of Pharmacokinetic Parameters: Age-Related

The above considerations may result in modifications of the absorption, distribution, metabolism, and excretion of the drugs (Table 5.1). Absorption can be reduced by decreased gastrointestinal motility, decreased splanchnic blood flow, decreased secretion of digestive enzymes, and mucosal atrophy. The volume of distribution (V_d) of drugs is a function of body composition and the concentration of plasma

Table 5.1 Changes of pharmacokinetic parameters, age-related

Parameter	Change	Effects
Absorption	Decreased	↓ Mucosal area
		↓ Splanchnic circulation
		↓ Gastric motility
		↓ Enzymatic secretion
Volume of distribution	Decreased: hydrophilic drugs	↓ Body water
	Increased: lipophilic drugs	↑ Body fat
		↓ Proteinemia
		↓ Hemoglobinemia
Hepatic drug metabolism	Decreased: phase I reactions	↓ Enzymes cytochrome P450 related
	Unchanged: phase II reactions	↓ Splanchnic flow
Excretion	Decreased: renal	↓ Glomerular filtration rate
	Unchanged: hepatic	

proteins. Fat content can double in the elderly, and intracellular water decreases. This leads to a decrease in the V_d of drugs that are distributed primarily to the body water, while that of lipid-soluble drugs increases. This can lead to changes in peak concentration and prolongation of the terminal half-life. Aging is often associated with a decreased albumin level and anemia. Cytotoxic drugs, which are often highly protein bound, such as paclitaxel and etoposide, could theoretically interact with other highly protein-bound drugs such as warfarin, which is routinely used for the prevention and treatment of thromboses in patients with cancer [11].

Anemia can be relevant in the case of treatment with drugs that bind heavily to red blood cells. The correction of anemia is beneficial, and anemia is the only component of V_d that can be manipulated. The liver is the main site of drug metabolism. Phase 1 metabolism occurs primarily via the CYP450 microsomal system, which consists of several isoenzymes. Phase 2 deals with conjugation reactions. The CYP450 system is made up of heme-based enzymes located in the liver, small bowel, kidneys, lungs, and brain. The potential for drug interactions is high, particularly with the CYP3A4 enzyme. This enzyme is inhibited by a variety of common medications and is involved in the metabolism of a variety of anticancer agents. The levels of CYP450 1A2 is 20–25 % lower in healthy elderly patients than in younger patients. Renal excretion is affected by the gradual decline in function with age. There is a decrease in the glomerular filtration rate (GFR) by approximately 1 ml/min for every year after the age of 40. The reduction in GFR is not reflected in an increase in serum creatinine, because of the simultaneous loss of muscle mass. If creatinine clearance (CrCl) is merely estimated in the elderly, this may lead to errors in dosing [3, 9, 10].

Guidelines for Dose Adjustment Related to Renal and Liver Function in the Elderly

The correlation of renal and liver function changes age-related on the pharmacokinetics is an important aspect in the dose adjustment of anticancer drugs (Tables 5.2, 5.3, 5.4, and 5.5) [4]. Dose adjustment related to the functionality of emunctory systems represents a very commonly used way to minimize toxic effects of drugs, as this approach compensates for the decline of emunctory functions associated with age, under either physiological conditions or associated with organ pathologies, particularly renal and liver ones. Therefore, it is crucial to know the clearance pathway of the administered drug.

Pharmacokinetic and Renal Function

A progressive decline in GFR is one of the most consistent findings of normal aging. The importance of GFR impairment in the management of older persons with cancer has been highlighted by Gelman and Taylor [12]. These authors

Table 5.2 Dose adjustment (%) for some urinary excreted cytostatic drugs according to creatinine clearance

	Excreted drug (%)	Creatinine clearance (ml/min)		
Cytostatic drug	As active metabolite or toxic	≤60	≤45	≤30
Bleomycin	62	0.70	0.60	–
Carboplatin	66	Calvert formula[a]		
Carmustine	43	0.80	0.75	–
Lomustine	50	0.75	0.70	–
Semustine	47	0.75	0.70	–
Cisplatin	30	0.75	0.50	–
Cytarabine	76	0.60	0.50	–
Dacarbazine	41	0.80	0.75	0.70
Fludarabine	44	0.80	0.75	0.65
Hydroxyurea	36	0.85	0.80	0.75
Ifosfamide	40	0.80	0.75	0.70
Melphalan	34	0.85	0.75	0.70
Methotrexate	77	Gelman and Taylor formula[b]		
Etoposide	32	0.85	0.80	0.75

[a]Calvert formula: carboplatin dosage (mg) = Area under curve (mg/ml × minute) × (glomerular filtration rate (ml/min) + 25)
[b]Gelman and Taylor formula: methotrexate dosage = dose × creatinine clearance l/70

Table 5.3 Some cytostatic drugs excreted by biliary route

Cytostatic drug	% of urinary excreted drug
Daunorubicin	<18
Doxorubicin	<10
Idarubicin, mitoxantrone	<10
Amsacrine	>10
Paclitaxel, docetaxel	<10
Vincristine, vinblastine	10–11
Vindesine, vinorelbine	13–14

Table 5.4 Cytostatic drugs with hepatic and extrahepatic inactivation

Cytostatic drug	% of urinary excreted drug as a drive or toxic metabolite
Chlorambucil	<1
Cyclophosphamide	16
Cytarabine	11
5-Fluorouracil	<10
Gemcitabine	<10
6-Mercaptopurin	21
Mitomycin C	5
Procarbazine	Not detected
Teniposide	<10
6-Thioguanine	Not detected

Table 5.5 Criteria for hepatic function and cytostatic drug adjustment (%)

Hepatic function	Thrombotest	AST (U/I)	Albumin (g/l)	Bilirubin (mg/dl)	Drug adjustment (%)
Good	>40	<51	>34	<1.2	100
Fair	25–39	51–200	28–34	1.2–3.0	50–75
Poor	<25	>200	>28	>3.0	25–50

treated 167 women affected by metastatic breast cancer with a combination of cyclophosphamide, methotrexate, and 5-fluorouracil. In women aged ≥65 years, the doses of cyclophosphamide and methotrexate were adjusted on the patients' GFR. The therapeutic response was similar in younger and older women, but the myelotoxicity was less severe in the older women. Kintzel and Dorr [13] calculated the dose adjustment with declining renal function for drugs whose parent compounds, active metabolites, or toxic metabolites are excreted through the kidneys. They based this calculation on the fraction of drug or drug metabolite undergoing renal excretion. The relative formula, in which the CrCl was calculated according to Cockroft and Gault formula [14], might be helpful to the busy practitioner. However, it should be pointed out that many of these adjustments were not tested in the clinical context.

Also the doses of methotrexate given by intravenous push may be adjusted according to the formula proposed by Gelman and Taylor. The Calvert formula [15] allows the practitioner to calculate the dose of carboplatin for the desired area under curve (AUC) based on age and serum creatinine. For other drugs, the dose adjustment proposed by Kintzel and Dorr [13] has been recommended:

Adjusted dose: (normal dose) + [f (K_f−1) +1] f = fraction excreted through the kidney, K_f = CrCl (in ml/min) divided by 120

Several drugs, such as etoposide, have a mixed hepatic and renal excretion. In these circumstances, a reduction of GFR of up to 25 ml/min does not seem to prevent adequate drug excretion, as long as biliary obstruction is not present.

Pharmacokinetic and Liver Function

Hepatic function is modified by aging but in several, and sometimes reciprocally, equilibrating ways: decreased blood flow, decreased albumin production, and decreased CYP450 function [16]. In general, biliary excretion seems to be unaffected by age. The half-life of doxorubicin and daunorubicin is not affected by age-related changes, whereas a high variability in the half-life of paclitaxel in older individuals is found. Paclitaxel and other taxanes are metabolized in the liver, and their metabolites are excreted through the bile; less than 10 % of the parent compound is found unchanged in the urine.

Chemotherapeutic Agents

Chemotherapy is the cornerstone of lung cancer treatment and mainly in the advanced stage disease. Several old and new drugs are still used in the clinical practice including the treatment of elderly patients. Many of them are excluded from the routinely use in this population due to safety concerns. However, several results showed that these drugs when studied specifically in the elderly population employing doses and regimens tailored to them can be administered safely with no lack of activity and efficacy [17–26] (Table 5.6).

Cisplatin

Cisplatin is used to treat various types of cancers including lung carcinomas. These platinum complexes react in vivo, binding to and causing cross-linking of deoxyribonucleic acid (DNA), which ultimately triggers apoptosis. The triphasic elimination shows that the half-life is 20–30 min, 48–67 min, and 24 h, respectively, during the initial, intermediate, and terminal infusion. Each of these steps is affected by the excretory function of kidney; through the renal elimination, about 90 % of the drug is removed. The following adjustments of dose have been reported in relation to the value of the CrCl: CrCl ≤60 ml/min, 75 % of the scheduled dose; CrCl ≤45 ml/min, 50 % of the scheduled dose. No data in the presence of CrCl ≤30 ml/min are available. The main toxicities include renal failure, hypomagnesemia, nausea and vomiting, peripheral neuropathy, myelosuppression, and hearing abnormalities. The nephrotoxicity requires particular caution in the use of the drug in the elderly population, although allowing adequate hydration to reduce the incidence of 5 % [27]. Studies exploring the pharmacokinetics of cisplatin in lung cancer patients of different ages have found that the drug concentration was increased for a more prolonged period of time in older individuals, indicating a decreased rate of drug elimination. Moreover, retrospective studies have documented an increase of nephrotoxicity in elderly patients [28, 29]. The use of amifostine seems to reduce the renal, neurological, acoustic, and bone marrow toxicity [30].

Carboplatin

It was introduced in the late 1980s. Carboplatin has a mechanism of action similar to cisplatin and is active in several cancers, as well. In contrast to cisplatin, its binding to plasma proteins is very limited, and therefore, dose reductions are not necessary in the presence of hypoalbuminemia. Its elimination takes place exclusively through the kidneys. Cockcroft-Gault's and Calvert's formulas allow the calculation of the dose according to renal function, to age, and to AUC [14, 15, 31]. The first

Table 5.6 Pharmacokinetic studies of some drugs and schedules for the treatment of lung cancer in the elderly

Author	No. of patients	Age distribution	Drug	Dose and schedule	Results
Lichtman et al. [17]	122	Cohort 1: $n=46$	Paclitaxel	Paclitaxel 175 mg/m^2 IV over 3 h every 3 weeks	Increasing age associated with increased AUC and decreased clearance
		Range: 55–64 Cohort 2: $n=44$ Range: 65–74 Cohort 3: $n=32$ Range: 75–86			Increased age associated with increased grade ≥3 neutropenia and lower absolute neutrophil count
Fidias et al. [18]	13	Median 76 Range 70–85	Paclitaxel	Paclitaxel 90 mg/m^2 IV over 1 h weekly for 6 weeks followed by a 2-week break	No difference in PK in this older cohort compared with historical data from younger patients
Smorenburg et al. [19]	23	Cohort 1: $n=8$	Paclitaxel	Paclitaxel 80 mg/m^2 IV over 1 h weekly for 3 weeks followed by a 1-week break	Older age associated with decreased clearance of unbound and total paclitaxel
		Median: 77 Range: 70–84 Cohort 2: $n=15$ Median: 54 Range: 22–69		Paclitaxel 100 mg/m^2 IV over 1 h weekly for 3 weeks followed by a 1-week break	Despite receiving a lower dose of paclitaxel, older patients experienced similar decreases in white blood cell and absolute neutrophil count compared with younger patients

(continued)

Table 5.6 (continued)

Author	No. of patients	Age distribution	Drug	Dose and schedule	Results
Bruno et al. [20]	640	Not specified	Docetaxel	Not specified	Small decrease in clearance with age (estimated at a 7 % decrease in clearance for a 71-year-old patient)
Hurria et al. [21]	19	Median 75 Range: 66–84	Docetaxel	Docetaxel 35 mg/m^2 IV over 1 h weekly for 3 weeks followed by a 1-week break	No association of age with docetaxel clearance
Minami et al. [22]	52	Cohort 1 $\geq$75: $n=27$	Docetaxel and cisplatin	Docetaxel 20 mg/m^2 IV over 1 h weekly for 3 weeks followed by a 1-week break	No association of age with clearance or volume distribution
		Median: 76		Docetaxel 35 mg/m^2 IV over 1 h weekly for 3 weeks followed by a 1-week break	Older patients received a lower dose of docetaxel and had a smaller AUC, but both groups had similar rates of neutropenia
		Range: 75–86 Cohort 2 <75: $n=25$ Median: 56 Range: 39–73 Both cohorts		Cisplatin 25 mg/m^2 IV weekly for 3 week followed by a 1-week break	
Sorio et al. [23]	10	Median 70 Range 66–81	Vinorelbine	Vinorelbine 30 mg/m^2 IV day 1 and 8 of every 3 week	No age-related difference in PK, no correlation between age, toxicity, and drug exposure

Gauvin et al. [24]	12	Mean 74 Range 65–79	Vinorelbine	Vinorelbine 20–30 mg/m^2 IV over 10 min weekly	Older age associated with decreased total clearance of vinorelbine. Increased AUC of vinorelbine correlated with increased hematologic toxicity
Miller et al. [25]	106	<50 ($n=6$) 50–59 ($n=29$) 60–69 ($n=42$) ≥70 ($n=29$)	Etoposide	Etoposide 50 mg/m^2/day orally for 21 days and cisplatin 33 mg/m^2/day IV for 3 days every 28 days for 6 courses	Older age associated with increased etoposide not bound to protein and etoposide concentrations
Ando et al. [26]	12	Median 79 Range 75–84	Etoposide	Etoposide 50 mg/day [Dose level 1 ($n=6$)] Etoposide 75 mg/day [Dose level 2 ($n=6$)]	No difference in PK in this older cohort in comparison to historical data from younger patients, older patients experienced greater myelosuppressive effects despite equivalent exposure

IV intravenous administration, *PK* pharmacokinetics, *AUC* area under curve

formula was derived to calculate a dosage based on patient CrCl, pretreatment platelet count, desired platelet nadir, and prior chemotherapy status, providing help in maintaining tolerable levels of myelosuppression in pretreated and untreated patients with variable levels of renal function [14]. The second formula is based on the demonstration of an inverse linear relationship between GFR and free platinum AUC at both low and high glomerular filtration levels. This formula allows to calculate the total dose of carboplatin in mg independently from body size:

$$\text{Dose (mg)} = \text{target AUC} \times (\text{GFR} + 25)$$

The latter formula suggests that in order to obtain the desired AUC, the dose not only must be decreased in patients with low renal function, but higher than standard doses may be required for patients with high renal clearance values. The AUC suggested for obtaining a manageable degree of myelosuppression is 5 and 7 mg/ml/min, respectively, for patients previously treated and untreated. This formula can be applied in both combination and high-dose therapy [15, 31].

Etoposide

Etoposide is an inhibitor of topoisomerase II used for the treatment of several malignancies. Etoposide can be administered both intravenously and orally.

Intravenously etoposide follows two-compartment pharmacokinetics with a terminal half-life of 4–8 h. There are reports of a third compartment with a much longer terminal half-life in some studies which have sampled patients for longer than 24 h. Renal clearance is 6–10 ml/min/m^2 accounting for approximately 30 % of the total clearance. Both AUC and peak plasma concentration increase in a linear fashion with increasing dose. There is no evidence of accumulation with repeated daily doses. Plasma protein binding in normal volunteers is 95 % but may be reduced in patients, an effect associated with albumin and bilirubin concentrations. Inter- and intrapatient variability in AUC is in the order of 25 and 10 %, respectively [32].

Peak concentrations appear 0.5–4 h after oral administration of etoposide with two-compartment pharmacokinetics and a terminal half-life of 4–8 h. The bioavailability of oral etoposide is approximately 50 % but decreases with doses larger than 200 mg. There is no evidence of accumulation with repeated daily or bid dosing and no change in bioavailability across a 15-day treatment period of 50 mg bid. There is considerable variability in AUC both within and between patients. Changes in bioavailability are more evident with oral administration [25].

The high (>90 %) plasma protein binding affects their greater toxicity in the presence of hypoalbuminemia. The following adjustments of the dose are recommended in relation to the degree of renal failure: 85 % of the total dose with CrCl ≤60 ml/min, 80 % with CrCl ≤45 ml/min, and 75 % with CrCl ≤30 ml/min. In elderly patients has suggested the use of the drug after modest reduction of its dosage and with careful monitoring of hematological parameters in the absence of organ failure. A poor performance status may be associated, in older patients, with a higher risk of dose-limiting toxicity of grade 4 including myelosuppression and stomatitis [25].

Vinorelbine

Vinorelbine is a semisynthetic vinca alkaloid approved for the treatment of several malignancies. The main pharmacokinetic parameters in man are described by a three-compartment model with a prolonged elimination phase (22–68 h). There is an excellent correlation at early times between radioimmunoassay (RIA) and total radioactivity. The plasma levels determined by RIA continued to decrease after 4 h, while radioactivity levels remained stable for a much longer time, indicating extensive formation of metabolites. High protein binding (80 %) is observed initially, decreasing to 50 % after 96 h. In most patients, a dose and/or time dependence was demonstrated. The neurotoxicity is lower than for other drugs of this class and myelotoxicity is the DLT. Its elimination is mainly via the bile in the feces. Dose changes are necessary in the presence of impaired liver function, with dose reduction of 50 and 75 % in the presence of bilirubin, respectively, values of 2–3 and >3 mg/dl [33]. The pharmacokinetic properties of the drug are similar in the youngest patient and in patients over 65 years old although some studies have documented age-related reduction of body clearance resulting in increased myelotoxicity [23].

Gemcitabine

Gemcitabine is a pyrimidine antagonist, and as the fluorouracil and other analogues of pyrimidines, the triphosphate analogue of gemcitabine replaces one of the building blocks of nucleic acids, in this case cytidine, during DNA replication. The process arrests tumor growth, as only one additional nucleoside can be attached to the "faulty" nucleoside, resulting in apoptosis. Its pharmacokinetic characteristics are partly related to age and sex with an increase in its half-life from 42 to 62 min and 49 to 73 min, respectively, in men and women over 60. Myelosuppression (neutropenia and thrombocytopenia) is the main toxicity. Dosage adjustments are recommended in the presence of abnormalities in liver function tests and kidney. In particular, in case of increase in bilirubin (≥1.6 mg/ml), it is necessary to reduce the initial dose to 800 mg/m^2 [34].

Taxanes

For taxanes, paclitaxel and docetaxel, the binding to plasma proteins is more than 90 % bound, making necessary changes in the dosages for elderly patients with hypoalbuminemia. Dose reductions are not indicated in presence of renal failure. Instead, their predominant biliary excretion is responsible for the increased toxicity in presence of liver failure [35].

Paclitaxel is mainly metabolized in the liver by the CYP3A4 and CYP3A5 subfamilies of CYP450 isoenzymes, and its elimination is mainly fecal and urinary. The concentration-time profile of paclitaxel was consistent with a three-compartment pharmacokinetic model, with a relatively slow γ-half-life of mean 5.8 h, which represents the slow efflux of paclitaxel from the peripheral compartment. The main toxicities of the drug are alopecia, peripheral neuropathy, and myelosuppression. In presence of abnormalities in liver function tests, the following changes in dose have been proposed: 135 mg/m^2 in presence of serum aspartate transaminase ≤2 times upper normal value and serum bilirubin ≤1.5, 75 mg/m^2 in presence of serum bilirubin of 1.6–3, and 50 mg/m^2 in the presence of bilirubin >3 mg/dl [35]. The clearance of paclitaxel decreases with increasing age without any apparent increase in side effects [17]. The weekly infusion allows to increase the tolerability without loss of effectiveness probably as a consequence of antiangiogenic effect. The association with platinum derivatives increases the severity of neuropathy which appears to be reduced by amifostine and probably also by glutamic acid [36].

Docetaxel differs from the chemical structure of paclitaxel for the presence of a hydroxyl functional group on carbon 10 and a tert-butyl carbamate ester on the phenylpropionate side chain instead of the benzyl amide of the paclitaxel molecule. The carbon 10 functional group change causes docetaxel to be more water soluble than paclitaxel. The concentration-time profile of docetaxel was consistent with a three-compartment pharmacokinetic model. An initial, relatively rapid decline, with an α-half-life of mean 4.5 min, is representative of distribution to peripheral compartments from the systemic circulation. A β-half-life of mean 38.3 min and a relatively slow γ-half-life of mean 12.2 h represent the slow efflux of docetaxel from the peripheral compartment. Like paclitaxel, docetaxel is mainly metabolized in the liver by the CYP3A4 and CYP3A5 subfamilies of CYP450 isoenzymes. The administration of the docetaxel with the strong CYP3A4 inhibitor ketoconazole has been shown to reduce docetaxel clearance, which may increase the odds of neutropenia. Similarly the concomitant use of docetaxel and dronedarone, a new antiarrhythmic drug alternative to amiodarone for a better safety profile, has been responsible of the first case of docetaxel overdose probably related to pharmacokinetic interaction with dronedarone and responsible of a fatal mucositis [37]. Even for this drug, changes in liver function may increase the hematologic toxicity and worsening morbidity with increased incidence of toxic deaths [38]. A dose reduction of 25 % was evaluated in the presence of abnormal values of transaminases and alkaline phosphatase also with normal levels of bilirubin. However, in patients with liver metastases and normal liver function, modifications of doses are not required [39]. Similar to paclitaxel, the weekly docetaxel schedule improves tolerability without reducing the effectiveness [40]. The water retention of moderate to severe grade appears after a cumulative dose of 800 mg/m^2 in the patients where a proper premedication has been performed [41].

Irinotecan

Irinotecan is a topoisomerase I inhibitor, which prevents DNA from unwinding. In chemical terms, it is a semisynthetic analogue of the natural alkaloid camptothecin. Its main use is in colon cancer, in combination with other chemotherapy agents [42]. However, it is also active in glioblastoma multiforme and in small cell lung cancer [43, 44]. Irinotecan is activated by hydrolysis to SN-38 which is then inactivated by glucuronidation by uridine diphosphate glucuronosyltransferase 1A1 (UGT1A1). The inhibition of topoisomerase I by the active metabolite SN-38 eventually leads to inhibition of both DNA replication and transcription. It can be administered weekly or biweekly according to schedules. The main toxicities were hematologic and gastrointestinal. The delayed diarrhea may be resulting from the accumulation of its metabolite SN-38 in the intestine. To relate the value of SN-38 in the bile with the severity of diarrhea has been proposed [45]. A retrospective analysis showed an increased incidence of delayed diarrhea in elderly patients [46], while no difference in response was observed based on patient's age [47]. A dose reduction in elderly patients >70 years with prior pelvic irradiation or with poor performance status is recommended [48].

Topotecan

Topotecan is a topoisomerase I inhibitor approved for the treatment of several malignancies [49]. About 40 % of the drug is eliminated through the kidneys with a half-life of approximately 3 h. Dose reductions are required in patients with moderate renal impairment. Dose schedule change on the values of CrCl in elderly patients is reported in Table 5.7. In the elderly patients, the most common side effects are myelosuppression and diarrhea [50].

Pemetrexed

Pemetrexed is a folate antimetabolites. It works by inhibiting three enzymes used in purine and pyrimidine synthesis: thymidylate synthase, dihydrofolate reductase, and glycinamide ribonucleotide formyltransferase [51]. Pemetrexed is indicated for

Table 5.7 Recommended adjustment of doses of topotecan in the presence of renal failure

Creatinine clearance (ml/min)	Few previous treatments	Many previous treatments
>60	1.5	1.5
40–59	1.5	1.0
20–39	0.75	0.5
<20	Not established	Not established

the treatment of pleural mesothelioma and non-squamous non-small cell lung cancer [52, 53]. Patients are required to be on folic acid and vitamin B12 supplementation when they are on pemetrexed therapy. In fact, this vitaminic supplementation reduced the frequency of adverse events. It is also recommended for patients to be on a steroid on the day prior, day of, and day after pemetrexed infusion to avoid skin rashes. Neutropenia is the DLT in the elderly patients. Studies have not demonstrated that pemetrexed inhibits the cytochrome P450 isoenzymes 3A4, 2D6, 2C9, or 1A2. Pemetrexed is mainly excreted in the urine, and 70–90 % of the dose is eliminated as unchanged drug within 24 h of the administered dose. In patients with normal renal function, the elimination half-life is 3.5 h. The half-life and exposure to the drug increase as renal function decreases. Patients with CrCl of 50 ml/min have a 54 % increase in pemetrexed AUC compared with patients with CrCl of 100 ml/min. No dosage adjustment is necessary for patients with a CrCl above 45 ml/min. Pemetrexed administration has not been studied in patients with a CrCl <45 ml/min and therefore should be avoided in this patient population [54].

Targeted Agents

The ability to identify and target specific molecular pathways for the treatment of lung cancer has been the main goal of researchers and clinicians for more than two decades. However, despite strong preclinical evidence from both in vitro assays and animal models, most of the agents evaluated in lung cancer patients to date have failed to improve any outcome. The two exceptions to this include blockade of the epidermal growth factor (EGF) pathway through inhibition of EGF receptor (EGFR) and inhibition of angiogenesis by targeting vascular endothelial growth factor (VEGF). To date, the only drugs employed in the clinical practice for the treatment of advanced non-small cell lung cancer are an anti-VEGF monoclonal antibody, the bevacizumab, and two small molecules EGFR tyrosine kinase inhibitors (TKIs), erlotinib and gefitinib.

Unfortunately, despite these drugs are commonly used in the elderly today, there are few data concerning the pharmacokinetics and pharmacodynamics specifically studied in this population.

Bevacizumab

Bevacizumab is an immunoglobulin G (IgG) composed of two identical light chains, consisting of 214 amino acid residues and two 453 residue heavy chains containing an N-linked oligosaccharide and has a molecular weight of approximately 149,000 Da [55]. The pharmacokinetics of bevacizumab were characterized in patients with various types of solid tumors. The doses tested were 0.1–10 mg/kg weekly in phase I, which yield a maximum concentration of 2.8–284 μg/mL and show a dose–response relationship; 3–20 mg/kg every 2 weeks or 3 weeks in phase II, 5 or 10 mg/kg every 2 weeks, and 7.5 or 15 mg/kg every 3 weeks in phase III [56]. In all clinical trials, bevacizumab was administered as an intravenous infusion. In non-small cell lung cancer first-line therapy, bevacizumab was investigated and registered, in combination with chemotherapy in two doses: 7.5 and 15 mg/kg on day 1 every 3 weeks [57]. Bevacizumab demonstrates linear pharmacokinetics over a dosage range of 3–10 mg/kg, a limited volume of distribution, and a low clearance. The serum half-life is 13–21 days [56]. Clearance appears to vary with sex, tumor burden, body weight, and albumin levels [58]. Males have a higher clearance and a larger volume of distribution than females after adjusting for body-weight differences. Patients with higher tumor burdens have a higher clearance than those with lower burdens. A 30 % change in body weight results in an 18 % change in clearance. Reduced albumin levels increase bevacizumab clearance. Despite the pharmacokinetic differences seen with sex, tumor burden, body weight, and albumin levels, response rates and toxic effects do not differ appreciably, and no dosage modifications are needed. There was no significant difference in the pharmacokinetics of bevacizumab in relation to age with no correlation between bevacizumab clearance and patient age (the median age was 59 years with 5th and 95th percentiles of 37 and 76 years) [58].

High levels of free VEGF are correlated with a poor prognosis and an increased risk of metastatic disease. In phase I study, bevacizumab given at single doses greater than 0.3 mg/kg completely suppressed free serum VEGF. Currently, there is no clear association among the dosage of bevacizumab, disease stability, and toxicity. However, a phase I trial found that bevacizumab-treated patients with stable disease had slightly higher baseline VEGF levels than bevacizumab recipients with progressive disease. The authors hypothesized that an elevated baseline VEGF level may indicate that the patient is a better candidate for bevacizumab therapy [56].

Retrospective analyses reported that elderly patients affected by advanced NSCLC and receiving bevacizumab, when compared to younger patients, experienced a higher incidence of severe grade toxicities such as neutropenia, melena, gastrointestinal bleeding, and proteinuria [57].

Erlotinib

Erlotinib is a small molecule administered orally daily with a molecular weight of 429,90 Da [59]. Phase I trials assessed the pharmacokinetics of erlotinib in volunteers and patients with advanced solid tumors showing that erlotinib is absorbed rapidly, with peak concentration achieved within 4 h, followed by a monophasic decline of approximately 9 h. Bioavailability of erlotinib was estimated at 59 % (95 % confidence interval, 55–63 %) in healthy humans and is highly protein bound (92–95 %) [60]. The bioavailability of erlotinib is increased by almost 100 % with the intake of food. A randomized, open-label, parallel-group study was conducted in 62 healthy male volunteers in order to evaluate the impact of food on its pharmacokinetics. This trial demonstrated a rise in erlotinib exposure after single- and multiple-dose administration of erlotinib with a high-fat, high-calorie meal [61]. The overall pharmacokinetic analysis stated that erlotinib should be taken ≥1 h before and 2 h after food [62, 63]. A phase I study of escalating daily oral doses of erlotinib showed that the MTD was 150 mg/day and the DLT was the acneiform rash and diarrhea. In this trial, the pharmacokinetics were dose independent with a large volume of distribution and moderate interpatient variability. Erlotinib was rapidly absorbed (time to maximum plasma concentration [t_{max}] was 2 ± 0 h), the mean maximum plasma concentration (C_{max}) was 2.12 ± 1.52 μg/ml, and plasma exposure (AUC_{0-24}) was 38.42 ± 29.55 μgh/l. The elimination half-life was 18.18 ± 5.74 h, and the steady state through concentration was 1.17 ± 0.50 μg/ml, which was reached in about 7 days. As a consequence, erlotinib at 150 mg/day was determined to be the MTD at which biologically relevant plasma levels were achieved and was therefore recommended for phase II trials [63]. Another phase I study evaluated, in 28 patients with refractory solid tumors, a weekly escalating dose of erlotinib without reaching an MTD, even after escalation to 1,600 mg/week. Pharmacokinetic analysis revealed that the target average plasma drug concentration exceeded at all dose levels [64]. Erlotinib is metabolized in the liver and excreted with its metabolites in the bile. Approximately 80 % of the metabolism of erlotinib occurs via cytochrome CYP3A4 and, to a lesser extent, via CYP1A2 and CYP1A1. The predominant metabolite is OSI-420. Potent inhibitors of CYP3A4, such as ketoconazole, can affect the metabolism of erlotinib, increasing the plasma exposure and potentially altering efficacy and tolerability. Erlotinib plasma exposure can be decreased by CYP3A4 inducers, such as rifampicin, or antiepileptics (phenytoin, carbamazepine, and barbiturates). Therefore, concomitant treatment with CYP3A4 inhibitors or inducers should be performed carefully [60]. If concurrent therapy with erlotinib and a strong CYP3A4 inducer is necessary, a dose increase of 50 mg po daily should be considered. Elevated concentrations of erlotinib may occur when it is given with CYP3A4 inhibitors. When tested with ketoconazole, erlotinib concentrations were decreased by 60–70 %. Dose decreases in increments of 50 mg should be considered, along with careful monitoring. The oral absorption of erlotinib is pH-dependent; decreases in erlotinib absorption may occur when it is given with antacids, H_2 blockers, and proton-pump inhibitors. Coadministration of erlotinib has been reported to enhance the carboplatin exposure and increase the serum concentration of phenytoin. When erlotinib is given with phenytoin, a decrease in erlotinib concentrations would be expected; in addition, an increase in phenytoin concentrations and toxicity has been reported with this combination [60]. Cigarette smoking induces CYP1A1 and 1A2 enzymes which attributes to the reduction in erlotinib exposure seen in current smokers with non-small cell lung cancer [65].

Considering that skin rash is one of the major adverse effects associated with erlotinib therapy, skin is an appropriate tissue to be used in erlotinib pharmacodynamics research. A study was conducted to determine the pharmacodynamic effects of erlotinib in normal skin tissue collected from 28 patients affected by solid tumors and treated with erlotinib, administered at doses ranging from 25 to 200 mg/day, in a phase I trial. The results of this study determined that erlotinib exhibits biologic effects in the normal epidermis of patients undergoing therapy which includes the agent. The expression of p27 appears to be the most apparent indicator [66].

No differences in erlotinib safety or efficacy were observed between younger and older patients both in retrospective and prospective studies. Erlotinib, being metabolized in the liver, showed a good safety profile also when administered to patients with chronic renal failure [67].

Gefitinib

Gefitinib is an orally administered low-molecular-weight, 446,90 Da, anilinoquinazoline. The inhibition of the EGFR and its related downstream process was achieved by gefitinib at the dosage of 250 mg/day, while the MTD, assessed in phase 1 trials, was 700 mg/day [68]. Pharmacokinetic studies, performed in healthy male volunteers aged 18–62 years, administered escalating doses from 1 to 100 mg daily for 3 days and evaluated also the effect of food intake after a single dose of 50 mg. These trials showed a C_{max} between 3 and 7 h after administration, with a terminal elimination half-life of 28 h. Because of its biological half-life of about 28 h, gefitinib is administered once in a day [69]. The C_{max} was decreased by 34 % with food ingestion, and the prolonged half-life suggested the feasibility of once-daily administration. Gefitinib is metabolized mainly by CYP3A4, while CYP3A5 and CYP2D6 are less involved. This is the reason why gefitinib metabolism can differ from patient to patient in consideration of interindividual variability of CYP3A4 expression and activity. Therefore, inducers or inhibitors of this cytochrome can also influence the pharmacokinetics of this drug [70]. Clinical studies showed that co-medication with a CYP3A4 inducer (rifampin) reduces exposure to gefitinib and co-medication with a CYP3A4 inhibitor (itraconazole) increases exposure to gefitinib in healthy men [71]. Similarly, patients who receive drugs that reduce CYP3A4, e.g., ketoconazole, itraconazole, fluconazole, erythromycin, clarithromycin, ritonavir, nelfinavir, nefazodone, as well as grapefruit juice, may need a lower dose of gefitinib to prevent side effect from increased levels of gefitinib. Gefitinib is unlikely to exert a clinically relevant effect on the pharmacokinetics of drugs that are dependent on CYP2D6-mediated metabolism for their clearance, but the potential to increase plasma concentrations should be considered if gefitinib is coadministered with CYP2D6 substrates that have a narrow therapeutic index or are individually dose titrated [72].

The pharmacodynamics of gefitinib were studied in two phase I trials in which the effects of gefitinib on EGFR-TK activity in cancer patients were evaluated [73]. Skin biopsies were obtained from 65 patients receiving escalating doses of daily oral gefitinib. The results showed that gefitinib inhibited EGFR activation and affects downstream receptor-dependent processes in vivo. These effects were profound at doses well below the one producing unacceptable toxicity, a finding that strongly supports pharmacodynamic assessments to select optimal doses instead of an MTD for definitive efficacy and safety trials [73].

Also for gefitinib, no differences were observed for safety and efficacy between younger and older patients. Gefitinib showed a good safety profile also when administered to patients with chronic renal failure, too [74].

Conclusions

Differences in pharmacokinetics between elderly and younger patients that occur are usually due to physiologic changes often associated with aging, such as changes in renal and liver function. However, end-organ dysfunction also affects pharmacokinetics, but this concern is not limited to the elderly. For drugs and drug metabolites that are excreted renally, caution should be exercised because even small changes in renal function can lead to significant toxicity. Despite increasingly widespread drug exposure with age, elderly patients did not have adverse outcomes with the standard dose. Moreover, drugs that do not have different pharmacokinetics in the elderly as compared to younger patients can have different toxicities. Frailty, performance status, and functional assessment are important factors to evaluate in treating elderly patients. These assessments in terms of pharmacodynamics are still in early stages for the elderly, and much research should be performed in this regard. An important direction of research concerning pharmacokinetics and, mainly, pharmacodynamics in the elderly is how to predict toxicity. It is difficult, in clinical practice, to predict the side effects a patient will experience. Incorporating a pharmacokinetic evaluation into geriatric assessment should help.

These concerns are much more when considering the targeted therapies. In fact, there is a paucity of data to help guide a physician on how to use these drugs in the elderly. Patients who are octogenarians are very different from patients who are 65 years old, and the former represent the most rapidly growing patient population in the developed countries. As consequence, it should be important to assess the pharmacokinetics of new biological agents in this population.

Overall, considering that the median age at diagnosis of lung cancer is 71 years, the regulatory agencies should require that all new drugs used to treat this cancer should be studied in this population.

References

1. Brocklehurst JC. Textbook of geriatric medicine and gerontology. New York: Churchill Livingstone; 1985.
2. Lynch T, Price A. The effect of cytochrome P450 metabolism on drug response, interactions, and adverse effects. Am Fam Physician. 2007;76:348–51.
3. Cova D, Balducci L. Cancer chemotherapy in the older patient. In: Balducci L, Lyman GH, Ershler WB, et al., editors. Comprehensive geriatric oncology. 2nd ed. London: Taylor and Francis; 2004. p. 463–88.
4. Tranchant B. Pharmacology of cytotoxic agents: guidelines for dose adaption. Acts of the 7th International Conference on Geriatric Oncology Cancer in the Elderly. Boston, 27–28 Sep 2002. p.127–8.

5. Borkowski JM, Duerr M, Donehower RC, et al. Relation between age and clearance rate of nine investigational anticancer drugs from phase I pharmacokinetics data. Cancer Chemother Pharmacol. 1994;33:493–6.
6. Meiner S. Polypharmacy in the elderly. Early intervention can prevent complications. Adv Nurse Pract. 1997;5:28–34.
7. Loadman PM, Bibby MC. Pharmacokinetics drug interactions with anticancer drugs. Clin Pharmacokinet. 1994;26:486–500.
8. McLeod HL. Clinically relevant drug-drug interactions in oncology. Br J Clin Pharmacol. 1998;45:539–44.
9. Skirvin JA, Lichtman SM. Pharmacokinetic considerations of oral chemotherapy in elderly patients with cancer. Drugs Aging. 2002;19:25–42.
10. Lichtman SM, Skirvin JA. Pharmacology of antineoplastic agents in older cancer patients. Oncology. 2000;14:1743–55.
11. Jørgensen TL, Hallas J, Land LH, et al. Comorbidity and polypharmacy in elderly cancer patients: the significance on treatment outcome and tolerance. J Geriatr Oncol. 2010;1:87–102.
12. Gelman RS, Taylor SG. Cyclophosphamide, methotrexate and 5 fluorouracil chemotherapy in woman more than 65 year old with advanced breast cancer. The elimination of age trends in toxicity by using doses based on creatinine clearance. J Clin Oncol. 1984;2:1406–14.
13. Kinzel PE, Dorr RT. Anticancer drug renal toxicity and elimination: dosing guidelines for altered renal function. Cancer Treat Rev. 1995;21:33–64.
14. Cockcroft DW, Gault MH. Prediction of creatinine clearance from serum creatinine. Nephron. 1976;16:31–41.
15. Calvert DH, Newell DR, Gumbrell LA, et al. Carboplatin dosage: prospective evaluation of a simple formula based on renal function. J Clin Oncol. 1989;7:1748–56.
16. Sotaniemi EA, Arranto AJ, Pelkonen O, et al. Age and cytochrome P450-linked drug metabolism in humans: an analysis of 226 subjects with equal histopathologic conditions. Clin Pharmacol Ther. 1997;61:331–9.
17. Lichtman SM, Hollis D, Miller AA, et al. Prospective evaluation of the relationship of patient age and paclitaxel clinical pharmacology: Cancer and Leukemia Group B (CALGB 9762). J Clin Oncol. 2006;24:1846–51.
18. Fidias P, Supko JG, Martins R, et al. A phase II study of weekly paclitaxel in elderly patients with advanced non-small cell lung cancer. Clin Cancer Res. 2001;7:3942–9.
19. Smorenburg CH, ten Tije AJ, Verweij J, et al. Altered clearance of unbound paclitaxel in elderly patients with metastatic breast cancer. Eur J Cancer. 2003;39:196–202.
20. Bruno R, Vivier N, Veyrat-Follet C, et al. Population pharmacokinetics and pharmacokinetic-pharmacodynamic relationships for docetaxel. Invest New Drugs. 2001;19:163–9.
21. Hurria A, Flemming M, Baker SD, et al. Pharmacokinetics and toxicity of weekly docetaxel in the elderly. Clin Cancer Res. 2006;12:6100–5.
22. Minami H, Ohe Y, Niho S, et al. Comparison of pharmacokinetics and pharmacodynamics of docetaxel and cisplatin in elderly and non-elderly patients: why toxicity increased in elderly patients? J Clin Oncol. 2004;22:2901–8.
23. Sorio R, Robieux I, Galligioni E, et al. Pharmacokinetics and tolerance of vinorelbine in elderly patients with advanced metastatic breast cancer. Eur J Cancer. 1997;33:301–3.
24. Gauvin A, Pinguet F, Culine S, et al. Bayesian estimate of vinorelbine pharmacokinetic parameters in elderly patients with advanced metastatic cancer. Clin Cancer Res. 2000;6:2690–5.
25. Miller AA, Rosner GL, Ratain MJ, et al. Pharmacology of 21-day oral etoposide given in combination with i.v. cisplatin in patients with extensive-stage small cell lung cancer: a cancer and leukemia group B study (CALGB 9062). Clin Cancer Res. 1997;3:719–25.
26. Ando M, Minami H, Ando Y, et al. Pharmacological analysis of etoposide in elderly patients with lung cancer. Clin Cancer Res. 1999;5:1690–5.
27. Daugaard G, Abildgaard U. Cisplatin nephrotoxicity. Cancer Chemother Pharmacol. 1998;25:1–9.
28. Thyss A, Saudes L, Otto J, et al. Renal tolerance of cisplatin in patients more than 80 years old. J Clin Oncol. 1994;12:2121–5.

29. Cubillo A, Cornide M, Lopez JL, et al. Renal tolerance to cisplatin in patients 70 years and older. Am J Clin Oncol. 2001;24:192–7.
30. Kemp G, Rose P, Lurain J, et al. Amifostine pretreatment for protection against cyclophosphamide-induced and cisplatin-induced toxicities: result of a randomized control trial in patients with advanced ovarian cancer. J Clin Oncol. 1996;14:2101–12.
31. Calvert AH, Egorin MJ. Carboplatin dosing formulae: gender bias and the use of creatinine-based methodologies. Eur J Cancer. 2002;38:11–6.
32. Joel SP, Shah R, Slevin ML. Etoposide dosage and pharmacodynamics. Cancer Chemother Pharmacol. 1994;34(Suppl):S69–75.
33. Robieux I, Sorio R, Borsetti E, et al. Pharmacokinetics of vinorelbine in patients with liver metastases. Clin Pharmacol Ther. 1996;59:32–40.
34. Venook AP, Egorin MJ, Rosner GL, et al. Phase I and pharmacokinetic trial of gemcitabine in patients with hepatic or renal dysfunction. Cancer and Leukemia Group B 9565. J Clin Oncol. 2000;18:2780–7.
35. Venook AP, Egorin MJ, Rosner GL, et al. Phase I and pharmacokinetic trial of paclitaxel in patients with hepatic dysfunction: cancer and leukemia group B 9264. J Clin Oncol. 1998;16:1811–9.
36. Vahdat L, Papadopoulos K, Lange D, et al. Reduction of paclitaxel–induced peripheral neuropathy with glutamine. Clin Cancer Res. 2001;7:1192–7.
37. Vodovar D, Mongardon N, Moachon L, et al. Severe docetaxel overdose induced by pharmacokinetic interaction with dronedarone. J Clin Oncol. 2011;29:e694–5.
38. Burris H. Optimal use of docetaxel (Taxotere): maximizing its potential. Anticancer Drugs. 1996;7(Supp 2):25–8.
39. Bruno R, Hille D, Riva A, et al. Population pharmacokinetics/pharmacodynamics of docetaxel in phase II studies in patients with cancer. J Clin Oncol. 1998;16:187–96.
40. Hainsworth JD, Burris HA, Litchy S, et al. Weekly docetaxel in the treatment of elderly patients with advanced nonsmall cell lung carcinoma. A Minnie Pearl Cancer Research Network Phase II Trial. Cancer. 2000;89:328–33.
41. Hainsworth JD, Burris HA, Erland JB, et al. Phase I trial of docetaxel administered by weekly infusion in patients with advanced refractory cancer. J Clin Oncol. 1998;16:2164–8.
42. Saltz LB. Irinotecan in the first-line treatment of colorectal cancer. Oncology (Williston Park). 1998;12:54–8.
43. Friedman HS, Petros WP, Friedman AH, et al. Irinotecan therapy in adults with recurrent or progressive malignant glioma. J Clin Oncol. 1999;17:1516–25.
44. Noda K, Nishiwaki Y, Kawahara M, et al. Irinotecan plus cisplatin compared with etoposide plus cisplatin for extensive small-cell lung cancer. N Engl J Med. 2002;346:85–91.
45. Kehrer DF, Sparreboon A, Verweij J, et al. Modulation of irinotecan-induced diarrhea by cotreatment with neomycin in cancer patients. Clin Cancer Res. 2001;7:1136–41.
46. Skirvin J, Relias V. Topoisomerase inhibitors: 2. Irinotecan. J Oncol Pharm Pract. 1998;4:103–16.
47. Rothenberg ML, Cox JV, DeVore RF, et al. A multicenter, phase II trial of weekly irinotecan (CPT-11) in patients with previously treated colorectal carcinoma. Cancer. 1999;85:786–95.
48. Rougier P, Van Cutsem E, Bajetta E, et al. Randomised trial of irinotecan versus fluorouracil by continuous infusion after fluorouracil failure in patients with metastatic colorectal cancer. Lancet. 1998;352:1407–12.
49. Relias V, Skirvin JA. Topoisomerase I inhibitors: 1. Topotecan. J Oncol Pharm Pract. 1997;3:173–85.
50. O' Reilly S, Armstrong DK, Grochow LB. Life-threatening myelosuppression in patients with occult renal impairment receiving topotecan (letter). Gynecol Oncol. 1997;67:329–30.
51. Shih C, Chen VJ, Gossetti LS, et al. LY231514, a pyrrolo[2, 3-d]pyrimidine-based antifolate that inhibits multiple folate requiring enzymes. Cancer Res. 1997;57:1116–23.
52. Manegold C. Pemetrexed (Alimta, MTA, multitargeted antifolate, LY231514) for malignant pleural mesothelioma. Semin Oncol. 2003;30 Suppl 10:32–6.
53. Rossi A, Ricciardi S, Maione P, et al. Pemetrexed in the treatment of advanced non-squamous lung cancer. Lung Cancer. 2009;66:141–9.

54. Hazarika M, White RM, Johnson JR, et al. FDA drug approval summaries: pemetrexed (Alimta). Oncologist. 2004;9:482–8.
55. Ferrara N, Hillan KJ, Gerber HP, et al. Discovery and development of bevacizumab, an anti-VEGF antibody for treating cancer. Nat Rev Drug Discov. 2004;3:391–400.
56. Gordon MS, Margolin K, Talpaz G, et al. Phase I safety and pharmacokinetics study of recombinant human anti-vascular endothelial growth factor in patients with advanced cancer. J Clin Oncol. 2001;19:843–50.
57. Gridelli C, Rossi A. Unanswered questions: monoclonal antibodies in the treatment of advanced non-small cell lung cancer. Oncology (Williston Park). 2010;24:1216–23.
58. Gaudreault J. Pharmacokinetics (PK) of bevacizumab (BV) in colorectal cancer. Clin Pharmacol Ther. 2001;69 Suppl 2:P25.
59. Pollack VA, Savage DM, Baker DA, et al. Inhibition of epidermal growth factor receptor-associated tyrosine phosphorylation in human carcinomas with CP-358,774: dynamics of receptor inhibition in situ and antitumor effects in athymic mice. J Pharmacol Exp Ther. 1999;291:739–48.
60. Hidalgo M, Bloedow D. Pharmacokinetics and pharmacodynamics: maximizing the clinical potential of erlotinib (Tarceva). Semin Oncol. 2003;30 Suppl 7:25–33.
61. Frohna P, Lu J, Eppler S, et al. Evaluation of the absolute oral bioavailability and bioequivalence of erlotinib, an inhibitor of the epidermal growth factor receptor tyrosine kinase, in a randomized, crossover study in healthy subjects. J Clin Pharmacol. 2006;43:282–90.
62. Smith J. Erlotinib: small-molecule targeted therapy in the treatment of non-small-cell lung cancer. Clin Ther. 2005;27:1513–34.
63. Hidalgo M, Siu LL, Nemunaitis J, et al. Phase I and pharmacologic study of OSI-774, an epidermal growth factor receptor tyrosine kinase inhibitor, in patients with advanced solid malignancies. J Clin Oncol. 2001;19:3267–79.
64. Karp DD, Ferrante KJ, Tensfeldt TG, et al. A phase I dose escalation study of epidermal growth factor receptor (EGFR) tyrosine kinase (TK) inhibitor CP-358,774 in patients (pts) with advanced solid tumours. Lung Cancer. 2000;29 Suppl 1:65 (Abstr. 208).
65. Hughes AN, O'Brien MER, Petty WJ, et al. Overcoming CYP1A1/1A2 mediated induction of metabolism by escalating erlotinib dose in current smokers. J Clin Oncol. 2009;27:1220–6.
66. Malik SN, Siu LL, Rowinsky EK, et al. Pharmacodynamic evaluation of the epidermal growth factor receptor inhibitor OSI-774 in human epidermis of cancer patients. Clin Cancer Res. 2003;9:2478–86.
67. Gridelli C, Maione P, Galetta D, et al. Safety profile of erlotinib in patients with advanced non-small cell lung cancer with chronic renal failure. J Thorac Oncol. 2007;2:96–8.
68. Nakagawa K, Tamura T, Negoro S, et al. Phase I pharmacokinetic trial of the selective oral epidermal growth factor receptor tyrosine kinase inhibitor gefitinib ('Iressa', ZD1839) in Japanese patients with solid malignant tumors. Ann Oncol. 2003;14:922–30.
69. Swaisland H, Laight A, Stafford L, et al. Pharmacokinetics and tolerability of the orally active selective epidermal growth factor receptor tyrosine kinase inhibitor ZD1839 in healthy volunteers. Clin Pharmacokinet. 2001;40:297–306.
70. McKillop D, McCormick AD, Millar A, et al. Cytochrome P450-dependent metabolism of gefitinib. Xenobiotica. 2005;35:39–50.
71. van Erp NP, Gelderblom H, Guchelaar HJ. Clinical pharmacokinetics of tyrosine kinase inhibitors. Cancer Treat Rev. 2009;35:692–706.
72. Swaisland HC, Ranson M, Smith RP, et al. Pharmacokinetic drug interactions of gefitinib with rifampicin, itraconazole and metoprolol. Clin Pharmacokinet. 2005;44:1067–81.
73. Albanell J, Rojo F, Averbuch S, et al. Pharmacodynamic studies of the epidermal growth factor receptor inhibitor ZD1839 in skin from cancer patients: histopathologic and molecular consequences of receptor inhibition. J Clin Oncol. 2002;20:110–24.
74. Rossi A, Maione P, Del Gaizo F, et al. Safety profile of gefitinib in advanced non-small cell lung cancer elderly patients with chronic renal failure: two clinical cases. Lung Cancer. 2005;47:421–3.

Chapter 6
Drug Interactions and Polypharmacy

Silvana Leo, Dario Cova, Antonio Rossi, and Lazzaro Repetto

Abstract Lung cancer is highly prevalent in senior adults. Older people are the greatest consumers of medications and healthcare resources in developed countries; this implies that patients are affected by different age-related conditions including one or more other serious chronic diseases, i.e., comorbidity, especially cardiovascular diseases, chronic obstruction pulmonary disease (COPD), or diabetes. Due to the presence of comorbidity, older adults are more likely to use an increased number of medications and at high risk for adverse drug events. Such condition is generally referred as "polypharmacy." Cancer-related therapy, adding new medications for both active cancer treatment and supportive therapy, further increases the risk of polypharmacy. Older oncologic patients with multiple comorbidities are at risk for adverse drug events associated with polypharmacy and drug–drug interactions due to patients' altered pharmacokinetic/pharmacodynamic status and the narrow therapeutic windows associated with antineoplastic agents. In clinical practice, it is difficult to separate the effects of cancer and its treatment or complications from the effects of comorbidity and polypharmacy. In response to this, geriatricians and oncologists have developed comprehensive geriatric assessment (CGA) tools for

S. Leo, MD
Onco-Geriatric Unit, Division of Medical Oncology,
Vito Fazzi Hospital, Lecce, Italy

D. Cova, MD
Emeritus Head of Oncogeriatrics, Department of Pharmacology,
School of Clinical Pharmacology, University of Milan, Milan, Italy

A. Rossi, MD
Division of Medical Oncology,
S.G. Moscati Hospital, Avellino, Italy

L. Repetto, MD, PhD (✉)
Department of Oncology, Sanremo Hospital – ASL 1 Imperiese,
Via G. Borea 56 – 18038, Sanremo (IM), Italy
e-mail: l.repetto@asl1.liguria.it

C. Gridelli, R.A. Audisio (eds.), *Management of Lung Cancer in Older People*,
DOI 10.1007/978-0-85729-793-8_6,

cancer patients. The CGA encompasses the evaluation of numerous clinical domains, including physical function, psycho-cognitive status, nutrition, social support, comorbidity, and in a minor percentage polypharmacy. CGA instruments are strongly recommended and predictive of mortality and morbidity for several chronic diseases and in different clinical settings. Cancer-specific CGA are currently being evaluated with the aim to individualize the treatment based on age-related conditions including comorbidity.

Keywords Drug interactions and polypharmacy in the elderly • Polypharmacy in the elderly • Lung cancer in the elderly • The elderly and drug interactions • Lung cancer and drug interactions in the elderly • Lung cancer comorbidities

Lung cancer is highly prevalent in senior adults. Older people are the greatest consumers of medications and healthcare resources in developed countries; this implies that patients are affected by different age-related conditions including one or more other serious chronic diseases, i.e., comorbidity, especially cardiovascular diseases, chronic obstruction pulmonary disease (COPD), or diabetes [1]. Due to the presence of comorbidity, older adults are more likely to use an increased number of medications and at high risk for adverse drug events. Such condition is generally referred as “polypharmacy.” Cancer-related therapy, adding new medications for both active cancer treatment and supportive therapy, further increases the risk of polypharmacy. Older oncologic patients with multiple comorbidities are at risk for adverse drug events associated with polypharmacy and drug–drug interactions due to patients’ altered pharmacokinetic/pharmacodynamic status and the narrow therapeutic windows associated with antineoplastic agents. In clinical practice, it is difficult to separate the effects of cancer and its treatment or complications from the effects of comorbidity and polypharmacy. In response to this, geriatricians and oncologists have developed comprehensive geriatric assessment (CGA) tools for cancer patients. The CGA encompasses the evaluation of numerous clinical domains, including physical function, psycho-cognitive status, nutrition, social support, comorbidity, and in a minor percentage polypharmacy. CGA instruments are strongly recommended [2] and predictive of mortality and morbidity for several chronic diseases and in different clinical settings [3, 4]. Cancer-specific CGA are currently being evaluated with the aim to individualized treatment based on age-related conditions including comorbidity (Table 6.1).

In the clinical practice, the large majority of lung cancer patients are elderly with comorbidity and polypharmacy which are not represented in clinical trials [5, 6]. Thus, evidence-based guidelines in this subset of patients are largely nonexistent. Studies reporting on polypharmacy in cancer patients are very few [7–9]. Conversely, the benefits and tolerance of commonly approved antineoplastic treatments are expected to be different in senior adults and particularly in those affected by polypharmacy. Thus, there is an extreme need to develop specific clinical tools to evaluate polypharmacy and assess the risk of drug interactions in the older cancer patients. This chapter addresses the issue of polypharmacy and potential drug–drug

Table 6.1 Components of the comprehensive geriatric assessment (CGA) relevant in the increased risk of drug interactions

CGA component	Test	Implications in cancer
Comorbid (coexisting) medical conditions	The Cumulative Illness Rating Scale (CIRS)	Increasing extent of comorbidity has been associated with parallel increases in cancer-specific and all-cause mortality in patients with breast cancer
Polypharmacy	Number of medications Appropriateness of medications Risk of drug interactions	Studies of older adults with cancer suggest an average of up to 9 medications per patient, with limited efforts to assess for drug–drug interactions with chemotherapy

interactions in older cancer patients and provides clinically relevant information of potential drug–drug interactions for the prescribing behavior of oncologists.

Comorbidity

The incidence of chronic disease and cancer increases with age, and the prevalence of comorbidities is especially high in elderly cancer patients [10, 11]. In a study of 7,600 cancer patients ≥55 years, those aged 55–64 had an average number of comorbid conditions of 2.9 compared with 4.2 comorbid conditions in patients ≥75 [12]. The most frequent chronic diseases are hypertension, heart failure, atrial fibrillation, coronary heart disease (CHD), stroke, COPD, thyroid dysfunction, dementia, diabetes, arthritis, and depression.

Comorbidity is frequently measured in terms of an index, scale, or total number of acute and/or chronic conditions. Comorbidity indexes are a way to substitute the number of comorbid conditions by a score that reflects the severity of the conditions and the prognosis impact on overall mortality. The ability of these scales to predict clinical outcomes in cancer patients is still under investigation [13].

A careful evaluation of comorbidity is strongly recommended in older cancer patients because the presence of comorbidities adds complexity to cancer management and it may influence life expectancy, prognosis, and treatment decisions and affect overall goals of care [14].

Comorbidity is increasingly recognized as a critical clinical issue in medical care, in part because it is an independent predictor of adverse outcomes, including quality of life (QoL), mortality, healthcare, disability, and complications of treatment beyond the effects of the individual conditions. Comorbidity impacts surgical decision making in oncology, such as the use of axillary clearance, radical prostatectomy, and resection for breast, prostate, and lung cancer, respectively. Similarly, comorbidity appears to affect the choice of chemotherapy in all types of cancer: colon, breast, and lung cancer [15–20]. Although this trend reflects studies suggesting greater chemotherapy-related toxicity among patients with comorbidity [21, 22], conflicting data does exist [23], and there is a need to further identify patients at higher risk of treatment-related toxicities in clinical trials and the ability to modify cancer treatment in patients with severe comorbidity.

Comorbidity and performance status (PS) >1 were important for survival and toxicity in an analysis of the National Cancer Institute of Canada Clinical Group Trials on over 1,200 NSCLC patients, elderly patients, whereas the age was prognostic only for toxicity but not for survival [22]. Conversely, in the Multicenter Italian Lung Cancer in the Elderly Study (MILES), comorbidity and activities of daily living (ADL) did not have a significant prognostic value for survival of elderly patients with advanced non-small cell cancer treated with chemotherapy [24]. In surgical series, Sawada et al. showed that elderly patients had worse PS and greater comorbidity than younger patients, but the same surgical procedure can be performed and similar outcomes can be expected for both perioperative mortality and long-term results as long as patients who are >75 years old have good PS and no or slight comorbidity [25].

Polypharmacy

Polypharmacy is the use of multiple drugs to manage disease states and is one of the most distinguishing factors differentiating care of older patients from the care of younger ones, as it is associated with the presence of comorbidity. A standard definition of "polypharmacy" does not exist. Polypharmacy has been defined in various ways; criteria such as taking more than three medications, taking unnecessary or redundant medications, or taking medications that confer a risk for adverse drug events (ADEs) have been proposed. Some researchers have simply defined it as the simultaneous use of multiple drugs [26]. The prevalence of polypharmacy in older adults ranges from 13 to 92 % with the wide range explained by the different definition of polypharmacy used in the studies [27], and it is reported that 39–50 % of patients over 65 years regularly take ≥5 drugs [28–30]. Elderly cancer patients have a substantial risk of polypharmacy, both because of increasing comorbidity with age and also because the complex treatment of cancer often includes multiple antineoplastic agents plus supportive care agents. A significant armamentarium of supportive care drugs is required to manage the physical sequelae of therapy-related toxicities (i.e., antiemetics, growth factors, antibiotics) and the emotional demands of recovery (i.e., antianxiety agents, antidepressants, antidiarrheals, sleep enhancers). In the advent of progressing or advanced cancer, yet another cadre of drugs is subsequently employed to manage distress and enhance comfort (analgesics, laxatives, appetite stimulants).

Only few studies evaluated the occurrence of polypharmacy in older cancer patients. The number of drugs was correlated with the average age of the patients, with the clinical setting in which patients were recruited, and if the patients were receiving or not receiving chemotherapy. In a study comparing age-related conditions in patients 65 years and older with and without cancer, we reported ≥3 comorbidities in 44 % of cancer patient and 89,6 % of noncancer patient. A total of 39,8 % of cancer patients assumed ≥2 drugs and 10,8 % ≥4 drugs, whereas 86,4 % of noncancer patients assumed ≥2 drugs and 54 % ≥4 [31].

The awareness of clinical oncologists on the potential risks associated with polypharmacy is unacceptably low. Sokol and Knudsen reported a series of older cancer patients, with mean age 78 years (range, 70–90 years) and with an average of three comorbid conditions; each patient received an average of nine medications. Cardiovascular drugs were the most common medications used to treat chronic conditions, while carboplatin and paclitaxel were the most frequently used chemotherapeutic agents. The authors observed, despite of the potential for drug–drug interactions, physicians made no adjustments to prescriptions [9]. Concomitant medications can directly interact with chemotherapy drugs, induce drug metabolism pathways, and change the pharmacodynamics of drugs, all of which can alter the effectiveness of the therapy. Riechelmann et al. analyzed prescription drug use by patients receiving chemotherapy and identified at least one potential drug interaction in 27 % of the patients [32].

Risk factors for polypharmacy include number and classes of drugs, multiple disease processes, disease severity, frailty, medication "hoarding," nondisclosure, and access to multiple healthcare providers. Polypharmacy is associated with adverse drug reactions, drug–drug interactions, nonadherence, and increased risk of hospitalization [29]. Comorbidity resulting in polypharmacy leads to an increased risk of interactions with antineoplastic drugs, resulting in an increased risk of toxicity and/or reduced effect of cancer treatment.

Although the polypharmacy has been associated with increases in healthcare cost, adverse drug events, and even mortality, there is no evidence of independent association between polypharmacy and an increased risk of mortality in cancer patients [27, 29].

An increasing number of medications are associated with an increased risk of drug-related complication, inappropriate medication use, and medication nonadherence. Older patients may fail to consume their medications as prescribed because of faulty memory, a lack of understanding about the treatments they are being given, and their importance or concerns about cost.

Nonadherence to the prescribed regimen may impact their treatment outcome; toxicity profiles may be altered (often heightened) as a result of altered pharmacodynamics. Drug interactions may be responsible for admission to the acute care setting and prolong the length of hospitalization. Additionally, overall treatment efficacy and ultimately patient survival may be compromised.

It has been reported that the risk of discrepancy between the prescribed and actually taken medications is associated with the number of outpatient medications, with hospitalization and mortality, and is more frequent in older patients [33, 34].

The prescribing physician and the number of prescribing physicians are the main risk factors for polypharmacy [35, 36]. There are little data on the use of "over-the-counter" (OTC) and "complementary and alternative medications" (CAM), even though their use is two times greater than prescription medication in older patients [37]. Many elderly use OTC drugs, which increases the risk of drug–drug interactions, especially as their prescribing doctor does not always know of this self-medication. In a study of 492 randomly selected 75-year-olds, 87 % used at least one prescribed drug and 72 % used OTC drugs. The average use was 4.2 prescribed drugs and 2.5 OTC drugs [38]. Elderly also use CAM. It seems that cancer patients may be more likely to take dietary supplements including herbal medicine than noncancer patients. In a large-scale American survey, 19 % of adults said they had used herbs in the previous 12 months [39]. One survey showed that more than 20 % of adults take prescription medications concomitantly with non-vitamin dietary supplements [40]. In one study, 218 patients ≥65 years with cancer were interviewed. Patients took an average of 4.4 medications, 3.2 were prescription drugs, while 1.2 were OTC drugs taken on a daily basis. Two-thirds of the OTC drugs were classified as vitamins or dietary supplements, 25 % were analgesics, and the remaining were laxatives, antacids, and others [41]. It has been reported that 26–63 % of older patients take at least one nonprescription medication including vitamin, mineral, herbal, complementary, or alternative medications and up to 50 % take two to four medications [42, 43]. These figures are likely to be higher in older individuals and in those with cancer. Patients prefer these "medications" because they are readily available, widely advertised, often cheaper, and presumed to be "safer" than prescription drugs. Often patients will not regard such products as "medication." Since nonprescription medications may increase the risk for drug interactions, they need to be accounted for when considering the total number of medication. The potential for ADEs rises dramatically when patients fail to disclose use of these products to their practitioners. Patients may not regard the product as "medicine," or they may not wish to share that they have sought alternative therapies to augment their medical regimens. Nondisclosure increases the potential for adverse effects because practitioners may attribute symptoms to disease rather than to the product(s). Further, the mechanism of action and the quality and purity of these products are often unknown. Although these agents are not classified as medications, they may have pharmacologic properties. For example, iron and calcium supplements may inhibit the absorption of quinolones and some antihypertensive agents. Mushroom powders, "popular" cancer treatments, are cleared hepatically and may increase toxicity of taxanes. Antioxidants may control free radical damage to cells; supplement overuse can lead to anorexia and decreased absorption. Patients should be asked specifically about OTC and CAM use, and all agents should be carefully reviewed to prevent drug–drug and drug–disease interactions.

At the moment, the definition of polypharmacy is shifting from the number of concomitant medications to more clinically relevant considerations, including the use of inappropriate medications and their associated risk of adverse effects.

The occurrence of polypharmacy in lung cancer patients is highlighted in the combined analysis [44] of three prospective trials, ELVIS (Elderly Lung Cancer

Vinorelbine Italian Study), MILES (both studies performed in patients aged ≥70 years), and GEMVIN3 (patients < 70 years old) [45–47] where a picture of the number and variety of supportive drugs assumed by patients with advanced NSCLC during chemotherapy is shown. The supportive drugs were divided into three categories: drugs against treatment side effects, against tumor symptoms, and against concomitant diseases (antidiabetics, cardiovascular system, drugs for benign prostatic hypertrophy, psycholeptics, psychoanaleptics, antivertigo preparations). Gastrointestinal drugs (45.7 %), corticosteroids (33.4 %), and analgesics (23.8 %) were the most frequently observed categories, in addition to vitamins, integrators, and mineral supplements. In order to avoid bias related to different chemotherapy, impact of age on supportive drugs was studied by comparing 184 adults (<70 years) vs. 219 elderly (≥70 years) patients treated with the same chemotherapy (gemcitabine plus vinorelbine in the MILES and GEMVIN3 studies). Overall, 306 out of 403 patients (76 %) received at least one supportive drug. The mean number of supportive drugs assumed by adult patients was 2.2 and that in the elderly patients 2.3 ($p = 0.75$). Polypharmacotherapy was frequent: patients assumed 2.43 drugs on average; 898 (75.8 %) assumed at least one supportive drug, 709 (59.8 %) two or more, and 538 (45.4 %) three or more. The number of drugs assumed was similar across different treatment arms. While there was no statistically significant difference between adults and the elderly for drugs against treatment side effects and drugs against symptoms, drugs for concomitant diseases were assumed by 7 % vs. 20 % ($p < 0.0001$) in adults and elderly patients, respectively. Among drugs for concomitant diseases, cardiovascular drugs were more frequently used in elderly than adults (16 % vs. 3 %).

An increased risk of drug-related complication is also due to the aging process. Moreover, older patients experience varying degrees of physiological changes that may affect the pharmacokinetic and pharmacodynamic properties of a drug, and clearance of many drugs is reduced in the elderly [30].

The age-related decline in hepatic and renal function also reduces their ability to metabolize and eliminate drugs and increases the potential for toxicity. These physiological declines coupled with comorbid conditions and the use of multiple drugs mean that medications eliminated by the renal route require dose adjustment [48]. Hepatic volume and blood flow and activity of the P450 microsomal enzyme pathway critical to metabolism of many drugs decrease with age. The most chemotherapy agents as other drugs are metabolized by the liver, and the polypharmacy increases competition for enzymatic activity and increases the risk for drug–drug interactions.

Drug Interactions

A drug interaction is defined as the pharmacological or clinical response to the administration or co-exposure of a drug with another substance that modifies the patient's response to the drug and can occur throughout the process of drug disposition

Table 6.2 Class of medication that interacts with chemotherapy

Drugs	Examples of interactions
Antacids	Antacids that contain aluminum and magnesium can increase the bioavailability of capecitabine
Antibiotics	Penicillin blocks the elimination of methotrexate (MTX) through renal tubular secretion, which results in elevated MTX levels
Anticoagulants	Altered coagulation has been reported in patients who have taken warfarin concurrently with capecitabine
Anticonvulsants	Carbamazepine has been reported to increase systemic clearance of teniposide
Antiemetics	Coadministration of ondansetron with cisplatin and cyclophosphamide can result in a decrease in systemic exposure to both cisplatin and cyclophosphamide
Antifungal agents	Ketoconazole inhibits the metabolism of irinotecan, which leads to an increase in exposure to SN-38 (the active metabolite of irinotecan)
Antiretroviral agents	Coadministration of delavirdine and saquinavir with paclitaxel has resulted in severe paclitaxel toxicity, which is possibly caused by CYP3A inhibition
Corticosteroids	Corticosteroids decrease the antitumor efficacy of aldesleukin
Herbal supplements	St. John's wort decreases the plasma concentration of imatinib and SN-38 (the active metabolite of irinotecan)
Nonsteroidal anti-inflammatory drugs (NSAIDs)	NSAIDs block the elimination of MTX through renal tubular secretion, which results in elevated MTX levels of cytochrome P450 subfamily 3A

as a result of endogenous and exogenous factors. In the past decades, the number of potential drug interactions with cytotoxic drugs has increased. In fact, in cancer treatment, a heterogeneous group of co-medications is used to treat underlying disease and manage adverse effects.

Older oncology patients with multiple comorbidities are at risk for adverse drug events associated with polypharmacy and drug–drug interactions due to patients' altered pharmacokinetic/pharmacodynamic status and the narrow therapeutic windows associated with antineoplastic agents. The number of medications, certain types of cancer, and the use of drug for comorbid conditions are all predictors of drug interactions, whereas functional status, gender, race, cognitive status, and literacy are predictors of inappropriate medication use in older population although not specifically investigated in older cancer patients.

The risk of drug interaction and related toxicity is correlated with the increased number of medications which is likely to increase with the number of comorbid conditions and advanced age. The estimated risk of experiencing a drug interaction is 50 % when a patient takes five medications and rises to nearly 100 % with seven medications [49–52]. Examples of drug interaction are shown in Table 6.2.

Table 6.3 Cytochrome P450 (CYP) substrates, inhibitors, and inducers

CYP	Substrates	Inhibitors	Inducers
CYP1A2	Caffeine	Ciprofloxacin	Cigarette smoke
	Propanolol	Fluoxetine	Phenobarbital
CYP2A6	Nicotine	Tranylcypromine	Barbiturates
	Coumarin	Methoxsalen	
CYO2C9	Ibuprofen	Miconazole	Ethanol
	Tolbutamide	Sulfamethoxazole	Carbamazepine
CYP2C19	Diazepam	Fluoxetine	Rifampin
	Omeprazole	Ritonavir	
CYP2D6	Codeine	Paroxetine	Pregnancy
	Haloperidol	Sertraline	
CYP2E1	Acetaminophen	Cimetidine	Ethanol
	Ethanol	Watercress	Isoniazid
CYP3A4/5	Bupropion	Grapefruit juice	Prednisone
	Lovastatin	Erythromycin	Phenytoin

The term "drug interaction" is most often used to describe drug–drug interactions, but there are various substances and/or factors that can alter the pharmacokinetics and/or pharmacodynamics of medications. These include food [53], nutritional supplements [54], formulation excipients, environmental factors (such as cigarette smoking), and herbal agents [55]. A potential interaction of herbal agents with prescribed drugs has been reported with the most common being between ginkgo and aspirin [56].

It is reported that 20–30 % of all adverse reactions to drugs are caused by interactions between drugs [57]. Drug interactions can be the result of pharmacokinetic, pharmacodynamic, or a combination of mechanisms. The majority of anticancer medicines used in the therapy of lung cancer patients are metabolized by cytochrome P450 (CYP450) enzymes [58]. The CYP450 system, a family of about 50 enzymes that metabolize many medications, is located primarily in the liver and to a lesser extent in the intestinal wall. Most medications are metabolized by six specific enzymes: CYP1A2, CYP2C9, CYP3A4, CYP2C19, CYP2D6, and CYP2E1. The first three enzymes have the most clinical significance. CYP3A4 metabolizes about 50 % of all medications. Genetic and interpersonal variations in the activity of enzyme systems account for some variability in rates of drug metabolism. Drug interactions involving the P450 isoforms generally are of two types: enzyme induction or enzyme inhibition. Any anticancer drug or other medicine which has been identified to be an inhibitor or inducer of CYP450 enzymes and used to treat cancer patients in combination with these drugs could lead to drug interaction (Table 6.3). Inhibitors block the activity of a particular CYP450 enzyme, while inducers increase CYP450 enzyme activity by increasing the amount of a CYP450 enzyme. As a consequence, a metabolic drug interaction occurs, thus altering the metabolism and elimination of one or both drugs [52, 59]. An inhibitory medication reduces the metabolism of another drug by a competitive mechanism: both drugs compete for the same pathway, and the clearance rate of one or both medications is slowed. Noncompetitive interactions occur when one medication irreversibly binds to or inactivates the metabolic enzyme, thus slowing

Table 6.4 Effect of food on the pharmacokinetics of orally administered anticancer agents

Anticancer agents	Effect of food	Pharmacokinetic parameters affected
Busulfan, fluorouracil, methotrexate, and topotecan	Delayed absorption (effect on rate)	Change in T_{max} and C_{max}
Altretamine, capecitabine, chlorambucil, estramustine, gefitinib, melphalan, and thioguanine	Decreased absorption (effect on extent)	Change in AUC and C_{max}
Erlotinib and tretinoin	Increased absorption (effect on extent and/ or rate)	Increase in AUC and usually C_{max} and/or T_{max}
Etoposide, imatinib, mercaptopurine, and temozolomide	Unaffected absorption (no effect on rate or extent)	No significant change in AUC and C_{max} [a]

AUC area under the concentration-time curve, C_{max} change in maximum plasma drug concentration, T_{max} time to reach C_{max}

[a]Concluded when 90 % confidence interval for the ratio of population geometric means between fed and fasted treatments, based on log-transformed data, fall within the equivalence limits of 80–125 % for AUC and C_{max}

clearance of other medications. These inhibitory enzymes can lead to excessively high concentrations of the second medication, leading to toxicity. Inhibitory interactions usually manifest fairly quickly, but the maximal effect of the interaction may not be seen until a new steady state has been reached. In a pharmacokinetic interaction, one medication alters the absorption, distribution, metabolism, or excretion of another medication. Even though many newer antineoplastic agents are administered orally, clinically significant drug interaction involving changes in absorption is infrequent. The majority of clinically significant interactions with these agents involve hepatic metabolism by the CYP450 system [49, 52]. Oral delivery necessitates careful consideration of the various factors that influence drug absorption because interactions with other orally administered substances such as food can lead to altered bioavailability. The net effect of food on the pharmacokinetics of an orally administered medication depends on the chemical properties of the drug and its formulation, gastrointestinal physiology, and the type and quantity of food [60]. Food delays gastric emptying, raises intestinal pH, increases hepatic blood flow, and slows gastrointestinal transit, so it can significantly affect the pharmacokinetic profile of some orally administered medications. Food–drug interactions can have four pharmacokinetic effects on the bioavailability of the orally administered anticancer agent: delayed, decreased, increased, or unaffected absorption [53]. Therefore, food–drug interactions are optimally managed by scheduling the oral administration of anticancer agents with reference to meal timing—before, during, or after a meal—to improve chemotherapy outcomes. The effects of food on the pharmacokinetics of other orally administered anticancer agents are summarized in Table 6.4, and more detailed information is available in a comprehensive review by Singh and Malhotra [53]. In addition to CYP enzymes, various other metabolic enzymes (e.g., glucuronosyltransferases) and transporters (e.g., P-glycoprotein [P-gp], organic anion transporting peptide [OATP], and multidrug resistance protein [MRP]) also play important roles in drug interactions and changes in systemic exposure [61].

Various additive pharmacodynamic interactions have been described. Increased renal toxicity has been observed when cisplatin is given with other nephrotoxic agents such as aminoglycosides [62]. Vinorelbine has been associated with new or worsening neuropathy in patients with previous or current exposure to paclitaxel although the underlying paclitaxel treatment might cause latent neuronal damage, which only becomes clinically apparent following vinorelbine administration [63]. Another type of drug interaction is a pharmacodynamic interaction sequence dependent that is observed when paclitaxel is infused before carboplatin and that results in decreased thrombocytopenia compared with carboplatin alone [64].

Thus, polypharmacy and its inherent complications are particularly prevalent in the elderly cancer population, and such individuals are at high risk of ADEs. Riechelmann et al. reported that 63 % of older cancer patient were at risk for adverse drug interaction with the majority receiving ≥8 drugs [51]. It was found that the mean number of ADEs increased approximately linearly with the number of drugs taken [26].

Toxic effects of medications and drug-related problems can have profound medical and safety consequences for older adults and economically affect the healthcare system. ADEs have been linked to preventable problems in elderly patients such as depression, constipation, falls, immobility, confusion, and hip fractures. Drug-related problems or drug toxic effects are responsible for 10 % and 20 % of all hospital admission over the age of 65 and 80 years, respectively [9, 65].

Toxic effects of polypharmacy can have profound medical and safety consequences for older adults. Published tools to assist in geriatric prescribing include the Beers criteria, the Medication appropriateness index (MAI), the Screening Tool of Older Persons' Potentially Inappropriate Prescriptions (STOPP), and the Screening Tool to Alert Doctors to the Right Treatment (START).

Beers criteria (based on two items) and the MAI (based on ten items) are the most frequently used instruments to evaluate potentially inappropriate prescriptions. This provides an important starting point to improve prescribing by limiting the use of medicines that pose a high risk of adverse effects in older people (Table 6.5). Despite some limits including the need of periodical update and poor consideration of specific aspect of polypharmacy and potential benefit in individual patients, Beers criteria are the most extensively evaluated in clinical studies [66].

Table 6.5 Medication appropriateness index and Beers criteria

Description	Measures
Medication appropriateness index is determined based on series of ten items, ranked on scale of 1–3	Ten items: indication, effectiveness, dosage, directions, drug–drug interaction, drug–disease interaction, duplication, duration, comparative cost
Beers criteria based on two components and their level of severity (low/high)	Two components: inappropriate drug class because of risk of toxicity, inappropriate because of potential drug–disease interaction

The Beers criteria consist of a list of "inappropriate" drugs for use in older patients because of either ineffectiveness or unnecessary high risk (where a safer alternative exists) and potential interaction of the drug with a concomitant disease or condition. Intervention studies showed that the use of review of medication usage significantly reduced adverse drug reactions in outpatients. The Beers criteria are the most commonly and internationally used criteria; they list 48 inappropriate medications for use in older adults and categorize them as always inappropriate, potentially inappropriate, or potentially inappropriate in certain circumstances. The criteria also include 20 diseases and conditions and medications to be avoided in older adults with these conditions. The Beers criteria have a number of limitations. Many of the Beers criteria drugs are not absolutely contraindicated, and the criteria do not consider polypharmacy, drug interactions, or underuse. Drugs are rated as associated with a high to low severity of adverse events [67, 68].

The MAI measures elements of appropriate prescribing as determined according to ten questions and assigns a numerical score to each drug. It does not list inappropriate medications but ranks a selected drug as indicated or not indicated [69].

Perhaps the most comprehensive criteria are the STOPP [70] and START [71]. A European consensus group defined the STOPP criteria, which list 65 potentially inappropriate prescribing practices in older adults categorized according to organ system. They include drug–drug and drug–disease interactions, drugs that affect older patients at risk for falls, and therapeutic duplication. The START criteria address underprescribing and list 22 evidence-based prescribing indications for older adults and categorize medications according to organ system.

Two studies adopted the Beers criteria to assess the risk of polypharmacy and drug interactions [7, 8]. Pharmacist-based interventions to review drug prescriptions evidenced polypharmacy in 21 and 11 % of the patients and a reduction in the number of the prescribed drugs in 53 and 50 % of the patients.

Prevention of drug interactions with anticancer drugs is of particular concern because of the narrow therapeutic indexes of anticancer agents and the potential for lethal side effects.

To prevent possible reactions, databases have been carried out to include agents interacting with CYP450 and to identify possible interactions with drugs used.

They were categorized as either (1) *clinically important interaction*, for which there is in vitro metabolic evidence and/or in vivo pharmacokinetic and clinical evidence that a drug–drug interaction occurs or could occur; (2) *potentially clinically important interaction*, for which there is a theoretical basis for an interaction, but for which experimental evidence is lacking; or (3) *unlikely interaction* for which there is either evidence against or no theoretical basis for an interaction [72].

The majority of anticancer medicines used in the therapy of lung cancer patients are metabolized by CYP450 enzymes. In the study of Song et al. [58], drugs which may cause drug interaction by affecting the CYP450 enzymes were frequently prescribed during the anticancer treatment of lung cancer patients. In fact to assess the potential burden of drug interaction in patients receiving treatment for lung cancer, this study examined utilization of agents interacting with CYP450 enzymes in lung cancer patients on anticancer therapy using the US MarketScan research database.

Table 6.6 Categories of clinical effects of drug interactions

Severity level and examples of clinical effects per category
A: Clinically irrelevant effect
Increase or decrease in drug level without consequences: tyrosine kinase inhibitors, sirolimus (active metabolite of temsirolimus), endoxifen (active metabolite of tamoxifen)
B: Temporary discomfort (<24–28 h)
Adjustment of coumarin dosage necessary by cytostatic anticancer agents
C: Longer-lasting discomfort (48–168 h)
Increase of phenytoin plasma concentration by certain anticancer agents
D: Long-lasting (>168 h) or permanent adverse effect
Decrease of plasma concentration/failure of carbamazepine, phenytoin, valproic acid by certain anticancer agents
E: Severe adverse effect
Increased risk of failure of life-saving therapy: decrease of cyclosporine by cyclophosphamide, failure of cladribine by lamivudine
Neuromuscular toxicity vinblastine/vincristine by itraconazole
Hepatic veno-occlusive disease by busulfan (by itraconazole–ketoconazole)
F: Multiorgan failure (busulfan and metronidazole)
Death (by combination of methotrexate and trimethoprim or co-trimoxazole)

These databases provide access to medical and prescription drug claims for privately insured individuals including patients over the age of 65 with Medicare supplemental coverage. Combination therapy with strong CYP450 enzyme inhibitors or inducers also occurred within approximately 28 and 4 % of anticancer treatment episodes, respectively.

A Dutch expert group [73] of hospital and community pharmacists, medical oncologists, internists, and clinical pharmacologists has systematically assessed the clinical significance of interactions among anticancer agents and co-medications and provided recommendations for management of clinically significant interactions. Accordingly, the expert group selected 38 interactions with different clinically relevance with anticancer agents and made recommendations for the management of these interactions (Table 6.6).

In the Netherlands, the results are adopted into the "G-Standaard," the electronic medication surveillance system of KNMP (Koninklijke Nederlandse Maatschappij Pharmacie) by doctors and pharmacists, in the hospital, the polyclinic, and the community. The G-Standaard is used for interaction surveillance before dispensing so that clinically relevant interactions can be identified and prevented from occurrence.

Medi-Span, a part of Wolters Kluwer Health, is the leading provider of prescription drug information and drug interaction database solutions for thousands of healthcare professionals worldwide. With more than 30 years experience, Medi-Span continues to offer authoritative adverse drug reactions information and drug contraindications data in a variety of formats, including clinical decision support and disease suite modules [74].

When initiating chemotherapy, individual response to toxicity and risk for ADEs should be monitored continuously. Each additional medication, including supportive therapies and growth factors, should be weighed carefully for benefit vs. risk of

ADEs in the context of the existing regimen. Regular review of all medication for redundancy and interactions and simplification is critical in the onco-geriatric clinical practice. Many drugs show clinically significant drug interactions, which represent a therapeutic challenge for the researcher, clinician, and patient. Clinicians should include an assessment of the use of herbal therapies, CAM, and OTC when taking medication histories given the high prevalence of use and potential hazards that can result from concomitant administration with anticancer agents. This is especially important because many patients do not consider it necessary to tell their doctor about their use of other products. This phenomenon is difficult to measure in practice and clinical trials.

Conclusion

Polypharmacy is an important issue in the elderly. Given that polypharmacy and the chronic use of multiple drugs are a reality for older patients with cancer and comorbidity, outcome data need to be generated and motivations/incentives be provided for physicians to optimize safe and effective supportive oncologic therapeutic. Patients with metastatic cancer continue to take drugs for prevention of comorbidities which are associated with side effects and inconvenience. The benefits of these drugs are likely to be minimal, and medication reviews should be undertaken to address their appropriateness [75]. Comorbidity seems the most obvious explanation of the high number of drugs taken by older people, but additional factors deserve consideration. Boost sales of the pharmaceutical industry advertising on mass media Internet, prescriptions by specialists, prescriptions by organ/disease specialists with early access to compassionate use. Self-prescription of drugs is sometimes favored by “receiving mail.” Moreover, both over-prescribing and improper prescribing have been reported and seem to contribute to the age-related increase in the prevalence of adverse drug reactions. The prevention and recognition of drug-related problems in elderly patients and other vulnerable populations is one of the major healthcare quality and safety issues for this decade. There are many ways to define medication-related problems in elderly patients, including the use of lists containing specific drugs to avoid in the elderly and appropriateness indexes applied by pharmacists or clinicians [76]. Due to the lack of standardize definition of polypharmacy and instrument to evaluate potential drug interaction, we recommend the routine careful review of the patient’s list of medications including the over-the-counter, herbal and complementary compounds, with indications and dosages. The potential risk of drug interactions need also to be assessed and the number of drugs reduced whenever is possible.

Patients with cancer could be receiving different cytotoxic agents as part of their cancer treatment medication to prevent side effects and medication for comorbid conditions (such as cardiovascular disease, gastrointestinal disorders, diabetes, respiratory illnesses). As cytotoxic drugs generally have a narrow therapeutic index, even a slight increase or decrease in cytotoxic activity caused by a drug interaction could result in excessive toxicity or reduced efficacy. Through increased awareness of the potential for drug interactions, physicians can minimize these risks by prescribing appropriate medications and by monitoring for signs of an interaction.

In the daily practice, it is recommended to routinely assess for each patient the prescribed medications' list as reported by the patient and the nonprescribed complimentary medications including eye/ear drops, herbal and homeopathic agents, vitamins, and nutritional compounds. Potential drug interactions can be identified using available web-based thesaurus allowing classification of drug interactions according to the level of severity. Training/education program for medical oncologists and the development of monitoring systems of drug treatments and their interactions/complications are recommended. The use of customs uniform, prospective and all-encompassing, possibly magnetic card, with all the patient's medical records should be exploited.

References

1. Janssen-Heijnen MLG, Maas HA, Houterman S, et al. Comorbidity in older surgical cancer patients: influence on patient care and outcome. Eur J Cancer. 2007;43:2179–93.
2. Extermann M, Chen H, Cantor AB, et al. Predictors of tolerance to chemotherapy in older cancer patients: a prospective pilot study. Eur J Cancer. 2002;38:1466–73.
3. Repetto L, Fratino L, Audisio RA, et al. Comprehensive geriatric assessment adds information to Eastern Cooperative Oncology Group performance status in elderly cancer patients: an Italian Group for Geriatric Oncology Study. J Clin Oncol. 2002;20:494–502.
4. Extermann M, Aapro M, Bernabei R, Task force on CGA of the International Society of Geriatric Oncology, et al. Use of the comprehensive geriatric assessment in older cancer patients: recommendations from the task force on CGA of the International Society of Geriatric Oncology (SIOG). Crit Rev Oncol Hematol. 2005;55:241–52.
5. Levy B, Kosteas J, Slade M, et al. Exclusion of elderly persons from health-risk behavior clinical trials. Prev Med. 2006;43:80–5.
6. Van Spall HG, Toren A, Kiss A, et al. Eligibility criteria of randomized controlled trials published in high-impact general medical journals: a systematic sampling review. JAMA. 2007;297:1233–40.
7. Flood KL, Carroll MB, Le CV, et al. Polypharmacy in hospitalized older adult cancer patients experience from a prospective, observational study of an oncology-acute care for elders unit. Am J Geriatr Pharmacother. 2009;7:151–8.
8. Lichtman SM, Boparai MK. Geriatric medication management: evaluation of pharmacist interventions and potentially inappropriate medication (PIM) use in older (≥65 years) cancer patients. J Clin Oncol. 2009;27(15S):484s (Abstr. 9507).
9. Sokol KC, Knudsen JF, Li MM. Polypharmacy in older oncology patients and the need for an interdisciplinary approach to side-effect management. J Clin Pharm Ther. 2007;32:169–75.
10. Jemal A, Bray F, Center MM, et al. Global cancer statistics. CA Cancer J Clin. 2011;61: 69–90.
11. Marengoni A, Rizzuto D, Wang H, et al. Patterns of chronic multimorbidity in the elderly population. J Am Geriatr Soc. 2009;57:225–30.
12. Yancik R. Cancer burden in the aged: an epidemiologic and demographic overview. Cancer. 1997;80:1273–83.
13. Extermann M. Measuring comorbidity in older cancer patients. Eur J Cancer. 2000;36: 453–71.

14. Piccirillo JF, Tierney RM, Costas I, et al. Prognostic importance of comorbidity in a hospital based cancer registry. JAMA. 2004;291:2441–7.
15. Meyerhardt JA, Catalano PJ, Haller DG, et al. Impact of diabetes mellitus on outcomes in patients with colon cancer. J Clin Oncol. 2003;21:433–40.
16. Hughes KS, Schnaper LA, Berry D, et al. Lumpectomy plus tamoxifen with or without irradiation in women 70 years of age or older with early breast cancer. N Engl J Med. 2004;351: 971–7.
17. Konety BR, Cowan JE, Carroll PR. Patterns of primary and secondary therapy for prostate cancer in elderly men: analysis of data from CaPSURE. J Urol. 2008;179:1797–803.
18. Yancik R, Wesley MN, Ries LAG, et al. Effect of age and comorbidity in postmenopausal breast cancer patients aged 55 years and older. JAMA. 2001;285:885–92.
19. Keating NL, Landrum MB, Klabunde CN, et al. Adjuvant chemotherapy for stage III colon cancer: Do physicians agree about the importance of patient age and comorbidity? J Clin Oncol. 2008;26:2532–7.
20. Blanco JAG, Toste IS, Alvarez RF, et al. Age, comorbidity, treatment decision and prognosis in lung cancer. Age Ageing. 2008;37:715–8.
21. Aparicio T, Desrame J, Lecomte T, et al. Oxaliplatin- or irinotecan-based chemotherapy for metastatic colorectal cancer in the elderly. Br J Cancer. 2003;89(8):1439–44.
22. Asmis TR, Ding K, Seymour L, et al. Age and comorbidity as independent prognostic factors in the treatment of non-small-cell lung cancer: a review of National Cancer Institute of Canada Clinical Trials Group trials. J Clin Oncol. 2008;26:54–9.
23. Moscetti L, Nelli F, Padalino D, et al. Gemcitabine and cisplatin in the treatment of elderly patients with advanced non-small cell lung cancer: impact of comorbidities on safety and efficacy outcome. J Chemother. 2005;17:685–92.
24. Maione P, Perrone F, Gallo C, et al. Pretreatment quality of life and functional status assessment predict survival of elderly patients with advanced non small cell lung cancer receiving chemotherapy: a prognostic analysis of the multicenter Italian lung cancer in the elderly study. J Clin Oncol. 2005;28:6865–72.
25. Sawada S, Komori E, Nogami N, et al. Advanced age is not correlated with either short-term or long-term postoperative results in lung cancer patients in good clinical condition. Chest. 2005;128:1557–63.
26. Viktil KK, Blix HS, Moger TA, et al. Polypharmacy as commonly defined is an indicator of limited value in the assessment of drug-related problems. Br J Clin Pharmacol. 2007;63: 187–95.
27. Maggiore RJ, Gross GP, Hurria A. Polypharmacy in older adults with cancer. Oncologist. 2010;15:507–22.
28. Jørgensen T, Johansson S, Kennerfalk A, et al. Prescription drug use, diagnoses, and healthcare utilization among the elderly. Ann Pharmacother. 2001;35:1004–9.
29. Onder G, Landi F, Liperoti R, et al. Impact of inappropriate drug use among hospitalized older adults. Eur J Clin Pharmacol. 2005;61:453–9.
30. Lichtman S. Pharmacokinetics and pharmacodynamics in the elderly. Clin Adv Hematol Oncol. 2007;5:181–2.
31. Repetto L, Venturino A, Vercelli V, et al. Performance status and comorbidity in elderly cancer patients compared to a young neoplastic and an elderly non-neoplastic population. Cancer. 1998;82:760–5.
32. Riechelmann RP, Tannock IF, Wang L, et al. Potential drug interactions and duplicate prescriptions among cancer patients. J Natl Cancer Inst. 2007;99:592–600.
33. Hustey FM, Wallis N, Miller J. Inappropriate prescribing in an older ED population. Am J Emerg Med. 2007;25:804–7.
34. Hughes CM. Medication non-adherence in the elderly: how big is the problem? Drugs Aging. 2004;21:793–811.
35. Green JL, Hawley JN, Rask KJ. Is the number of prescribing physicians an independent risk factor for adverse drug events in an elderly outpatient population? Am J Geriatr Pharmacother. 2007;5:31–9.

36. Tamblyn RM, McLeod PJ, Abrahamowicz M, et al. Do too many cooks spoil the broth? Multiple physician involvement n medical management of elderly patients and potentially inappropriate drug combinations. CMAJ. 1996;154:1177–84.
37. Colt HG, Shapiro AP. Drug-induced illness as a cause for admission to a community hospital. J Am Geriatr Soc. 1989;37:323–6.
38. Barat I, Andreasen F, Damsgaard EM. The consumption of drugs by 75-year-old individuals living in their own homes. Eur J Clin Pharmacol. 2000;56:501–9.
39. Kennedy J. Herb and supplement use in the US adult population. Clin Ther. 2005;27: 1847–58.
40. Gardiner P, Graham RE, Legedza ATR, et al. Factors associated with dietary supplement use among prescription medication users. Arch Intern Med. 2006;166:1968–74.
41. Corcoran ME. Polypharmacy in the older patient with cancer. Cancer Control. 1997;4: 419–28.
42. Slone Epidemiology Center. Patterns of medication use in the United States: of medication use in the United States: Slone Epidemiology Center at Boston University. 2006. Available http://www.bu.edu/slone/SloneSurvey/sloneSurvey.htm. Accessed Sept 20 2009.
43. Qato DM, Alexander GC, Conti RM, et al. Use of prescription and over-the counter medications and dietary supplements among older adults in the United States. JAMA. 2008;300:2867–78.
44. Di Maio M, Perrone F, Gallo C, et al. Supportive care in patients with advanced non-small-cell lung cancer. Br J Cancer. 2003;89:1013–21.
45. Gridelli C. The ELVIS trial: a phase III study of single-agent vinorelbine as first-line treatment in elderly patients with advanced NSCLC. Oncologist. 2001;6:4–7.
46. Gridelli C, Perrone F, Gallo C, et al. Chemotherapy for elderly patients with advanced non-small cell lung cancer: Multicenter Italian Lung cancer in the Elderly Study (MILES) phase III randomized trial. J Natl Cancer Inst. 2003;95:362–72.
47. Gridelli C, Gallo C, Shepherd FA, et al. Gemcitabine plus vinorelbine compared with cisplatin plus vinorelbine or cisplatin plus gemcitabine for advanced non–small-cell lung cancer: a phase III trial of the Italian GEMVIN Investigators and the National Cancer Institute of Canada Clinical Trials Group. J Clin Oncol. 2003;21:3025–34.
48. Lichtman SM, Wildiers H, Chatelut E, et al. International Society of Geriatric Oncology (SIOG) Chemotherapy Taskforce: evaluation of chemotherapy in older patients-an analysis of the medical literature. J Clin Oncol. 2007;25:1832–43.
49. Jørgensen TL, Hallas J, Land LH, et al. Comorbidity and polypharmacy in elderly cancer patients: the significance on treatment outcome and tolerance. J Geriatr Oncol. 2010;1: 87–102.
50. Girre V, Arkoub H, Puts MTE. Potential drug interactions in elderly cancer patients. Crit Rev Oncol Hematol. 2011;78:220–6.
51. Riechelmann RP, Moreira F, Smaletz O, et al. Potential for drug interactions in hospitalized cancer patients. Cancer Chemother Pharmacol. 2005;56:286–90.
52. Blower P, de Wit R, Goodin S, et al. Drug-drug interactions in oncology: why are they important and can they be minimized? Crit Rev Oncol Hematol. 2005;55:117–42.
53. Singh BN, Malhotra BK. Effects of food on the clinical pharmacokinetics of anticancer agents: underlying mechanisms and implications for oral chemotherapy. Clin Pharmacokinet. 2004;43:1127–56.
54. Sparreboom A, Cox MC, Acharya MR, et al. Herbal remedies in the United States: potential adverse interactions with anticancer agents. J Clin Oncol. 2004;22:2489–503.
55. Damery S, Gratus C, Grivie R, et al. The use of herbal medicines by people with cancer: a cross-sectional survey. Br J Cancer. 2011;104:927–33.
56. Dergal JM, Gold JL, Laxer DA, et al. Potential interactions between herbal medicines and conventional drug therapies used by older adults attending a memory clinic. Drugs Aging. 2002;19:879–86.
57. Kuhlmann J, Muck W. Clinical-pharmacological strategies to assess drug interaction potential during drug development. Drug Saf. 2001;24:715–25.

58. Song X, Varkera H, Eichelbaumb M, et al. Treatment of lung cancer patients and concomitant use of drugs interacting with cytochrome P450 isoenzymes. Lung Cancer. 2011;74:103–11.
59. Lynch T, Price A. The effect of cytochrome P450 metabolism on drug response, interactions, and adverse effects. Am Fam Physician. 2007;76:348–51.
60. Goodin S. Oral chemotherapeutic agents: understanding mechanisms of action and drug interactions. Am J Health Syst Pharm. 2007;64:S15–24.
61. Dresser GK, Bailey DG, Leake BF, et al. Fruit juices inhibit organic anion transporting polypeptide-mediated uptake to decrease the oral availability of fexofenadine. Clin Pharmacol Ther. 2002;71:11–20.
62. Christensen ML, Stewart CF, Crom WR. Evaluation of aminoglycoside disposition in patients previously treated with cisplatin. Ther Drug Monit. 1989;11:631–6.
63. Parimoo D, Jeffers S, Muggia FM. Severe neurotoxicity from vinorelbine-paclitaxel combinations. J Natl Cancer Inst. 1986;88:1079–80.
64. Huizing MT, Giaccone G, van Warmerdan LJ, et al. Pharmacokinetics of paclitaxel and carboplatin in a dose-escalating and dose-sequencing study in patients with non-small-cell lung cancer. The European Cancer Centre. J Clin Oncol. 1997;15:317–29.
65. Legrain S. Prescription to elderly patients: reducing underuse and adverse drug reactions and improving adherence. Bull Acad Natl Med. 2007;191:259–69.
66. Beers MH, Ouslander JG, Rollingher I, et al. Explicit criteria for determining inappropriate medication use in nursing home residents: UCLA Division of Geriatric Medicine. Arch Intern Med. 1991;151:1825–32.
67. Fick DM, Cooper JW, Wade WE, et al. Updating the Beers criteria for potentially inappropriate medication use in older adults: results of a US consensus panel expert. Arch Intern Med. 2003;163:2716–24.
68. Vinks TH, Egberts TC, de Lange TM, et al. Pharmacist-based medication review reduces potential drug-related problems in the elderly: the SMOG controlled trial. Drugs Aging. 2009;26:123–33.
69. Hanlon JT, Schmader KE, Samsa GP, et al. A method for assessing drug therapy appropriateness. J Clin Epidemiol. 1992;45:1045–51.
70. Gallagher P, O'Mahony D. STOPP (Screening Tool of Older Person's Potentially Inappropriate Prescriptions): application to acutely ill elderly patients and comparison with Beers' criteria. Age Ageing. 2008;37:673–9.
71. Barry PJ, Gallagher P, Ryan C, et al. START (screening tool to alert doctors to the right treatment)an evidence-based screening tool to detect prescribing omissions in elderly patients. Age Ageing. 2007;36:632–8.
72. Davies SJC, Eayrs S, Pratt P, et al. Potential for drug interactions involving cytochromes P450 2D6 and 3A4 on general adult psychiatric and functional elderly psychiatric wards. Br J Clin Pharmacol. 2004;57:464–72.
73. Jansman F, Reyners AKL, van Roon EN, et al. Consensus-based evaluation of clinical significance and management of anticancer drug interactions. Clin Ther. 2011;33(3):305–14.
74. Medi-Span®. Indianapolis(IN): Medi-Span®. Master drug data base v2.5 (MDDB®). Available from: http://www.medispan.com/master-drug-database.aspx. Cited 29 Sep 2008.
75. Cashman J, Wright J, Ring A. The treatment of comorbidities in older patients with metastatic cancer. Support Care Cancer. 2010;18:651–5.
76. Hanlon JT, Landsman PB, Cowan K, et al. Physician agreement with pharmacist suggested drug therapy changes for elderly out patients. Am J Health Syst Pharm. 1996;53:2735–7.

Part III
Diagnostics

Chapter 7
Selection of Appropriate Surgery for Early Lung Cancer

Michael T. Jaklitsch and Weston Sacco

Abstract There are almost twice as many cases of lung cancer today as there were in 1980. There were an estimated 161,670 deaths related to lung cancer in the USA in 2010, which is more than any other cancer. Lung cancer is most commonly found in the elderly, with the 60–79-year-old range being the most prevalent. Eighty to eighty-five percent of primary lung tumors are non-small cell lung cancer (NSCLC) and, if caught in the early stages, can be treated surgically. The disease is more likely to be surgically resectable in the older patient population. Correspondingly, the percent of cancer in stage I also increases with age. There has also been a move toward minimally invasive surgery, new instruments and optics, and the use of VATS; the surgical field is ever evolving and the intricacies of each procedure are ever expanding. These advances have significantly improved surgical outcomes and recovery. In fact, VATS has dramatically reduced postop death in the elderly with stage I lung cancer.

Keywords Early lung cancer in the elderly • Lung cancer in the elderly • Elderly and lung cancer • Non-small cell lung cancer in the elderly • Lobectomy in the elderly • Limited resection of lung in the elderly

Case Study

Mr. Smith is an 82-year-old man diagnosed with non-small cell lung cancer. Noteworthy points in his history include a 35-pack-year smoking history and having had an MI 15 years ago. He quit smoking 7 years ago and walks the two blocks

M.T. Jaklitsch, MD (✉)
Department of Surgery, Harvard Medical School,
Boston, MA, USA
e-mail: mtjaklitsch@partners.org

W. Sacco, BS
Tulane University School of Medicine, New Orleans, LA, USA

C. Gridelli, R.A. Audisio (eds.), *Management of Lung Cancer in Older People*,
DOI 10.1007/978-0-85729-793-8_7, © Springer-Verlag London 2013

between his home and the park once a day. Mr. Smith is a retired middle school history teacher. He wife passed away 5 years ago leaving him as the primary caretaker of his daughter, age 50, who is severely mentally and physically handicapped. His insurance and finances are such that he has a visiting nurse who comes once a week to help care for his daughter. He is estranged from his other son, age 53.

Upon physical examination, Mr. Smith's BMI is 24 and FEV1 is 1.7 liters. He is able to walk up two flights of stairs without assistance. After further cardiac and pulmonary evaluation, surgery is deemed a viable treatment option. However, Mr. Smith is concerned about the care of his daughter. He asks for help weighing his life expectancy without the surgery versus the recovery time and degree to which he is expected to recovery functionally after the surgery.

In addition to deciding whether to have surgery or not, a complete staging of his cancer was done through a series of chest CTs, MRIs, and brain scans. It was determined that the tumor was stage I and approximately 2 cm in diameter. The surgeon now must weigh the patient's risk factors, the attributes of the tumor, and his own experience to determine whether to perform a limited resection or a lobectomy.

Introduction

There are almost twice as many cases of lung cancer today as there were in 1980. There were an estimated 161,670 deaths related to lung cancer in the USA in 2010, which is more than any other cancer. Lung cancer is most commonly found in the elderly, with the 60–79-year-old range being the most prevalent [1–3]. Eighty to eighty-five percent of primary lung tumors are non-small cell lung cancer (NSCLC) and, if caught in the early stages, can be treated surgically. And the older the patient, the higher the likelihood that the disease is surgically resectable [4]. Correspondingly, the percent of cancer in stage I also increases with age [5].

There has also been a move toward minimally invasive surgery, new instruments and optics, and the use of VATS; the surgical field is ever evolving and the intricacies of each procedure are ever expanding [6]. These advances have significantly improved surgical outcomes and recovery. In fact, VATS has dramatically reduced postop death in the elderly with stage I lung cancer [7–11].

Deciding the best treatment course for one's patient is hardly ever a cut and dry decision.

This decision gets even more complicated in the ever-evolving field of thoracic surgical oncology where any sort of "standard" treatment for NSCLC does not yet guarantee a complication and disease-free outcome. So, as is the case in any field with any disease, a physician treating NSCLC must continually evaluate the treatment options available with the most current data.

There are multiple surgical options available for the treatment of lung cancer including pneumonectomy, lobectomy, segmentectomy, wedge sampling, radiofrequency ablation, and cryotherapy ablation. The use of these options varies with functional age such that it may be decided that a patient with preserved function have an anatomic resection whereas a seriously impaired patient may have local ablation. In this chapter, we will limit our discussion to the surgical treatment of

NSLC in the elderly, more specifically, the choice to perform surgery or not and then the choice of performing between a limited resection and a lobectomy.

In order to make such a decision, three items must be evaluated. The first of these is the patient's risk factors. This category includes any factors which may predispose the patient to adverse surgical complications such as advanced age, pulmonary and cardiac health, BMI, previous surgeries, and the stage of the cancer. The second item to be considered is the patient and the patient's family's expectations for the surgery. This includes working with the patient and his family to determine how best to strike a balance between longevity and the patient's own definition of a satisfactory quality of life. The third item involves considering the previous two items as well as the trends corresponding to the available treatment options in order to choose the treatment option most likely to achieve the patient's goals.

It is this third item that is perhaps the most difficult task on the part of the physician. Unfortunately, in the surgical treatment of NSCLC in the elderly, there is no single universally agreed upon procedure. Both limited resection and lobectomies are currently in use. It is the goal of this chapter to assist the reader in addressing each of the three aforementioned items through an analysis of present trends in the evaluation and surgical treatment of NSCLC in the elderly.

Evaluating a Patient's Risk Factors

Lung surgery causes a great physiological insult as well as removes lung tissue, thus potentially decreasing lung function. So it is crucial to take note of any factors which may prohibit or caution a surgeon to proceed with the operation. This is especially true of the elderly population which may have more comorbidities than the general population. The elderly may also not have as rapid or as complete postsurgical recovery as younger individuals might. As perhaps expected, overall, older patients have an increased risk of death after lung surgery [5, 12]. The elderly are also more likely to aspirate, suffer from kyphosis, have decreased excursion of their lower ribs, and depend more heavily on their diaphragms to breathe. These may all contribute to the increased respiratory risk factors associated with the elderly. Despite these trends, it is imperative that one does not include or rule out a patient for a procedure simply on the basis of the patient's age. There is far too much variation in the physical condition and resiliency between patients of advanced age to not evaluate each elderly patient on a case-by-case basis regardless of his specific age.

A discussion with the patient and, when appropriate, the patient's family is of the utmost importance. One controversial consideration, however, is how much about the patient's condition the patient wants to or should be told. Upon examination and further testing, a physician likely has a general approximation of the implications of the patient's condition. Lung cancer, especially at advanced stages, is not a diagnosis any patient wants to receive. However, if it is the case, 88 % of patients would like to know that [13]. So despite the negative psychological effects of hearing such news, in the majority of cases, it is better to tell the patient, even if the patient's condition is such that his treatment options are limited to palliative care. Yet, in accord with the physician's ethical viewpoints on the matter and hospital policy, the physician may consider his phrasing of the news carefully, though accurately, depending on the perceived opinion of the patient.

Important factors to take note of in the taking of the patient's history are a history of smoking, significant weight loss, other previous lung or cardiac disease, other comorbidities, and prior surgeries. While taking the patient's history, one can often get a sense of the patient's cognitive and functional level without asking about it directly. So while taking the history, it is important to ask oneself several questions, such as the following: How often must the questions be repeated? Does the patient seem to understand the situation? Can the patient recall your discussion on subsequent patient visits? Can the patient restate what new information the physician is telling him in his own words? Must a family member answer questions on behalf of the patient? With these questions considered, the number of questions relating to the patient's cognitive status may be limited as the information gathered would be redundant.

After taking the patient's history, a thorough physical exam should ensue. Patients should also "undergo chest X-ray, electrocardiogram, a room air arterial blood gas, pulmonary function tests, basic laboratory work and a complete staging evaluation" [14]. For proper staging evaluation, the patient must be thoroughly checked for possible metastasis through a chest CT, PET scans, brain scans, and cervical mediastinoscopy [14]. Stage I tumors may be greater than 3 cm, but do not invade into the surrounding tissue [15]. Stage II tumors have invaded into part, but not all, of the lung [15]. Stage III are greater than 7 cm and/or have invaded beyond the lung but still within the chest cavity [15]. Stage IV have metastasized even further and more extensively than stage II [15].

An assessment of the patient's cardiac and pulmonary status is a crucial step in considering any operation of this magnitude. Further noninvasive testing should be pursued in patients with a history of claudication or angina. And the use of beta-blockers must also be considered to prevent postoperative atrial fibrillation which is linked to increased length of hospital stay, mortality, and other postoperative complications [16].

Exercise tolerance can be evaluated using two tests which are both highly predictive of postoperative complications: the 6-min walk test and the patient's ability to climb two flights of stairs. The 6-min walk test evaluates how far a patient can walk in 6 min with the normal being over 1,400 ft. For the stairs test, 82 % of those unable to climb two flights of stairs have a postoperative cardiopulmonary complication in a high-risk surgery [17].

The forced expiratory volume expired in 1 s (FEV1) should be evaluated via spirometry. An FEV1 greater than 1 L is a good indication that the patient may safely undergo surgery unless other tests indicate otherwise [18]. Through a thorough history, physical examination, cancer staging, and cardiac and pulmonary evaluation, the patient's risk factors for proceeding with a surgery can be assessed.

What Are Important Outcomes?

The first step in determining the patient's goals for his quality of life post surgery is to establish where the patient is functionally at present. Two important measures can be used to determine the functional status of an elderly patient. First are the activities of daily living (ADLs). These include tasks required to take care of oneself in bathing, dressing, using the restroom, motility, and feeding. The second measure is the instrumental activities of daily living (IADLs). These measure an individual's ability to manage the world outside of oneself and perhaps even be a part of the community. This may include using public transportation, cooking, and shopping.

After establishing a baseline, it is important to talk with the patient and the patient's family to discuss how the surgery may lower the patient's functional status and the expected length of recovery time. For an elderly patient, the potential for increasing the length of life that surgery may bring may or may not outweigh the loss in functional status. It may also depend upon the degree of functional status that the patient is willing to lose. For example, independently performing basic self-caring tasks may be more important to some than to others.

This is a very delicate discussion, and the decision to proceed with the surgery should not be made with haste. The patient, physician, and family must consider not only the patient's definition of an acceptable quality of life but also the ability for the patient to handle any responsibilities he may have and how he will receive postoperative care. Consider Mr. Smith from the clinical vignette at the beginning of this chapter.

Three of the most important outcomes to consider for patients contemplating surgery as a treatment option are nursing home admission, functional impairment, and death 1 year after surgery. One year post diagnosis, deficit in functional status, death, and composite nursing home admission or death were significantly increased in patients with NSCLC who did not undergo surgery. One year after diagnosis, of those patients who underwent surgery, 3 % were admitted to a nursing home, 12 % died, and 5 % reported that they could not perform their usual activities. This is compared to the patients who did not pursue the surgical option of which 4 % were admitted to a nursing home, 45 % died, and 13 % reported that they could not perform their usual activities [1]. It is important to note that these individuals were not randomly chosen to undergo surgery or not to undergo surgery. Rather, this study indicates that patients who both are healthy enough to undergo surgery and then do undergo surgery have better outcomes than those patients who either are not healthy enough for surgery and/or choose not to undergo surgery.

Therefore, it is desirable to identify patients who are fit to undergo surgery so that they may benefit from an increased likelihood of better outcomes. In order to do so, it is important to understand the trends of which patients tend to have better postsurgical outcomes. These include trends in age, stage of the disease, income, and education level. Better outcomes are significantly related to younger patients, patients with less severe comorbidities, stage I disease rather than stage II or III, a higher income, and a high school degree or better [1]. Of particular importance is that the rate of nursing home admission and death 1 year after surgery markedly increases after age 75 [1]. And patients with a college degree were found to be three times less likely to be admitted to a nursing home or report being severely functionally impaired 1 year after the surgery than patients who had less than a high school education [1].

Though 1 year post surgery death, severe functional impairment, and nursing home admission are important outcomes to consider, it is of vital importance to not make any assumptions about a patient's expectations and views on these or any other potential adverse outcomes. The patient and, when appropriate, the patient's family should be included in this discussion and given proper time to make an informed decision.

Lobectomy Versus Limited Resection

Early stage NSCLC can be treated surgically through a lobectomy or a limited resection. A lobectomy is the removal of an entire lobe of the lung, whereas a limited resection removes a subunit of the lobe. When removing a cancer, one want to make sure to remove all the cancerous cells to decrease the risk of subsequent metastases. On the other hand, removing excessive may be detrimental to lung function which may impact many aspects of the patient's health. An elderly patient already has reduced lung elasticity and function as compared to the younger population. So the goal would be to remove as little of the lung as possible while ensuring that you removed as much of the cancerous cells as possible. And it is these conflicting goals which drive the argument for lobectomy or for limited resection.

The concerns in performing a limited resection over a lobectomy are well founded. There is up to three times the locoregional recurrence rate with limited resection as compared to lobectomy [19]. There is also a higher death rate associated with limited resection as compared to lobectomy [19]. However, if the patients are selected properly, there is no significant difference in survival rate or recurrence between the two procedures [20–25]. Therefore, if patients are able to be properly evaluated for lobectomy or limited resection, then the recurrence and mortality rate can be kept stable while having the potential for preserving more of the lung function.

Presently, a perfect algorithm for deciding whether to perform a lobectomy or a limited resection does not exist. However, there are many visible trends in which circumstances tend to be associated with one procedure over the other. These trends include demographics, physician-associated factors, and the physical condition of the patient being evaluated. An evaluation of these trends may elucidate which procedure is most appropriate under which conditions.

Demographic Factors

Lung cancer is predominantly a disease which presents in the elderly. Among this age demographic, there does not seem to be a strong correlation between age and the type of procedure performed [2]. There is also no correlation with race or ethnicity [2]. One interesting finding is that though having a college degree is associated with limited resection, income does not have a significant correlation to one procedure over the other [2].

What to do with demographic trends of this nature is unclear. Without understanding the social or medical root of such trends, it should make one hesitant to factor in such information when making a decision on the treatment course.

Physician-Associated Factors

One intriguing trend is that limited resection is more likely to be performed by a thoracic surgeon than a general surgeon [2]. Though one should hesitate to make conclusions based upon this trend, it does open the door for much speculation. Perhaps a thoracic surgeon, having likely seen a proportionately greater number of NSCLC cases, has had enough cases to notice a trend of more positive outcomes with limited resection. Perhaps the limited resection requires more experience to perform as locating the correct subsection of lung is more difficult than locating the correct lobe to remove. Perhaps with lobectomy being the more standard procedure, a thoracic surgeon has enough focused expertise to be at the forefront of a trend toward limited resection over lobectomy. This conjecture is supported by the fact that surgeons who tended to perform more limited resections were more likely to enroll patients in clinical trials and be a part of a National Cancer Institute–designated cancer center [2].

A trend has also been found with the procedure type and the type of insurance payment plan. There tends to be a higher reimbursement for lobectomies ($1537–1642) over limited resection ($808–1491) [2]. This trend correlates with a higher incidence of lobectomies in a fee-for-service insurance payment plan vs. a non-fee-for-service payment plan [2]. An idealist may hope that this correlation is coincidental or that the two procedures are so similar in outcomes that fees may be taken into account. But perhaps it is best that surgeons do not take insurance coverage into account when making such a decision, especially since many other considerations exist.

Patient History and Condition Factors

The most clinically relevant trends to evaluate in the determination of whether to undergo a limited resection or a lobectomy are the patient history, physical, and characteristics of the tumor itself. The tumors associated with limited resection tend to be smaller and of an earlier stage than those treated by lobectomy [2]. However, the exact threshold tumor size for a limited resection varies depending on the source [19, 26–28]. A limited resection is far more likely to remove all of the cancerous cells if the tumor is small and less invasive. Therefore, one can limit the risk of recurrence while preserving more of the lung.

Preference for a limited resection is also associated with comorbidities and other factors which may increase the risk of negative surgical outcomes and an already decreased lung function. For example, a limited resection is more likely in patients with other lung disease, a history of stroke, a history of smoking, advanced age, obesity, and a history of heart failure [2]. In a surgery of this magnitude, one must be sure that the patient's heart and vessels can withstand the surgical insult and the ensuing decrease in function and circulation during recovery. Therefore, heart and vascular disease should be evaluated as well as a history of smoking which could impact both. Obesity is a consideration because it may decrease the maximum lung capacity, especially when lying down as in during a surgery and recovery. A limited resection removes less of the lung and thus preserves more lung function than a lobectomy. So it would make sense that one may not want to remove an entire lobe of the lung in a patient with decreased lung function.

Outcomes

The final consideration in the decision to proceed with a lobectomy or a limited resection is the outcomes associated with each. Overall, morbidities associated with each procedure are comparable [2, 19]. However, the 5-year survival rate is lower in limited resections. This trend may be associated with increased recurrence, yet it may also be attributed to the increased risk factors associated with patients who undergo a limited resection instead of a lobectomy.

Again, it is necessary to determine which outcomes are important to the patient and surgeon. And in cases where creating such a definition is impossible or inappropriate, one may use outcomes considered important by the general population [29]. These may include death after 1 year, nursing home admission, and severe functional impairment as mentioned previously or other outcomes such as a risk to one's independence, hospital stay length, and recovery time. However, these too may vary on a case-by-case basis. Perhaps the patient is already in a nursing home and already requires a nurse for most of his activities of daily life. That patient may have a different opinion on which outcomes are important than, say, Mr. Smith, who is highly functional for his age and must consider the well-being of his daughter in addition to his own well-being. Therefore, it appears as though the choice in procedure, like any of the trends in this chapter, is decided through a combination of multiple factors on a case-by-case basis.

Summary

In choosing the best treatment option for one's patients, one must carefully evaluate numerous factors. These factors include patient history, comorbidities, physical exam, demographics, patient's viewpoints, and trends found within one's field. The surgical treatment of non-small cell lung cancer in the elderly is no exception. First, one must make the decision of whether to perform surgery at all, based on a balancing of expectations and likelihoods. If surgery is deemed the best treatment option, one must then decide whether to perform a limited resection or a lobectomy. The latter decision is where future studies will likely illuminate a more concrete path. In the meantime, it is imperative for all trends to be analyzed and considered so that the surgeon chooses an option that is best for the patient as determined by the patient's own definition of their best outcome.

References

1. Billmeier S, Ayanian J, He Y, Jaklitsch M, Rogers S. Predictors of nursing home admission, severe functional impairment or death one year after surgery for non-small cell lung cancer. J Surg Res. 2012;172(2):276.
2. Billmeier S, Ayanian J, Zaslavsky A, Nerenz D, Jaklitsch M, Rogers S. Predictors and outcomes of limited resection for early stage non-small cell lung cancer. J Natl Cancer Inst. 2011; 103(21):1621–9.
3. Jemal DVM A, Siegel R, Xu J, Ward E. Cancer statistics, 2010. CA Cancer J Clin. 2011;61: 133–4.
4. O'Rourke MA, Feussner JR, Feigl P, Laszlo J. Age trends of lung cancer stage at diagnosis. Implications for lung cancer screening in the elderly. JAMA. 1987;258(7):921–6.
5. Mery CM, Pappas AN, Bueno R, Colson YL, Linden P, Sugarbaker DJ, et al. Similar long-term survival of elderly patients with non-small cell lung cancer treated with lobectomy or wedge resection within the surveillance, epidemiology, and end results database. Chest. 2005;128(1):237–45.
6. Jaklitsch MT, DeCamp Jr MM, Liptay MJ, Harpole Jr DH, Swanson SJ, Mentzer SJ, et al. Video-assisted thoracic surgery in the elderly. A review of 307 cases. Chest. 1996;110(3): 751–8.
7. McKenna Jr RJ. Lobectomy by video-assisted thoracic surgery with mediastinal node sampling for lung cancer. J Thorac Cardiovasc Surg. 1994;107(3):879–81; discussion 881–2.
8. Roviaro G, Varoli F, Rebuffat C, Vergani C, Maciocco M, Scalambra SM, et al. Videothoracoscopic staging and treatment of lung cancer. Ann Thorac Surg. 1995;59(4): 971–4.
9. Yim AP, Ko KM, Chau WS, Ma CC, Ho JK, Kyaw K. Video-assisted thoracoscopic anatomic lung resections. The initial Hong Kong experience. Chest. 1996;109(1):13–7.
10. Jaklitsch MT, DeCamp Jr MM, Liptay MJ, Harpole Jr DH, Swanson SJ, Mentzer SJ, et al. Video-assisted thoracic surgery in the elderly. A review of 307 cases. Chest. 1996;110(3): 751–8.
11. Asamura H, Nakayama H, Kondo H, Tsuchiya R, Naruke T. Video-assisted lobectomy in the elderly. Chest. 1997;111(4):1101–5.
12. Shamji FM, Ginsberg RJ, Cooper JD, Spratt EH, Goldberg M, Waters PF, et al. Open window thoracostomy in the management of postpneumonectomy empyema with or without bronchopleural fistula. J Thorac Cardiovasc Surg. 1983;86(6):818–22.
13. Ajaj A, Singh MP, Abdulla AJ. Should elderly patients be told they have cancer? Questionnaire survey of older people. Br Med J. 2001;323:1160.
14. Billmeier S, Jaklitsch M. Pulmonary surgery for malignant disease in the elderly. Principles and practice of geriatric surgery. New York: Springer; 2011.
15. Rodriguez CP. Treatment implications of the new lung cancer staging system. Cleve Clin J Med. 2012;79 Suppl 1:eS7–10.

16. Roselli EE, Murthy SC, Rice TW, Houghtaling PL, Pierce CD, Karchmer DP, et al. Atrial fibrillation complicating lung cancer resection. J Thorac Cardiovasc Surg. 2005;130(2): 438–44.
17. Girish M, Trayner Jr E, Dammann O, Pinto-Plata V, Celli B. Symptom-limited stair climbing as a predictor of postoperative cardiopulmonary complications after high-risk surgery. Chest. 2001;120(4):1147–51.
18. Jaklitsch M, Billmeier S. Preoperative evaluation and risk assessment for elderly thoracic surgery patients. Thorac Surg Clin. 2009;19(3):301–12.
19. Ginsberg RJ, Rubinstein LV. Randomized trial of lobectomy versus limited resection for T1 N0 non-small cell lung cancer. Lung Cancer Study Group. Ann Thorac Surg. 1995;60(3):615–22; discussion 622–3.
20. Koike T, Yamato Y, Yoshiya K, Shimoyama T, Suzuki R. Intentional limited pulmonary resection for peripheral T1 N0 M0 small-sized lung cancer. J Thorac Cardiovasc Surg. 2003; 125(4):924–8.
21. Okada M, Yoshikawa K, Hatta T, Tsubota N. Is segmentectomy with lymph node assessment an alternative to lobectomy for non-small cell lung cancer of 2 cm or smaller? Ann Thorac Surg. 2001;71(3):956–60; discussion 961.
22. Keenan RJ, Landreneau RJ, Maley Jr RH, Singh D, Macherey R, Bartley S, et al. Segmental resection spares pulmonary function in patients with stage I lung cancer. Ann Thorac Surg. 2004;78(1):228–33; discussion 228–33.
23. Martin-Ucar AE, Nakas A, Pilling JE, West KJ, Waller DA. A case-matched study of anatomical segmentectomy versus lobectomy for stage I lung cancer in high-risk patients. Eur J Cardiothorac Surg. 2005;27(4):675–9.
24. Wisnivesky JP, Henschke CI, Swanson S, Yankelevitz DF, Zulueta J, Marcus S, et al. Limited resection for the treatment of patients with stage IA lung cancer. Ann Surg. 2010; 251(3):550–4.
25. Kodama K, Doi O, Higashiyama M, Yokouchi H. Intentional limited resection for selected patients with T1 N0 M0 non-small-cell lung cancer: a single-institution study. J Thorac Cardiovasc Surg. 1997;114(3):347–53.
26. Okada M, Koike T, Higashiyama M, Yamato Y, Kodama K, Tsubota N. Radical sublobar resection for small-sized non-small cell lung cancer: a multicenter study. J Thorac Cardiovasc Surg. 2006;132(4):769–75.
27. Miller DL, Rowland CM, Deschamps C, Allen MS, Trastek VF, Pairolero PC. Surgical treatment of non-small cell lung cancer 1 cm or less in diameter. Ann Thorac Surg. 2002; 73(5):1545–50; discussion 1550–1.
28. Ohta Y, Oda M, Wu J, Tsunezuka Y, Hiroshi M, Nonomura A, et al. Can tumor size be a guide for limited surgical intervention in patients with peripheral non-small cell lung cancer? Assessment from the point of view of nodal micrometastasis. J Thorac Cardiovasc Surg. 2001;122(5):900–6.
29. Cykert S, Kissling G, Hansen CJ. Patient preferences regarding possible outcomes of lung resection. Chest. 2000;117(6):1551–9.

Part IV
Non Small-Cell Lung Cancer: Treatment of Early Stages

Chapter 8
Surgery: Indications and Issues

Lorenzo Spaggiari and Domenico Galetta

Abstract Surgery in elderly patients affected by NSCLC is safe and feasible when careful preoperative respiratory and cardiac studies have been carried on. The surgical treatment is not to be denied in an elderly patient due to age per se, but when a major contraindication to surgery has been recognized. The long-term survival for elderly patients with early-stage lung cancer treated by anatomical pulmonary resection is comparable to the survival rate of younger patients, as demonstrated by several studies. Nowadays studies in elderly patients have demonstrated that pneumonectomy, extended surgical procedure, and preoperative induction chemotherapy are major risk factors for an increased postoperative morbidity and mortality rate. Anyway, in our opinion, the proper selected elderly patient with NSCLC should be treated in the same way as the younger one, with anatomical pulmonary resection and radical lymphadenectomy. In fact, we believe that implementing preoperative cardiologic studies and redefining selective respiratory criteria specifically for elderly improve surgical results.

Keywords Non-small cell lung cancer in the elderly • Surgery for NSCLC in the elderly • Elderly with NSCLC • Postoperative management after surgery in NSCLC • Patient selection for surgery for NSCLC in the elderly

L. Spaggiari, MD, PhD
Division of Thoracic Surgery, European Institute of Oncology,
Via Ripamonti 435, Milan, Italy

School of Medicine, University of Milan, Milan, Italy
e-mail: lorenzo.spaggiari@ieo.it

D. Galetta, MD, PhD (✉)
Division of Thoracic Surgery, European Institute of Oncology,
Via Ripamonti 435, Milan, Italy
e-mail: domenico.galetta@ieo.it

C. Gridelli, R.A. Audisio (eds.), *Management of Lung Cancer in Older People*,
DOI 10.1007/978-0-85729-793-8_8, © Springer-Verlag London 2013

The general age of the population in our society is tending upward. The percentage of the population in the USA who are aged 65 years or older in 2012 is 13.5 %, and it is estimated to be 20.5 % in 2050 [1]. The percentage of people 65 years or older is even greater in 2012 in European countries such as Germany (20.7 %), Italy (20.5 %), and the UK (16.9 %) [1]. These percentages will also increase in the projections of the United States Census Bureau for the 2050 for European people 65 years or older: 30.1 % for Germany, 31.0 % for Italy, and 23.6 % for the UK [1].

Non-small cell lung cancer (NSCLC) is the leading cause of cancer-related death in people older than 65 years in Western countries in both men and women [2]. Improvements in medical care have led to an increase in the mean expectancy of life, so that the number of people older than 65 years living with lung cancer is estimated to double before 2050 [3].

Unfortunately, the majority of NSCLC patients have advanced or metastatic disease at the time of diagnosis [4], and treatment options are often limited to palliative measures for symptomatic control and offer only a modest survival benefit compared with best supportive care. However, those presenting with early-stage disease (I, II, and subsets of stage IIIA NSCLC according to the 7th version of TNM staging [5]) have the potential to undergo curative surgical resection [6, 7].

Advances in anesthetic management and surgical technique have enabled surgeons to include increasing numbers of elderly patients in surgical series. Recent British Thoracic Society Guidelines have emphasized the fact that patient age at presentation should no longer influence access to radical surgery [8]. Despite this change in attitude, age often negatively influences treatment decisions, thereby potentially limiting curative surgical options for older population groups [9, 10]. However, several studies support that surgical treatment of NSCLC in the elderly is feasible and that age itself is not a contraindication for surgical intervention [11–18], even in octogenarians [19–21].

During the past decade there has been a revolution in the development of minimally invasive chest surgery (Fig. 8.1) with smaller incisions and dramatic reductions in operative risk. These improvements have reopened an old debate of whether limited thoracoscopic wedge resection (Fig. 8.2) has a role as an adequate cancer treatment. Elderly patients with lung cancer may benefit the most from this new technique.

We analyze the recent evidences for optimal treatment of elderly patients with resectable NSCLC, focusing on surgery, by outlining the reasons for this restrictive surgical approach and determining the best strategy for the surgical treatment of this population.

Physiologic Changes with Age

Old age is associated with impairment of respiratory function. Physiologic changes of the respiratory system associated with aging include reduced chest wall compliance with stiffening of calcified costal cartilages, diminished

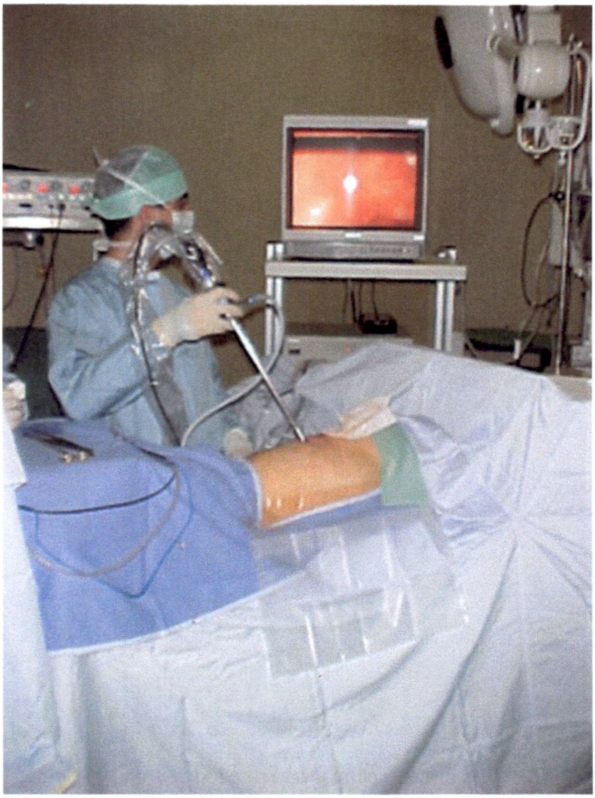

Fig. 8.1 Video-assisted thoracoscopic surgery is a new and widely used technique for resection of NSCLC. In this figure, the surgeon is performing a thoracoscopic lung resection

diaphragmatic excursion, and narrowing of the intervertebral disk space. A reduction of lung elastic recoil with loss of alveolar architecture produces a decreased alveolar gas exchange surface. Progressive atrophy creates weakness of the respiratory musculature. The loss of lung elastic recoil and decreased lung compliance diminished negative intrapleural pressure, which prevents reopening of small airways, resulting in air trapping and inadequate ventilation. Functionally, this manifests in a gradual decline of vital capacity and partial pressure of oxygen with an increased residual volume. The decline in motor power of the accessory muscles and stiffening of the chest wall also result in a declining forced expiratory volume in 1 s (FEV_1). Physiologic changes in lung mechanics make elderly patients particularly sensitive to narcotics and muscle relaxants. Additionally, elderly patients are at increased risk for respiratory tract infections due to waning immune responses [22]. Smoking in particular has been shown to cause bronchial mucociliary dysfunction [23], which has been associated with increased susceptibility to infection [24].

Increasing age is also associated with declines in other organ systems: there is a decline in the glomerular filtration rate, an increased incidence of heart disease, and an increased incidence of cognitive dysfunction [25].

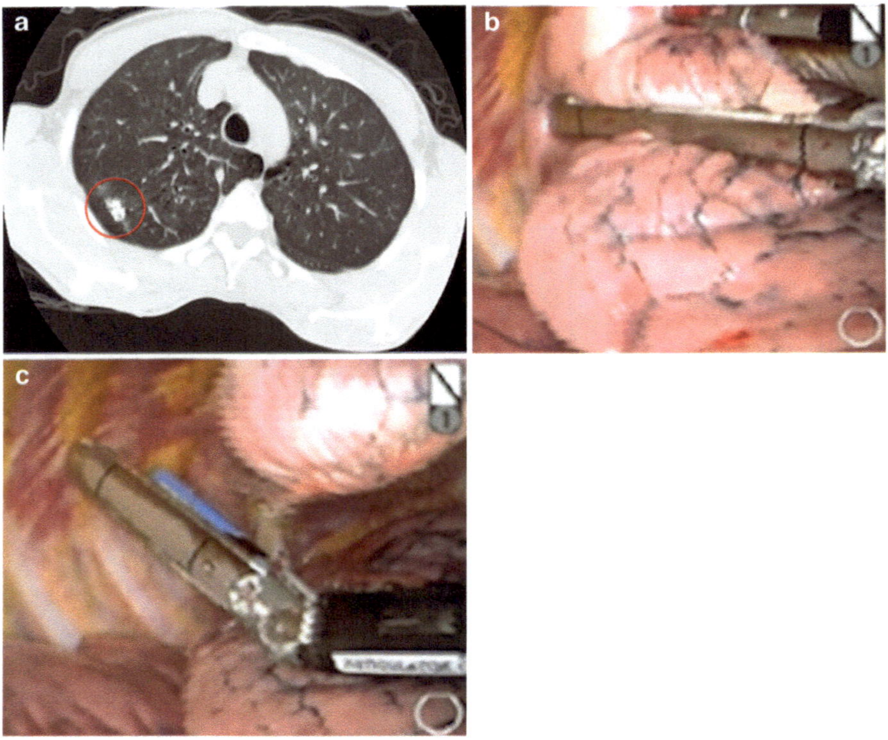

Fig. 8.2 Less invasive pulmonary resection performed by video-assisted thoracoscopic surgery for a small, peripheral lung nodule in a 74-year-old patients (**a**, encircled lesion). The pulmonary nodule is removed by a limited or wedge parenchymal resection by using mechanical stapler (**b**, **c**)

Some histological differences have been observed in lung cancer between elderly and young patients. Elderly patients have a lower incidence of adenocarcinoma and a higher incidence of squamous cell tumors, which have a better long-term prognosis. Furthermore, lung cancer in elderly patients seems to show clinically reduced growth rate and metastatic potential, with an apparently inverse relationship between stage and age [26].

Selection of Surgical Candidates

A careful selection of elderly patients who can be treated surgically is mandatory in order to decrease postoperative morbidity and mortality rate. Before planning surgery you should be confident to have a good life expectancy, characterized by an increase in the expected survival time with an acceptable postoperative mortality rate and a not deteriorated postsurgical quality of life. These objectives can be achieved through an appropriate preoperative study, which includes an accurate TNM staging of the disease and of a proper cardiorespiratory risk assessment.

Several preoperative risk factors are associated with morbidity and mortality during the hospital stay after major resection. Tumor stage, performance status, and weight loss are the most accepted preoperative prognostic predictive factors for patients considered fit for surgery [27]. Other important factors are the general status, the nutrition, the presence of a neurologic history, other comorbidities (i.e., diabetes, hepatic or renal disorders), and the social and familiar status.

All patients must have a detailed assessment based on history, symptoms, and signs of chronic lung or heart disease. Chest x-ray, electrocardiogram, arterial blood gas analysis, pulmonary function tests, and biochemical and hematological tests are helpful in screening potential surgical patients.

Preoperative TNM Staging

The preoperative assessment of the stage according to the TNM staging system [5] is of paramount importance for every patient affected by NSCLC and in particular for elderly patients. A total-body computer tomography (CT) scan and a positron emission tomography (PET) scan must be performed. Every suspect lymph nodal localization must be biopsied using endobronchial ultrasound-guided fine needle aspiration (EBUS-FNA) [28] or mediastinoscopy for paratracheal, pretracheal, and top subcarinal nodes (stations #2R, #4R, #2L, #4L, #3, and #7) according to the mediastinal lymph node map [5]. Endoscopic ultrasound-guided fine needle aspiration (EUS-FNA) [29], video-assisted thoracoscopy [30], or left anterior mediastinotomy [31] can be used to identify and biopsy lymph nodes in posterior aortopulmonary window (#5), subcarinal nodes (#7), paraesophageal nodes (#8), and inferior pulmonary ligament nodes (#9). Supraclavicular suspect localizations must be investigated through echo-guided needle biopsy or Daniels' surgical biopsy [30].

Preoperative Cardiorespiratory Evaluation

Functional Respiratory Study

The respiratory evaluation of an elderly patient who should undergo pulmonary resection has to be carefully conducted. Accurate respiratory functional study must be performed, including spirometry and arterial blood gas analysis, and for patients with borderline spirometry or PaO_2 findings, further examinations can be useful, such as regional pulmonary ventilation and perfusion studies, the 6-min walking test, or the stair-climbing test [32].

A preoperative FEV_1 of 55 % or lower and PaO_2 of 60 mmHg or lower have proven to be significantly related to an increment of the morbidity rate in patients aged 70 years or older [33]. For people aged 80 years or older, some authors suggested more severe criteria as compared to those used for younger patients (preoperative FEV_1 ≥50 %, predictive postoperative forced vital capacity ≥50 %) [34].

Patients with severely compromised pulmonary function – detected with spirometry (FEV1 <1 L) – may have a higher incidence of perioperative complications than patients with normal respiratory function, but their survival does not seems to be affected [35].

New method of risk assessment is thus being developed to supplement the existing ones. Simplicity, reproducibility, and cost-effectiveness must be taken into account when searching for reliable means of assessing operative risk.

Several clinical and experimental investigations have shown that pulmonary diffusion capacity for carbon monoxide is a highly reliable and inexpensive test for pulmonary function. The measurement of carbon monoxide uptake from alveolar gas is a unique, noninvasive way of assessing pulmonary vascular function, specifically the functional volume of the pulmonary capillary bed [36].

There is little correlation between predicted postoperative diffusing capacity and predicted postoperative FEV_1, so these values should be determined independently when estimating operative risk. The predicted postoperative diffusing capacity and predicted FEV_1 are calculated by multiplying the raw observed values with the percentage of lost lung parenchyma: right upper lung, 15 %; right middle lung, 10 %; right lower lung, 25 %; left upper lung, 25 %; and left lower lung, 25 %.

We recommend that all elderly patients with suspected lung cancer have a preoperative evaluation including the previous cited exams and for those patients with abnormality in pulmonary evaluation should either undergo rehabilitation and reassessment or be evaluated by more sophisticated tests such as oxygen uptake during exercise or a pulmonary ventilation and perfusion scan. All thoracic surgery candidates should be advised about smoking cessation before surgery. Physical chest therapy and optimization of bronchodilator therapy should be suggested during the preoperative period.

Functional Cardiac Study

Elderly patients have a higher incidence of cardiovascular complications after surgical resection of lung cancer [37]. For these reasons, all elderly patients who are candidates for lung surgery must have a detailed cardiovascular clinical history and an electrocardiogram. Patients can then be divided into subgroups according to the presence or absence of known coronary disease and cardiac functional status. If there is no history of coronary artery disease, myocardial infarction, or congestive heart failure and the electrocardiogram does not show abnormality, no further tests are required and the patient can be considered a suitable candidate for surgery. Patients with previous myocardial infarction or congestive heart failure should undergo echocardiography to evaluate ejection fraction. Those with a history of coronary artery disease or previous coronary artery bypass graft surgery should undergo an exercise stress test to evaluate cardiac function.

High-risk patients can then be treated preoperatively with anti-ischemic and antihypertensive therapy. After surgery more intensive monitoring and treatment can be given.

Surgical Treatment

According to the literature, there is evidence that patients with early-stage lung cancer can benefit from a surgical approach [38]. Patients with untreated or palliated early-stage NSCLC have an average life expectancy of 1.5 years [39], whereas individuals in their 80s have a 50 % chance of living 5–9 more years [40]. Because elderly patients are more likely to have earlier stage disease at diagnosis than younger patients [34], it is notable that the older age group is less likely to be treated surgically, despite a lower survival rate being observed using curative chemoradiotherapy [41]. Moreover, when surgery is performed in elderly patients, there is a higher percentage of nonanatomic resection, often not justified by preoperative respiratory functional findings [42]. A high long-term survival rate of 82 % at 5 years has been found in a group of stage IA elderly patients treated surgically with an anatomical resection of the disease [43].

The recent introduction of minimally invasive techniques (video-assisted thoracoscopic surgery) or, for example, the use of smaller incision (a small lateral muscle-sparing thoracotomy instead of larger posterolateral muscle-dividing incision) along with improvement in anesthesiology led to a reduction of operative risk and to a quicker recovery and discharge [44].

Elderly patients with lung cancer who have pulmonary resection via thoracotomy have a higher incidence of postoperative mortality than younger patients. The Lung Cancer Study Group found that patients aged 70 years or older had a 30-day postoperative mortality of 7.1 % compared with 1.3 % for patients younger than 60 years and 4.1 % for those aged between 60 and 69 [45]. More recently, other studies of elderly patients undergoing surgical resection of NSCLC have been reported (Table 8.1) showing low morbidity and mortality rates among elderly patients during the past decade [15, 37, 43, 46–50].

Although in the past years lobectomy has been the standard of care for early-stage lung cancer in patients able to tolerate this procedure, lung-sparing procedures such

Table 8.1 Selected series of elderly patients operated on for NSCLC

Ref.	No. of patients	Age range (years)	Stage I *n* (%)	Morbidity *n* (%)	Mortality *n* (%)
Cerfolio et al. [15]	191	70–74	111 (58)	38 (19)	5 (2.4)[a]
	121	75–79	77 (66)	35 (29)	2 (1.6)[a]
	51	80+	43 (84)	10 (20)	1 (2)[a]
Morandi et al. [37]	85	70–88	48 (56)	41 (48)	1 (1)
Port et al. [43]	61	80–87	44 (72)	23 (38)	1 (1.6)
Naunheim et al. [46]	40	80–88	35 (87)	18 (45)	6 (15)
Jack et al. [47]	79	70–85	57 (72)	20 (26)	3 (4)
Broch et al. [48]	68	80–87	41 (60)	45 (66)	6 (8.8)
Blokbas et al. [49]	110	75–79	42 (47)	43 (39)	4 (3.6)
	47	80–90	18 (38)	17 (36)	2 (4.3)
Fanucchi et al. [50]	82	80–87	43 (52)	24 (309)	2 (2.4)

[a]Operative mortality

as anatomic segmentectomy or wedge resection (Fig. 8.2) are becoming more common in the treatment of NSCLC [51, 52], particularly in elderly patients [44].

Lung-sparing procedures enable the preservation of pulmonary function and decrease operative morbidity and mortality in patients with NSCLC [52]. However, the long-term effects of such procedures on survival and recurrence are controversial. In the multi-institution randomized trial of the Lung Cancer Study Group experience [53] comparing limited resection with lobectomy in patients with T1 N0 NSCLC, there was no significant overall difference in postoperative complications and mortality. However, patients who had limited resections had a higher incidence of recurrence than patients who had lobectomies ($p=0.02$) even if there was no difference in terms of survival between the two groups.

In another multi-institution study [54] analyzing patients with T1 N0 NSCLC who underwent different procedures (lobectomy, open wedge resection, video-assisted thoracoscopic surgery, and wedge resection), patients who had lobectomy had a higher incidence of operative mortality, postoperative complications, and length of staying hospital than patients who had more limited resections.

Limited resections seem to be promising for elderly patients with lung cancer because of their higher prevalence of stage I disease and the potential reduction in postoperative complications. For the first year after surgery, limited resections are not associated with increased risk of recurrence or death, thus potentially benefiting elderly patients with lower life expectancy than younger patients. Although there is not enough data to suggest the use of limited resections in every patient with early-stage lung cancer, these procedures are reasonable alternatives for elderly patients with high operative risk, cardiopulmonary impairment, and other comorbid diseases.

Although pneumonectomy has been considered a useful surgical procedure for the treatment of locally advanced lung cancer, its use in the elderly population has been rarely reported because the rate of complications (cardiac and respiratory) in this population remains high [55, 56].

The value of radical lymphadenectomy has been extensively debating over the last 10 years, the majority of the more recent studies supporting the importance of this procedure in order to achieve better results [34, 42]. Anyway, radical lymphadenectomy is associated with an increase in postoperative morbidity (due to bleeding, phrenic and laryngeal nerve injuries, chylothorax), and so some authors prefer to avoid this technique in highly vulnerable patients [13].

Intraoperative and Postoperative Management

Intraoperative management should provide a minimization of anesthetic stress, and a continuous monitoring with electrocardiogram, arterial line, temperature, urine production, end tidal carbon dioxide, and pulse oximetry is mandatory [34, 42]. Attention must be paid to careful positioning of the patient due to the increased frequency of joint limitation and musculoskeletal alteration in elderly people [34]. Because elderly patients are often affected by chronic obstructive pulmonary disease, preoperative and postoperative respiratory physiotherapy is of paramount importance in order to obtain better postoperative recovery [57, 58]. A well-addressed physiotherapy program can lead to a reduction of hospital stay and decrease of postoperative complications such as atelectasis and pneumonia [59].

The control of postoperative pain is extremely important, and a proper analgesia can improve respiratory function and stimulate a productive cough. The use of thoracic epidural analgesia has been recently associated with lower mortality and postoperative respiratory complications [59]. Intraoperative administration of local anesthetics (anesthesiology blocking of intercostal nerves) can be used to reduce perioperative pain and so the need for drug administration, while a recent study focused on the use of an intercostal nerve catheter with patient-controlled analgesia in order to effectively control the postoperative pain [60].

Discussion

Surgery in elderly patients affected by NSCLC is safe and feasible when careful preoperative respiratory and cardiac studies have been carried on. The surgical treatment is not to be denied in an elderly patient due to age per se, but when a major contraindication to surgery has been recognized. The long-term survival for elderly patients with early-stage lung cancer treated by anatomical pulmonary resection is comparable to the survival rate of younger patients, as demonstrated by several studies. Nowadays studies in elderly patients have demonstrated that pneumonectomy, extended surgical procedure, and preoperative induction chemotherapy are major risk factors for an increased postoperative morbidity and mortality rate. Anyway, in our opinion, the properly selected elderly patient with NSCLC should be treated in the same way as the younger one, with anatomical pulmonary resection and radical lymphadenectomy. In fact, we believe that implementing preoperative cardiologic studies and redefining selective respiratory criteria specifically for elderly improve surgical results.

When comorbidities are present or a patient is 80 years or older, there is evidence that a nonanatomic resection can be performed without affecting long-term results. Pneumonectomies or extended resections should be reserved for properly selected patients.

References

1. US Census Bureau. International database. http://www.census.gov/population/international/data/idb/region.php. Accessed 1 Nov 2012.
2. Jemal A, Siegel R, Xu J, et al. Cancer statistics, 2010. CA Cancer J Clin. 2010;60:277–300.
3. Simmonds MA. Cancer statistics, 2003: further decrease in mortality rate, increase in persons living with cancer. CA Cancer J Clin. 2003;53:4.

4. Yang P, Allen MS, Aubry MC, et al. Clinical features of 5,628 primary lung cancer patients: experience at Mayo Clinic from 1997 to 2003. Chest. 2005;128:452–62.
5. Rami-Porta R, Bolejak V, Goldstraw P. The new tumor, node, and metastasis staging system. Semin Respir Crit Care Med. 2011;32(1):44–51.
6. NCCN Clinical Practice Guidelines in Oncology. V.1.2013. Non-small cell lung cancer. http://www.nccn.org/professionals/physician_gls/pdf/nscl.pdf. Accessed 2 Dec 2012.
7. Scott WJ, Howington J, Feigenberg S, et al. Treatment of non-small cell lung cancer stage I and stage II: ACCP evidence-based clinical practice guidelines (2nd edition). Chest. 2007;132(3 Suppl):234S–42.
8. Lim E, Baldwin D, Beckles M, et al. Guidelines on the radical management of patients with lung cancer. Thorax. 2010;65(Suppl3):iii1–27.
9. Sigel K, Bonomi M, Packer S, et al. Effect of age on survival f clinical stage I non-small cell lung cancer. Ann Surg Oncol. 2009;16:1912–7.
10. Cykert S, Iworth-Anderson P, Monroe MH, et al. Factors associated with decisions to undergo surgery among patients with newly diagnosed early-stage lung cancer. JAMA. 2010;303:2368–76.
11. Mery CM, Pappas AN, Bueno R, et al. Similar long-term survival of elderly patients with non-small cell lung cancer treated with lobectomy or wedge resection within the surveillance, epidemiology, and end results database. Chest. 2005;128:237–45.
12. Ciriaco P, Zannini P, Carretta A, et al. Surgical treatment of non-small cell lung cancer in patients 70 years of age or older. Int Surg. 1998;83:4–7.
13. Thomas P, Piraux M, Jacques LF, et al. Clinical patterns and trends of outcome of elderly patients with bronchogenic carcinoma. Eur J Cardiothorac Surg. 1998;13:266–74.
14. Yamamoto K, Padilla AJ, Calvo MV, et al. Surgical results of stage I non-small cell lung cancer: comparison between elderly and younger patients. Eur J Cardiothorac Surg. 2003;23:21–5.
15. Cerfolio RJ, Bryant AS. Survival and outcomes of pulmonary resection for non-small cell lung cancer in the elderly: a nested case–control study. Ann Thorac Surg. 2006;82:424–9.
16. Dyszkiewicz W, Pawlak K, Gasiorowsli L. Early post-pneumonectomy complications in the elderly. Eur J Cardiothorac Surg. 2000;17:246–50.
17. Spaggiari L, Scanagatta P. Surgery of non-small cell lung cancer in the elderly. Curr Opin Oncol. 2007;19:84–91.
18. Goodgame B, Viswanathan A, Zoole J, et al. Risk of recurrence of resected stage I non-small cell lung cancer in elderly patients as compared with younger patients. J Thorac Oncol. 2009;4:1370–4.
19. Dominguez-Ventura A, Cassivi SD, Allen MS, et al. Lung cancer in octogenarians: factors affecting long-term survival following resection. Eur J Cardiothorac Surg. 2007;32:370–4.
20. Okami J, Higashiyama M, Asamura H. Pulmonary resection in patients aged 80 years or over with clinical stage I non-small cell lung cancer: prognostic factors for overall survival and risk factors for postoperative complications. J Thorac Oncol. 2009;4:1247–53.
21. Matsuoka H, Okada M, Sakamoto T, et al. Complications and outcomes after pulmonary resection for cancer in patients 80 to 89 years of age. Eur J Cardiothorac Surg. 2005;28:380–3.
22. Meyer KC. Lung infections and aging. Ageing Res Rev. 2004;3:55–67.
23. Verra F, Escudier E, Lebargy F, et al. Ciliary abnormalities in bronchial epithelium of smokers, ex-smokers, and nonsmokers. Am J Respir Crit Care Med. 1995;151:630–4.
24. Salathe M, O'Riordan TG, Wanner A. Treatment of mucociliary dysfunction. Chest. 1996;110:1048–57.
25. Marcantonio ER, Goldman L, Mangione CM, et al. A clinical prediction rule for delirium after elective noncardiac surgery. JAMA. 1994;271:134–9.
26. Teeter SM, Holmes FF, McFarlane MJ. Lung carcinoma in the elderly population: influence of histology on the inverse relationship of stage to age. Cancer. 1987;60:1331–6.
27. Harpole Jr DH, Herndon 2nd JE, Young Jr WG, et al. Stage I non-small cell lung cancer: a multivariate analysis of treatment methods and patterns of recurrence. Cancer. 1995;76:787–96.
28. Ost DE, Ernst A, Lei X, et al. Diagnostic yield of endobronchial ultrasound-guided transbronchial needle aspiration: results of the AQuIRE Bronchoscopy Registry. Chest. 2011;140:1557–66.

29. Caddy G, Conron M, Wright G, et al. The accuracy of EUS-FNA in assessing mediastinal lymphadenopathy and staging patients with NSCLC. Eur Respir J. 2005;25:410–5.
30. Sihoe A, Yim AP. Lung cancer staging. J Surg Res. 2004;117:92–106.
31. Carbognani P, Rusca M, Spaggiari L, et al. Mediastinoscopy, thoracoscopy and left anterior mediastinotomy in the diagnosis of N2 non small cell lung cancer. J Cardiovasc Surg (Torino). 1996;37:177–8.
32. Brunelli A, Sabbatini A, Xiume' F, et al. Inability to perform maximal stair climbing test before lung resection: a propensity score analysis on early outcome. Eur J Cardiothorac Surg. 2005;27:367–72.
33. Ciriaco P, Casiraghi M, Calori G, et al. Lung resection for cancer in patients with coronary arterial disease: analysis of short term results. Eur J Cardiothorac Surg. 2002;22:35–40.
34. Dexter EU, Jahamgir N, Kohman LJ. Resection for lung cancer in the elderly patient. Thorac Surg Clin. 2004;14:163–7.
35. Roberts JR, Chang A, Slovis B. Severely compromised pulmonary function does not increase perioperative mortality after pulmonary lobectomy in a high volume center. Chest. 1999;116:370S.
36. MacIntyre NR. Diffusing capacity of the lung for carbon monoxide. Respir Care Clin N Am. 1997;3:221–33.
37. Morandi U, Stefani A, Golinelli M, et al. Results of surgical resection in patients over the age of 70 years with non-small cell lung cancer. Eur J Cardiothorac Surg. 1997;11:432–9.
38. Rami-Porta R, Ball D, Crowley J, et al. The IASLC Lung Cancer Staging Project: proposals for the revision of the T descriptors in the forthcoming (seventh) edition of the TNM classification for lung cancer. J Thorac Oncol. 2007;2:593–602.
39. National Cancer Institute. SEER cancer statistics review 1973–1997. Bethesda: National Cancer Institute; 2000.
40. Anderson R. United States life tables, 1997. Natl Vital Stat Rep. 1999;47:1–38.
41. Okamoto T, Maruyama R, Shoji F, et al. Clinical pattern and treatment outcome of elderly patients in clinical stage IB/II non-small cell lung cancer. J Surg Oncol. 2004;87:134–8.
42. Jaklitsch MT, Mery CM, Audisio RA. The use of surgery to treat lung cancer in elderly patients. Lancet Oncol. 2003;4:463–71.
43. Port JL, Kent M, Korst RJ, et al. Surgical resection for lung cancer in the octogenarian. Chest. 2004;126:733–8.
44. Jaklitsch MT, Pappas-Estocin A, Bueno R. Thoracoscopic surgery in elderly lung cancer patients. Crit Rev Oncol Hematol. 2004;49:165–71.
45. Ginsberg RJ, Hill LD, Eagan RT, et al. Modern thirty-day operative mortality for surgical resections in lung cancer. J Thorac Cardiovasc Surg. 1983;86:654–8.
46. Naunheim KS, Kesler KA, D'Orazio SA, et al. Lung cancer surgery in octogenarian. Eur J Cardiothorac Surg. 1994;8:453–6.
47. Jack CI, Lye M, Lesley F, et al. Surgery for lung cancer: age alone is not a contraindication. Int J Clin Pract. 1997;51:423–6.
48. Broch MV, Kim MP, Hooker CM, et al. Pulmonary resection in octogenarians with stage I non-small cell lung cancer: a 22-year experience. Ann Thorac Surg. 2004;77:271–7.
49. Blokbas S, Beqiri S, Bergmann T, et al. Pulmonary resection of non-small cell lung cancer: is survival in the elderly not affected by tumor stage after complete resection? Ann Thorac Cardiovasc Surg. 2008;56:476–81.
50. Fanucchi O, Ambrogi MC, Dini P, et al. Surgical treatment of non-small cell lung cancer in octogenarians. Interact Cardiovasc Thorac Surg. 2011;12:749–53.
51. Miller JI, Hatcher Jr CR. Limited resection of bronchogenic function. Ann Thorac Surg. 1987;44:340–3.
52. Pastorino U, Valente M, Bedini V, et al. Limited resection for stage I lung cancer. Eur J Surg Oncol. 1991;17:42–6.
53. Ginsberg RJ, Rubinstein LV. Randomized trial of lobectomy versus limited resection for T1N0 non-small cell lung cancer. Lung Cancer Study group. Ann Thorac Surg. 1995;60:615–22.

54. Landrenau RJ, Sugarbaker DJ, Mack MJ, et al. Wedge resection versus lobectomy for stage I (T1 N0 M0) non-small cell lung cancer. J Thorac Cardiovasc Surg. 1997;113:691–8.
55. Mizushima Y, Noto H, Sugiyama S, et al. Survival and prognosis after pneumonectomy for lung cancer in the elderly. Ann Thorac Surg. 1997;64:193–8.
56. Leo F, Scanagatta P, Baglio P, et al. The risk of pneumonectomy over the age of 70. A case–control study. Eur J Cardiothorac Surg. 2007;31:780–2.
57. Cesario A, Ferri L, Galetta D, et al. Pre-operative pulmonary rehabilitation and surgery for lung cancer. Lung Cancer. 2007;57:118–9.
58. Cesario A, Ferri L, Galetta D, et al. Post-operative respiratory rehabilitation after lung resection for non-small cell lung cancer. Lung Cancer. 2007;57:175–80.
59. Licker MJ, Widikker I, Robert J, et al. Operative mortality and respiratory complications after lung resections for lung cancer: impact of chronic obstructive pulmonary disease and time trends. Ann Thorac Surg. 2006;81:1830–7.
60. Wildgaard K, Petersen RH, Hansen HJ, et al. Multimodal analgesic treatment in video-assisted thoracic surgery lobectomy using an intraoperative intercostal catheter. Eur J Cardiothorac Surg. 2012;41:1072–7.

Chapter 9
Is There a Role for Postoperative Radiotherapy in Elderly Patients with Early-Stage Non-small Cell Lung Cancer?

Nicolas Girard and Françoise Mornex

Abstract Surgery is the standard treatment of early-stage non-small cell lung cancer (NSCLC). The risk of locoregional tumor recurrence after complete surgical resection is estimated to be as high as 10, 20, and 40 % for stage I, stage II, and stage III tumors, respectively. In this setting, the potential benefits and harms of postoperative radiotherapy have been considerably debated worldwide since the mid-1980s. The main objective of postoperative radiotherapy is to reduce the risk of local and locoregional recurrence and ultimately increase the survival of patients. Some clinical trials reported such survival benefit with postoperative radiotherapy, while other studies did not confirm this finding. Given the limited amount of data in the indexed literature about the role of postoperative radiotherapy after complete resection of early-stage NSCLC in elderly patients, this chapter will first present the available evidence about postoperative radiotherapy in the general population.

Keywords Postoperative radiotherapy in older patients • Radiotherapy in older patients • Lung cancer in older patients • Selection of elderly patients for radiotherapy in lung cancer • Non-small lung cancer in the elderly

Surgery is the standard treatment of early-stage non-small cell lung cancer (NSCLC) [1–3]. The risk of locoregional tumor recurrence after complete surgical resection is estimated to be as high as 10, 20, and 40 % for stage I, stage II, and stage III tumors,

N. Girard, MD, PhD
Respiratory Medicine Department and UMR 754,
Louis Pradel Hospital, Hospices Civils de Lyon, Claude Bernard University, Lyon, France
e-mail: nicolas.girard@chu-lyon.fr

F. Mornex, MD, PhD (✉)
Radiation Oncology Department and EMR 3738,
Centre Hospitalier Lyon Sud, Hospices Civils de Lyon, Claude Bernard University, Lyon, France
e-mail: francoise.mornex@chu-lyon.fr

C. Gridelli, R.A. Audisio (eds.), *Management of Lung Cancer in Older People*, DOI 10.1007/978-0-85729-793-8_9, © Springer-Verlag London 2013

respectively [1, 4]. In this setting, the potential benefits and harms of postoperative radiotherapy have been considerably debated worldwide since the mid-1980s. The main objective of postoperative radiotherapy is to reduce the risk of local and locoregional recurrence and ultimately increase the survival of patients. Some clinical trials reported such survival benefit with postoperative radiotherapy, while other studies did not confirm this finding [5–9]. Given the limited amount of data in the indexed literature about the role of postoperative radiotherapy after complete resection of early-stage NSCLC in elderly patients, this chapter will first present the available evidence about postoperative radiotherapy in the general population.

General Context of Postoperative Radiotherapy in NSCLC

The current recommendations and guidelines about postoperative radiotherapy after complete resection of NSCLC are mostly based on the PORT meta-analysis that was initiated by the UK Medical Research Council Cancer Trials Office and initially published in 1998; the meta-analysis was subsequently updated in 2008 by the Cochrane Collaboration [10, 11]. Overall, data from 11 prospective trials evaluating the effect of postoperative radiotherapy after complete resection of stage I to III NSCLC were analyzed. Collectively, these studies included a total of 2,343 patients. Median follow-up was 4.4 years. Results in the global population indicated a detrimental effect of postoperative radiotherapy on overall survival, with an 18 % increase in the risk of death corresponding to an estimated absolute mortality increase of 5 % at 2 years: overall survival rate was 58 % for patients not treated with postoperative radiotherapy vs. 53 % for patients who had received postoperative radiotherapy. Subgroup analyses suggested that the adverse effect of postoperative radiotherapy was limited to stage I–II disease, while the survival difference was not significant for stage III tumors. The numerous limitations of these results have largely been debated. The major criticism has been the inclusion in the meta-analysis of older trials that were initiated in the mid-1960s, at a time when radiation delivery used cobalt-60 machines, hypofractionated schemes, and single radiation field. The modalities of radiation delivery were highly heterogeneous from one study to another, with total doses ranging from 30 to 60 Gy in 10–30 daily fractions.

The technical optimization of medical radiotherapy that occurred over the past 15 years has been linked with the development of computed tomography scan, together with the availability of computerized radiation planning and delivery devices, allowing three-dimensional conformation of the radiation field, leading to a better focalization of the ballistics and better sparing of normal tissues from radiation-induced toxicities. A strong assumption is that these improvements may prevent treatment-induced deaths and then would unmask a putative benefit of postoperative radiotherapy after complete resection of NSCLC. Ultimately, the recent demonstration of the better survival of patients receiving adjuvant chemotherapy led to minimize the interest for postoperative radiotherapy, in both the routine care and the investigational setting [12].

More recently, data – both retrospective and prospective – have emerged that may actually lead to reconsider the use of modern radiotherapy techniques, especially in stage

IIIA-N2 NSCLC [13–17]. In the ANITA adjuvant chemotherapy trial, postoperative radiotherapy was recommended, in a nonrandomized fashion, for patients with N-positive tumor involvement [17]. Recommended total doses were 45–60 Gy using a standard fractionation scheme. Of the 840 patients accrued in the trial, 232 received postoperative radiotherapy, including 33 % of the 433 patients randomized in the observation arm and 22 % of the 407 patients randomized in the postoperative chemotherapy arm. The survival of patients with stage N2 disease was increased after postoperative radiotherapy, no matter postoperative chemotherapy was delivered or not: The 5-year overall survival was 47 % for patients receiving postoperative chemoradiation vs. 34 % for patients treated with postoperative chemotherapy alone, 21 % for patients treated with postoperative radiotherapy alone, and 17 % for patients receiving no postoperative treatment. Median overall survival was even doubled with postoperative radiotherapy: 47 months vs. 23 months in the chemotherapy arm and 23 months vs. 13 months in the observation arm. These data, obtained in a prospective cohort of patients, of course selected based on the inclusion criteria of the trial, strongly support the use of postoperative radiotherapy. Interestingly, for patients with N1 disease, 5-year overall survival was longer for irradiated patients in the observation arm – 43 % with postoperative radiotherapy vs. 31 % without postoperative radiotherapy – but lower in the postoperative chemotherapy arm, 40 % with postoperative radiotherapy vs. 56 % without postoperative radiotherapy.

A recent analysis of the Surveillance, Epidemiology and End Results (SEER) database included 7,465 patients with stage II–III completely resected NSCLC, who were treated between 1988 and 2002 [13]. Median follow-up was 3.5 years. No survival benefit was identified at multivariate analysis in the global population; however, while postoperative radiotherapy had a detrimental effect in patients with N0 and N1 disease (5-year overall survival was 31 and 30 % after postoperative radiotherapy vs. 41 and 32 % without radiotherapy, respectively), the overall survival of patients with N2 disease was significantly higher after postoperative radiotherapy (5-year overall survival, 27 % vs. 20 % without postoperative radiotherapy; HR = 0.855; 95 % CI, 0.762–0.959; $p = 0.0077$).

These findings are consistent with the signal of the previous meta-analysis, suggesting that the potential role of postoperative radiotherapy may be limited to patients with N2 disease. Based on these data, most groups currently recommend postoperative radiotherapy to be delivered only to patients with stage IIIA-N2 NSCLC that, contrary to N0–N1 tumors, bear a high risk of local and regional recurrence that radiation is supposed to reduce [2, 3].

Postoperative Radiotherapy in the Elderly Population

Current Evidence

Even more limited data exist in the literature regarding the role of postoperative radiotherapy in elderly patients. In the PORT meta-analysis, the majority of trials had strict inclusion and exclusion criteria, selecting younger patients with no age-related comorbidities. Subgroup analyses presented in the last available update for the Cochrane Collaboration showed no differential survival effect of postoperative radiotherapy among any group of patients defined by age (trend $p=0.34$) [11]. Of note, in the group of patients aged 65 years or more, the hazard ratio was 1.30 (95 % CI, 1.04–1.60) toward a nonsignificant detrimental effect of postoperative radiotherapy, contrary to what was observed in other age groups.

A large number of elderly patients actually receive postoperative radiotherapy. A recent analysis of the SEER database evaluated the survival of patients aged 65 years or more, after complete resection of stage IIIA-N2 NSCLC, depending on whether postoperative radiotherapy was delivered or not [18]. A total of 1,307 patients, treated from 1992 to 2005, were included in the study; the vast majority of patients (86 %) had a lobectomy, and a significant proportion of patients (32 %) received adjuvant chemotherapy. The first finding of this study is that 710 (54 %) patients actually received postoperative radiotherapy, including 43 % of the patients aged more than 75 years old. However, the frequency in the use of postoperative radiotherapy after complete resection of stage I–IIIA NSCLC is lower than that observed in younger patients. Analyzing SEER data from 22,953 patients based on TNM stage and patient age, other authors showed that compared to a reference population aged 30–49 years, the relative odds ratio for patients aged 65–79 years to receive postoperative radiotherapy was 0.59 (95 % CI, 0.45–0.77) for N0 disease, 0.46 (95 % CI, 0.35–0.61) for N1 disease, and 0.46 (95 % CI, 0.32–0.65) for N2 disease, meaning that postoperative radiotherapy is delivered almost two times less in elderly patients [14].

Regarding the effect of postoperative radiotherapy on the survival of elderly patients, the most recent analysis of the SEER database analysis failed to identify any benefit on overall survival [18]. In the cohort of 1,307 patients aged 65 years or more who had undergone complete resection of stage IIIA-N2 NSCLC from 1992 to 2005, the survival of patients was not impacted by postoperative radiotherapy (HR = 1.11; 95 % CI, 0.97–1.27). Subgroup analyses conducted in the subsets of patients receiving postoperative chemotherapy or not, optimized radiation treatment planning or not, or treated at different times led to similar conclusions. These results contradict the most recent data obtained in the general population and suggest that elderly patients even at high risk of tumor recurrence may not benefit from postoperative radiotherapy.

One must keep in mind that all these SEER database data, although less prone to selection biases compared to prospective trials, may be affected by referral biases, potential confounding influence of practicians and patients preferences, baseline characteristics, and practice patterns. Moreover, comparisons among different cohorts are difficult, as information about comorbidities, adjuvant chemotherapy or surgical morbidities, doses, and fractionation is not consistently available.

Current Recommendation

A systematic review and expert consensus about the treatment of NSCLC in elderly patients has been conducted by the European Organisation for Research and

Treatment of Cancer "Elderly Task Force" and "Lung Cancer Group" and the International Society for Geriatric Oncology [19]. Given the absence of evidence in the literature, routine postoperative radiotherapy is not recommended in elderly patients after complete resection of stage I–IIIA NSCLC. This statement is consistent with that of other groups for the global population of patients with completely resected NSCLC [2, 3, 20, 21].

Considerations for Routine Practice

For routine practice, postoperative radiotherapy has then not been evaluated in population-based studies focusing on radiotherapy principles for elderly patients with lung cancer [22]. Eligibility for thoracic surgery is highly restricted for these patients and requires careful evaluation of cardiopulmonary functions, using pulmonary function tests (spirometry, arterial gas measurement, and CO transfer evaluation), exercise tolerance testing, pulmonary ventilation gammagraphy, cardiac stress testing, and echocardiography [23]. One assumption may be that once surgery is considered feasible, even in elderly patients, the whole treatment strategy should follow recommendations and standards, including individualized discussion of postoperative radiotherapy based on tumor pathological stage.

Data from the literature clearly show that chronological age alone actually does not help to select patients for postoperative radiotherapy, as (1) overall survival data look to be similar to the global population with debated benefit even for high-risk patients with N2 disease and (2) population-based studies report on the use of postoperative radiotherapy in a significant proportion of patients. The major consideration is then, rather than age, the importance of associated medical disorders that may increase both the operative morbidity rate and the risk of radiation-induced toxicity. The length of hospital stay after lung cancer surgery may also preclude postoperative radiotherapy to be delivered in a timely schedule [24, 25]. Quality of life in the immediate postsurgical period may be considerably altered, leading to misevaluate the potential benefit of subsequent postoperative radiotherapy. Overall, available data based on subgroup analyses from general population studies may likely be biased in favor of the treatment, as only healthy enough elderly patients are included in those analyses.

Age also increases the risk of radiation-induced toxicities on normal tissues. Especially, cardiac toxicity may be a concern. An SEER database analysis was conducted to evaluate the heart disease-related mortality after complete resection of early-stage NSCLC in 6,148 patients, 3,589 (58 %) of whom treated with postoperative radiotherapy and 2,559 (42 %) not treated with postoperative radiotherapy [26]. Interestingly, 20 % of patients in the postoperative radiotherapy group and 30 % of patients in the no-postoperative-radiotherapy group were aged over 70 years. Results indicate that postoperative radiotherapy was associated with increased heart disease-related mortality (HR = 1.30; 95 % CI, 1.04–1.61; $p = 0.0193$). Age was identified at multivariate analysis as being associated with an even higher risk of toxicity (HR = 1.05; 95 % CI, 1.04–1.07; $p < 0.001$). It is nowadays unclear whether dosimetric constraints should be adapted when treating elderly patients in a postoperative setting, for which tissue constraints do usually not represent a significant issue given the modest doses – 50–54 Gy – delivered [27–29].

As recommended by geriatric oncology groups, elderly patients should undergo systematic geriatric assessment before determining the optimal therapeutic strategy, including discussion of surgery and radiotherapy [30]. Regarding postoperative radiotherapy, our recommendation would be to evaluate the usefulness of such assessment after surgery before postoperative treatment strategy is determined, to provide with criteria that may help to better select elderly patient who may benefit from postoperative radiotherapy.

To conclude, as for the global population of NSCLC patients, the role of postoperative radiotherapy after complete resection of early-stage NSCLC in elderly patients is yet to be determined. Data suggesting a potential role for stage IIIA-N2 tumors in the general population may not be applicable to the treatment of elderly patients. In this subset of patients, the role of surgery is actually debated as well, and definitive chemoradiation may represent an alternative as well as induction chemotherapy that offers the advantage to provide with a window of observation that would help to better select these patients for subsequent treatment [31, 32].

Elderly patients are eligible for the ongoing LungART trial (NCT00410683), an international multicenter study that randomly evaluates the delivery of postoperative radiotherapy after complete resection of stage IIIA-N2 NSCLC. The trial aims at including 700+ patients, with no upper age limit, to have an 80 % power to detect a 10 % improvement – from 30 to 40 % – in 3-year recurrence-free survival. This promising trial will be the first to include modern radiotherapy techniques with strict quality control, allowing a reevaluation of postoperative radiotherapy not only in the general population but also in elderly patients.

Overall, the management of elderly patients with postoperative radiotherapy after NSCLC surgical resection remains challenging and represents a typical clinical situation for which multidisciplinary consensus between radiation oncologists, medical oncologists, surgeons, and geriatrists is mandatory to determine the optimal strategy that will provide patients with survival and quality of life benefit.

References

1. Goldstraw P, Crowley J, Chansky K, International Association for the Study of Lung Cancer International Staging Committee; Participating Institutions, et al. The IASLC Lung Cancer Staging Project: proposals for the revision of the TNM stage groupings in the forthcoming (seventh) edition of the TNM Classification of malignant tumours. J Thorac Oncol. 2007; 2:706–14.
2. Ettinger DS, Akerley W, Bepler G, NCCN Non-Small Cell Lung Cancer Panel Members, et al. Non-small cell lung cancer. J Natl Compr Canc Netw. 2010;8:740–801.
3. Crinò L, Weder W, van Meerbeeck J, ESMO Guidelines Working Group, et al. Early stage and locally advanced (non-metastatic) non-small-cell lung cancer: ESMO Clinical Practice Guidelines for diagnosis, treatment and follow-up. Ann Oncol. 2010;21S5:v103–15.

4. Marcus PM, Bergstralh EJ, Fagerstrom RM, et al. Lung cancer mortality in the Mayo Lung Project: impact of extended follow-up. J Natl Cancer Inst. 2000;92:1308–16.
5. Van Houtte P, Rocmans P, Smets P, et al. Postoperative radiation therapy in lung cancer: a controlled trial after resection of curative design. Int J Radiat Oncol Biol Phys. 1980;6:983–6.
6. The Lung Cancer Study Group. Effects of postoperative mediastinal radiation on completely resected stage II and stage III epidermoid cancer of the lung. N Engl J Med. 1986;315:1377–81.
7. Debevec M, Bitenc M, Vidmar S, et al. Postoperative radiotherapy for radically resected N2 non-small-cell lung cancer (NSCLC): randomised clinical study 1988–1992. Lung Cancer. 1996;14:99–107.
8. Stephens RJ, Girling DJ, Bleehen NM, et al. The role of post-operative radiotherapy in non-small-cell lung cancer: a multicentre randomised trial in patients with pathologically staged T1-2, N1-2, M0 disease. Medical Research Council Lung Cancer Working Party. Br J Cancer. 1996;74:632–9.
9. Lafitte JJ, Ribet ME, Prévost BM, et al. Postresection irradiation for T2 N0 M0 non-small cell carcinoma: a prospective, randomized study. Ann Thorac Surg. 1996;62:830–4.
10. Burdett S, Stewart L, PORT Meta-analysis Group. Postoperative radiotherapy in non-small-cell lung cancer: update of an individual patient data meta-analysis. Lung Cancer. 2005;47:81–3.
11. PORT Meta-analysis Trialists Group. Postoperative radiotherapy for non-small cell lung cancer. Cochrane Database Syst Rev. 2005;2:CD002142.
12. Pignon JP, Tribodet H, Scagliotti GV, LACE Collaborative Group, et al. Lung adjuvant cisplatin evaluation: a pooled analysis by the LACE Collaborative Group. J Clin Oncol. 2008;26:3552–9.
13. Lally BE, Zelterman D, Colasanto JM, et al. Postoperative radiotherapy for stage II or III non-small-cell lung cancer using the surveillance, epidemiology, and end results database. J Clin Oncol. 2006;24:2998–3006.
14. Bekelman JE, Rosenzweig KE, Bach PB, et al. Trends in the use of postoperative radiotherapy for resected non-small-cell lung cancer. Int J Radiat Oncol Biol Phys. 2006;66:492–9.
15. Sawyer TE, Bonner JA, Gould PM, et al. Effectiveness of postoperative irradiation in stage IIIA non-small cell lung cancer according to regression tree analyses of recurrence risks. Ann Thorac Surg. 1997;64:1402–7.
16. Machtay M, Lee JH, Shrager JB, et al. Risk of death from intercurrent disease is not excessively increased by modern postoperative radiotherapy for high-risk resected non-small-cell lung carcinoma. J Clin Oncol. 2001;19:3912–7.
17. Douillard JY, Rosell R, De Lena M, Adjuvant Navelbine International Trialist Association, et al. Impact of postoperative radiation therapy on survival in patients with complete resection and stage I, II, or IIIA non-small-cell lung cancer treated with adjuvant chemotherapy: the adjuvant Navelbine International Trialist Association (ANITA) Randomized Trial. Int J Radiat Oncol Biol Phys. 2008;72:695–701.
18. Wisnivesky JP, Halm EA, Bonomi M, et al. Postoperative radiotherapy for elderly patients with stage III lung cancer. Cancer. 2012;118(18):4478–85.
19. Pallis AG, Gridelli C, van Meerbeeck JP, et al. EORTC Elderly Task Force and Lung Cancer Group and International Society for Geriatric Oncology (SIOG) experts' opinion for the treatment of non-small-cell lung cancer in an elderly population. Ann Oncol. 2010;21:692–706.
20. Pisters KM, Evans WK, Azzoli CG, Cancer Care Ontario, American Society of Clinical Oncology, et al. Cancer Care Ontario and American Society of Clinical Oncology adjuvant chemotherapy and adjuvant radiation therapy for stages I-IIIA resectable non small-cell lung cancer guideline. J Clin Oncol. 2007;25:5506–18.
21. Okawara G, Ung YC, Markman BR, Lung Cancer Disease Site Group of Cancer Care Ontario's Program in Evidence-Based Care, et al. Postoperative radiotherapy in stage II or IIIA completely resected non-small cell lung cancer: a systematic review and practice guideline. Lung Cancer. 2004;44:1–11.

22. Koning CC, Aarts MJ, Struikmans H, et al. Mapping use of radiotherapy for patients with non-small cell lung cancer in the Netherlands between 1997 and 2008. Clin Oncol (R Coll Radiol). 2012;24:e46–53.
23. Gonzalez-Aragoneses F, Moreno-Mata N, Simon-Adiego C, et al. Lung cancer surgery in the elderly. Crit Rev Oncol Hematol. 2009;71:266–71.
24. Weinmann M, Jeremic B, Toomes H, et al. Treatment of lung cancer in the elderly. Part I: non-small cell lung cancer. Lung Cancer. 2003;39:233–53.
25. Blanchard EM, Arnaoutakis K, Hesketh PJ. Lung cancer in octogenarians. J Thorac Oncol. 2010;5:909–16.
26. Lally BE, Detterbeck FC, Geiger AM, et al. The risk of death from heart disease in patients with nonsmall cell lung cancer who receive postoperative radiotherapy: analysis of the Surveillance, Epidemiology, and End Results database. Cancer. 2007;110:911–7.
27. Balducci L, Cohen HJ, Engstrom PF, National Comprehensive Cancer Network, et al. Senior adult oncology clinical practice guidelines in oncology. J Natl Compr Canc Netw. 2005;3: 572–90.
28. Bayman N, Alam N, Faivre-Finn C. Radiotherapy for lung cancer in the elderly. Lung Cancer. 2010;68:129–36.
29. Emami B, Lyman J, Brown A, et al. Tolerance of normal tissue to therapeutic irradiation. Int J Radiat Oncol Biol Phys. 1991;21:109–22.
30. Maas HA, Janssen-Heijnen ML, Olde Rikkert MG, et al. Comprehensive geriatric assessment and its clinical impact in oncology. Eur J Cancer. 2007;43:2161–9.
31. van Meerbeeck JP, Kramer GW, European Organisation for Research and Treatment of Cancer-Lung Cancer Group, et al. Randomized controlled trial of resection versus radiotherapy after induction chemotherapy in stage IIIA-N2 non-small-cell lung cancer. J Natl Cancer Inst. 2007;99:442–50.
32. Albain KS, Swann RS, Rusch VW, et al. Radiotherapy plus chemotherapy with or without surgical resection for stage III non-small-cell lung cancer: a phase III randomised controlled trial. Lancet. 2009;374:379–86.

Chapter 10
Is There a Role for Neoadjuvant Chemotherapy in Older Patients?

Alejandro Navarro and Enriqueta Felip

Abstract No clinical trial specifically assesses the value of neoadjuvant chemotherapy directed to elderly population. Elderly patients with cancer often present with medical and physiological challenges, and it is crucial to carefully evaluate functional and psychological status in order to decide on the best approach. A multidisciplinary assessment is essential in the selection of elderly patients who may benefit from a more aggressive multimodality treatment which is at present reserved for younger patients.

Keywords Neoadjuvant chemotherapy in older patients • Chemotherapy in older patients • Lung cancer in older patients • Selection of elderly patients for neoadjuvant chemotherapy • Non-small lung cancer in the elderly

Lung cancer remains the leading cause of cancer-related mortality in most countries worldwide [1]. More than 80 % of all newly diagnosed cases of lung cancer are non-small cell lung cancer (NSCLC). The cornerstone of treatment for early-stage NSCLC is radical surgery. Unfortunately, the majority of patients present with locally advanced or metastatic disease at diagnosis, with only 15–20 % of tumors being resected, and even when this potentially curative approach is used, overall survival does not exceed 40 % at 5 years [2]. To improve this outcome, preoperative and postoperative approaches are needed. The potential role of chemotherapy in the adjuvant setting has been studied over the last two decades. The LACE meta-analysis provides evidence in favor of adjuvant cisplatin-based chemotherapy in patients with resected stage II and III disease, and, at present, adjuvant cisplatin-based chemotherapy is the standard of care in this group of patients [3]. Several randomized

A. Navarro, MD • E. Felip, MD, PhD (✉)
Oncology Department, Vall d'Hebron
University Hospital, Barcelona, Spain
e-mail: efelip@vhebron.net

C. Gridelli, R.A. Audisio (eds.), *Management of Lung Cancer in Older People*,
DOI 10.1007/978-0-85729-793-8_10, © Springer-Verlag London 2013

trials have analyzed the contribution made by neoadjuvant chemotherapy in patients with non-metastatic disease, but although its role is still considered controversial, neoadjuvant treatment is the preferred choice in stage IIIA-N2 patients [4].

The number of elderly patients diagnosed with lung cancer is substantial. The median age of lung cancer patients at diagnosis has been slowly increasing and is now aged 69 years; 47 % of patients are at least 70 years old at the time of diagnosis, and 14 % of cases occur in octagenerarians [5]. Approximately 70 % of lung cancer deaths in the USA occur in patients older than 65 years.

Unfortunately, elderly patients are generally excluded from clinical trials using chemotherapy, and the exact role of neoadjuvant treatment in the elderly population is yet to be established.

Neoadjuvant Randomized Trials in the General Population

Even when NSCLC is diagnosed at early stage, overall survival (OS) rates for patients tend to be poor. The need to improve survival rates in these patients prompted research exploring the role of systemic therapy in resectable NSCLC. In the 1990s, several trials were conducted to clarify the potential role of neoadjuvant chemotherapy followed by surgery or radiation in patients with stage III NSCLC.

Two small randomized trials comparing neoadjuvant platinum-based chemotherapy followed by surgery versus surgery alone in stage IIIA had an impact on clinical practice. Roth et al. evaluated the efficacy of three cycles of cisplatin/etoposide/cyclophosphamide followed by surgery versus surgery alone in patients with potentially resectable clinical stage IIIA [6, 7]. Additional three cycles of chemotherapy were administered after surgery to patients who achieved radiological response. Following an interim analysis, the trial was closed after a total of 60 patients were randomized because of survival benefit in favor of the neoadjuvant arm, resulting in a 64-month median survival versus 11 months for the surgery alone arm. However, after a median follow-up of 82 months, median OS was 21 and 14 months in the neoadjuvant and the surgery alone arms, respectively, without statistical significance.

Rosell et al. conducted a similar trial to evaluate the efficacy of three cycles of mitomycin/ifosfamide/cisplatin followed by surgery versus surgery alone in patients with clinical stages I to IIIA [8, 9]. Both arms received postoperative radiotherapy. The study was closed after recruitment of 60 patients when an interim analysis was performed. It showed survival benefit for the neoadjuvant arm with a median survival of 22 and 10 months, in favor of the neoadjuvant arm in comparison with the control arm. The poor outcome of patients treated with immediate surgery is worth mentioning here.

In 2001, Depierre et al. reported results from a phase III randomized trial to evaluate the efficacy of induction mitomycin/ifosfamide/cisplatin chemotherapy in resectable stages IB, II, and IIIA [10, 11]. A total of 355 patients were randomized to surgery alone or combined modality therapy consisting of two cycles of neoadjuvant chemotherapy followed by surgery and even two additional cycles of adjuvant chemotherapy for patients who achieved benefit from induction setting. Postoperative mortality was 7 % in the neoadjuvant chemotherapy arm and 5 % in the surgery alone arm ($p=0.38$). Median survival was 37 months in the neoadjuvant arm and 26 months in the surgery alone arm without statistically significant differences. An update of this study was reported at the ASCO meeting in 2010 [12]. With a median follow-up of 13.8 years, the 10-year survival rate was 20.8 % for the surgery alone arm and 29.4 % for the neoadjuvant arm ($p=0.12$). When a multivariate analysis was performed, neoadjuvant chemotherapy (HR=0.78, 95 % CI=0.61–0.99, $p=0.038$), age, and the T and N status significantly correlated with OS. The 10-year recurrence-free survival rate was 38.2 % in the surgery alone arm and 54.6 % in the neoadjuvant arm ($p=0.001$). The mortality rate from second primary cancer was 6.9 % in the surgery alone arm and 5 % in the neoadjuvant arm. In a subgroup analysis, the 10-year survival rate for patients with stage I and II disease was 23.1 % in the surgery alone arm and 37.6 % in the neoadjuvant arm ($p=0.04$), although there was no significant difference in survival for patients with stage IIIA. The authors concluded that although neoadjuvant chemotherapy did not significantly increase long-term survival, an 8 % survival benefit in favor of neoadjuvant chemotherapy remained stable beyond 10 years.

The Southwest Oncology Group (SWOG) trial S9900 was a phase III randomized trial designed to evaluate the efficacy of induction paclitaxel/carboplatin chemotherapy [13]. It was closed prematurely in 2004 after evidence in favor of adjuvant chemotherapy was observed. A total of 354 patients with clinical stage IB, II, and IIIA NSCLC (excluding superior sulcus and N2 disease) were included before closure of the study and randomly assigned to receive three cycles of chemotherapy followed by surgery or immediate surgery. Mediastinoscopy was performed whenever the mediastinal lymph node size exceeded 1 cm. Of the patients randomized to chemotherapy, 79 % completed three cycles of chemotherapy, and 41 % achieved radiographic response. Complete resection was possible in 94 % of patients in the neoadjuvant chemotherapy group versus 89 % in the control arm. With a median follow-up of 53 months, median survival was 75 versus 46 months, in favor of the neoadjuvant chemotherapy arm. Although the use of neoadjuvant chemotherapy was associated with a 19 % reduction in the risk of death, this difference was not statistically significant.

The European Intergroup trial MRC-LU 22 EORTC-08012 NVALT-2 included a total of 519 patients with resectable early-stage NSCLC who were randomized to either surgery alone or three cycles of platinum-based chemotherapy followed by surgery [14]. Choice of chemotherapy regimen and intensity of preoperative staging were performed according to the policy of each center. This trial was also prematurely closed because of slowing accrual. Of the patients randomized to chemotherapy, 75 % completed three cycles of chemotherapy, and 49 % had radiographic response. The rate of complete resection was similar in both groups, 81 % in the neoadjuvant arm versus 79 % in the control arm. With a median follow-up of 41 months, median survival was 54 versus 55 months, respectively.

In 2008, at the ASCO meeting, Berz et al. reported a study designed to determine whether using a dose-intense weekly paclitaxel (80 mg/m^2) in combination with carboplatin in the neoadjuvant setting would increase the pathologic complete response rate in patients with stage IB–IIIA NSCLC [15]. Twenty patients were enrolled, of whom 17 were stage IB, one was IIB, and two were IIIA. All patients completed the planned neoadjuvant treatment. Finally, 17 patients underwent complete resection, either lobectomy [14] or pneumonectomy [3], without significant postsurgical complications. The pathologic complete response rate by intent to treat was 16 %, and no patient progressed during neoadjuvant treatment.

In 2009, at the ASCO meeting, Westeel et al. reported data about IFCT 0002, a phase III study in resectable NSCLC comparing preoperative and perioperative chemotherapy approaches with two different regimens: gemcitabine/cisplatin and paclitaxel/carboplatin [16]. Between 2001 and 2005, 528 patients with a stage I–II NSCLC were randomized to four different arms. Ninety-day postoperative mortality was 4.9 % for the preoperative arms and 4.2 % for the perioperative arms. In an intent-to-treat analysis, 3-year survival was 67.8 and 68.6 %, respectively ($p=0.96$). Survival did not differ with the regimen used.

The NATCH study, a multicenter, phase III study, was designed to evaluate the potential role of neoadjuvant chemotherapy in resectable NSCLC in comparison to an adjuvant approach [17]. This study enrolled 624 patients with clinical early-stage (stage IA with tumor size >2 cm, IB, II, or T3N1) resectable NSCLC who were randomized to surgery alone versus neoadjuvant chemotherapy followed by surgery versus surgery followed by adjuvant chemotherapy. Patients in the neoadjuvant and adjuvant chemotherapy arms received three cycles of carboplatin/paclitaxel. The primary end point was 5-year disease-free survival (DFS). Median DFS was not significantly different among the three arms (28, 32, and 24 months in the surgery, neoadjuvant, and adjuvant arms, respectively). The 5-year DFS rate was also similar among the three groups, and no significant difference in median OS was observed. It is noteworthy that almost 50 % of the patients had stage I disease. The rate of resection, types of surgery, and postoperative mortality were similar across treatment groups. Ninety-seven percent of patients in the neoadjuvant arm, and 66 % of those in the adjuvant chemotherapy group received the planned three cycles. An exploratory analysis showed that the patients with clinical stage II and T3N1 disease derived the greatest benefit from neoadjuvant chemotherapy.

In the recently published CHEST trial, chemotherapy-naïve patients with stage IB, II, and IIIA NSCLC were randomized to surgery alone or neoadjuvant chemotherapy with cisplatin/gemcitabine followed by surgery [18]. This trial was closed earlier than planned with a total of 270 patients accrued, of which 55 % were stage IB/IIA. Response rate to neoadjuvant chemotherapy was 35 %. The results of this trial seem to favor the neoadjuvant arm for OS (HR = 0.63, CI = 0.43–0.92, $p=.02$). A statistically significant impact of neoadjuvant chemotherapy on outcomes was observed in the stage IIB/IIIA subgroup (3-year DFS rate = 36.1 % versus 55.4 %, $p=.002$). No evidence of treatment-by-histology interaction effect was reported.

Two meta-analyses from data of randomized trials in early-stage NSCLC are of interest. Berghmans et al. reported data from six randomized trials, published between 1990 and 2003, including 590 patients [19]. The addition of neoadjuvant chemotherapy to surgery was associated with a nonsignificant improvement in OS (HR=0.65, CI=0.41–1.04).

Burdett et al. examined data from seven randomized trials, published between 1990 and 2005, including 988 patients [20]. Neoadjuvant chemotherapy was found to improve survival (HR=0.82, CI=0.69–0.97), with an absolute benefit of 6 % at 5 years.

Finally, recently presented preliminary results from a systematic review and meta-analysis of individual patient data from 13 randomized trials reported that neoadjuvant chemotherapy was associated with an improvement in survival in operable patients with 5 % absolute benefit at 5 years (HR=0.88, p=0.025) [21].

Neoadjuvant Chemotherapy in Elderly Patients

Neoadjuvant chemotherapy is still considered an experimental modality of treatment in elderly NSCLC patients mainly because randomized trials, including those mentioned above, rarely include elderly patients. In current practice, the elderly are often deliberately excluded from participation in clinical trials in general and particularly from neoadjuvant trials. Furthermore, to our knowledge, there is no randomized trial of neoadjuvant chemotherapy specifically designed for this population. The underrepresentation of the elderly population is relevant because treatment recommendations for lung cancer are obtained from clinical trials. Clinical data obtained in a younger population cannot be automatically extrapolated to the great majority of nonselected elderly patients.

A retrospective analysis of all patients (not only those receiving neoadjuvant chemotherapy) enrolled in SWOG trials between 1993 and 1996 showed that only 25 % of patients were 65 years old or older, although this age group in fact represents 60 % of the total number of lung cancer patients [22].

At the 2001 ASCO meeting, Iacobelli et al. reported results of a small study designed to evaluate the tolerability and activity of the cisplatin/epirubicin/vinorelbine (PEV) regimen given preoperatively in patients with stage IIIAN2 NSCLC [23]. Patients received PEV for three cycles followed by thoracotomy. Of the 21 patients who entered the study, 15 of whom were 70 years or older, 18 were evaluable. The response rate in the whole patient population was 55 % and thoracotomy was conducted in 12 (66 %), nine of whom (75 %) achieved complete resection. Ten patients were alive at a median follow-up of 14 months. Of eight deaths, seven were from recurrent disease and one was unrelated. The authors supported the hypothesis that PEV could be a reasonable option for locally advanced NSCLC, particularly in elderly patients. However, the small sample size of the study does not allow us to draw clear conclusions.

Results of a study by D'Angelillo et al. reported at the 2004 ASCO meeting aimed to clarify the feasibility of multimodality treatment including surgery in elderly patients [24]. Patients were 65 years old or older, ECOG 0–1, with confirmed NSCLC and deemed unresectable for stage IIIA or IIIB disease or resectable only by a pneumonectomy. They were treated according to a combined chemotherapy-radiation protocol. Response rate to induction treatment was 72.6 %. Fifty-three patients were considered operable, and 37 (69.8 %) were radically resected. Median survival was 20.3 months for the whole study population and 30.4 months for patients who underwent surgical resection. According to the multivariate analysis, surgery was the major statistically influencing parameter for survival. The authors concluded that elderly patients with good performance status and without comorbidities should be considered for multimodality treatment.

In the absence of phase II–III data of neoadjuvant chemotherapy in elderly population, treatment decisions should be made according to each individual patient's characteristics and clinical condition. Discussion by tumor committee members of the management of each case is the best approach for all patients and particularly for elderly patients.

Selection of Elderly Patients for Neoadjuvant Treatment

Major frequency of multiple comorbidities and physiologic organ failure mean that the elderly tolerate chemotherapy worse than their younger counterparts. The prevalence of comorbid conditions in the elderly population is approximately twice as high as in the general population [25]. The most significant coexisting pathologies for patients with lung cancer are cardiovascular and pulmonary diseases, which are common among long-term cigarette smokers.

In the elderly there are physiologic changes such as increased body fat, less total body water and reduced renal and hepatic function reserves, and the decline in the glomerular filtration rate can reduce the excretion rate of commonly employed cytotoxic therapies [26].

These factors may have pharmacokinetic implications for drug disposition that lead to pharmacodynamic consequences. There is also an increased likelihood of drug-drug interactions and treatment-related toxicities in the elderly, who often need several other medications.

Moreover, presence of a geriatric syndrome is common, in which most functional reserve is exhausted. Generally, for these NSCLC patients, chemotherapy should be avoided. To plan treatment of such patients, a multidimensional geriatric evaluation including not only comorbidity assessment but also functional, nutritional, and mental status is required [27, 28].

The main clinical data on chemotherapy for elderly patients with NSCLC come from advanced disease, the most frequent presentation at diagnosis. Phase II and III trials specifically designed for elderly patients suggest that single-agent chemotherapy with third-generation agents may be considered the standard treatment in this population [29–43].

The study recently published by Quoix et al. evaluating the potential benefit of doublet chemotherapy over single-agent in elderly patient with advanced NSCLC reported a significant benefit in median OS and 1-year OS for those patients treated with a doublet combination [43]. Median overall survival was 10.3 months for doublet chemotherapy and 6.2 months for monotherapy (HR=0.64, CI=0.52–0.78, $p<.0001$); 1-year survival rates were 44.5 and 25.4 %, respectively. As expected, more toxicity was observed in the doublet combination arm. As a result of these findings, a doublet platinum combination emerged as a good treatment approach to the elderly patient with good ECOG PS and functional reserve and without relevant medical comorbidities.

According to the recent ASCO recommendations, there is no evidence to support the use of a specific first-line chemotherapy drug or combination based on age alone [44]. Older patients may experience more toxicity from cytotoxic chemotherapy than younger patients but may garner an equal amount of benefit. However, the benefit is largely limited to patients with good ECOG PS (0–1) and is less clear in patients with an ECOG PS of 2.

At the 2010 ESMO Consensus Conference in lung cancer, the experts agreed that platinum-based chemotherapy is preferred in fit elderly patients with ECOG PS 0–1 and adequate organ function and single-agent third-generation drugs are preferred in unfit elderly patients [45].

Postoperative Potential Complications in Elderly Patients

Concerns regarding increased postoperative morbidity and mortality result in a reluctance to offer curative surgery for very elderly patients with early-stage disease. One of the main issues in the treatment of the elderly population is how the aggressive combined modality approach affects patients' quality of life after the completion of treatment.

In 2009, Rivera et al. published a study with the aim to evaluate the impact of neoadjuvant chemotherapy on pulmonary function tests in resectable early-stage NSCLC [46]. It was seen that in the preoperative setting, the administration of neoadjuvant chemotherapy was safe in regard to lung toxicity, with DLCO being the most commonly affected pulmonary function test parameter following chemotherapy. It is crucial, in patients treated with neoadjuvant chemotherapy, to repeat pulmonary function tests, including DLCO, after chemotherapy treatment and before surgery.

A recent published case–control study was performed by French investigators to compare postoperative morbidity of patients over 75 years old who received neoadjuvant chemotherapy with that of younger ones [47]. Data from 1,510 patients were prospectively obtained from January 2005 to December 2009. Only 81 patients were older than 75 years. To compare patients with similar characteristics, they were matched according to gender, American Society of Anesthesia (ASA) score, ECOG PS, FEV1, and histological subtype of the tumor. Surgical treatment, postoperative morbidity, mortality rates, and length of stay were compared. No significant difference in surgical procedure was observed between the two groups ($p=0.07$); pneumonectomy was performed in 15 % ($n=12$) of patients aged 75 years or over in comparison to 28 % ($n=23$) in younger patients and lobectomy in 65 % ($n=53$) versus 54 % ($n=44$), respectively. There was no difference in the extension of mediastinal lymphadenectomy between the groups.

Elderly patients had more postoperative complications ($p = 0.04$), and they were more severe. However, there was no significant difference in postoperative mortality at 30, 60, and 90 days between the study groups. Finally, length of in-hospital stay was longer in the elderly group (14.9 days versus 11.9 days, $p < 0.001$).

Summary

No clinical trial specifically assesses the value of neoadjuvant chemotherapy directed to elderly population. Elderly patients with cancer often present with medical and physiological challenges, and it is crucial to carefully evaluate functional and psychological status in order to decide on the best approach. A multidisciplinary assessment is essential in the selection of elderly patients who may benefit from a more aggressive multimodality treatment which is at present reserved for younger patients.

References

1. Jemal A, Siegel R, Ward E, et al. Cancer statistics, 2009. CA Cancer J Clin. 2009;59:225–49.
2. Nesbitt JC, Putnam Jr JB, Walsh GL, et al. Survival in early-stage non-small cell lung cancer. Ann Thorac Surg. 1995;60:466–72.
3. Pignon JP, Tribodet H, Scagliotti GV, et al. Lung adjuvant cisplatin evaluation (LACE): a pooled analysis by the LACE Collaborative Group. J Clin Oncol. 2008;26:3552–9.
4. Crino L, Weder W, Meerbeeck JV, Felip E. Early stage and locally advanced (non-metastatic) non-small-cell lung cancer: ESMO Clinical Practice Guidelines for diagnosis, treatment and follow-up. Ann Oncol. 2010;21(Supplement 5):v103–15.
5. Owonikoko TK, Ragin CC, Belani CP, et al. Lung cancer in elderly patients: an analysis of the Surveillance, Epidemiology, and End Results Database. J Clin Oncol. 2007;25:5570–7.
6. Roth JA, Fosella F, Komaki R, et al. A randomized trial comparing perioperative chemotherapy and surgery with surgery alone in resectable stage IIIa non-small cell lung cancer. J Natl Cancer Inst. 1994;86:673–80.
7. Roth JA, Atkinson EN, Fossella T, et al. Long-term follow-up of patients enrolled in a randomized trial comparing perioperative chemotherapy and surgery with surgery alone in resectable stage IIIA non-small-cell lung cancer. Lung Cancer. 1998;21:1–6.
8. Rosell R, Gomez-Codina J, Camps C, et al. A randomized trial comparing preoperative chemotherapy plus surgery with surgery alone in patients with non-small-cell lung cancer. N Engl J Med. 1994;330:153–8.
9. Rosell R, Gomez-Codina J, Camps C, et al. Preresectional chemotherapy in stage IIIA non-small-cell lung cancer: a 7-year assessment of a randomized controlled trial. Lung Cancer. 1999;26:7–14.
10. Depierre A, Milleron B, Moro-Sibilot D, et al. Pre-operative chemotherapy followed by surgery compared with primary surgery in resectable stage I (except T1N0), II and IIIA non-small cell lung cancer. J Clin Oncol. 2002;20:247–53.
11. Depierre A, Westeel V, Milleron B, et al. 5 year results of the French randomized study comparing preoperative chemotherapy followed by surgery and primary surgery in resectable stage I (except T1N0), II and IIIA non-small cell lung cancer. Lung Cancer. 2003;41 Suppl 2:S62. Journal article/abstract.

12. Westeel V, Milleron BJ, Quoix EA, et al, on behalf of the Intergroupe Francophone de Cancerologie Thoracique. Long-term results of the French randomized trial comparing neoadjuvant chemotherapy followed by surgery versus surgery alone in resectable non-small cell lung cancer (Abstract 7003). J Clin Oncol. 2010;28 (15 May 20 Suppl).
13. Pisters KMW, Vallieres E, Crowley JJ, et al. Surgery with or without preoperative paclitaxel and carboplatin in early-stage non-small-cell lung cancer: Southwest Oncology Group Trial S9900, an intergroup, randomized, phase III trial. J Clin Oncol. 2010;28:1843–9.
14. Gilligan D, Nicolson M, Smith I, et al. On behalf of the trial collaborators. Preoperative chemotherapy in patients with resectable non-small cell lung cancer: results of the MRC LU22/NVALT 2/EORTC 08012 multicentre randomised trial and update of systematic review. Lancet. 2007;369:1929–37.
15. Berz D, Birbbaum A, Dipetrillo TA, et al. Neoadjuvant carboplatin and weekly paclitaxel in stage Ib-III non-small cell lung cancer (NSCLC): a Brown University Oncology Group (BrUOG) phase II study. J Clin Oncol, 2008 ASCO Annual Meeting Proceedings (Post-Meeting Edition). Vol 26, No 15S (May 20 Supplement), 2008: 18502.
16. Westeel V, Milleron B, Quoix E, et al. Results of the IFCT 0002 phase III study comparing a preoperative and a perioperative chemotherapy (CT) with two different CT regimens in resectable non-small cell lung cancer (NSCLC). J Clin Oncol, 2009 ASCO Annual Meeting Proceedings (Post-Meeting Edition).Vol 27, No 15S (May 20 Supplement), 2009: 7530.
17. Felip E, Rosell R, Maestre JA, et al. Preoperative chemotherapy plus surgery versus surgery plus adjuvant chemotherapy versus surgery alone in early-stage non-small cell lung cancer. J Clin Oncol. 2010;28:3138–45.
18. Scagliotti GV, Pastorino U, Vansteenkiste JF, et al. Randomized phase III study of surgery alone or surgery plus preoperative cisplatin and gemcitabine in stages IB to IIIA non-small cell lung cancer. J Clin Oncol. 2012;30:172–8.
19. Berghmans T, Paesmans M, Meert AP, et al. Survival improvement in resectable non-small cell lung cancer with (neo)adjuvant chemotherapy: results of a meta-analysis of the literature. Lung Cancer. 2005;49:13–23.
20. Burdett S, Stewart L, Rydzewska L, et al. A systematic review and meta-analysis of the literature: chemotherapy and surgery versus surgery alone in non-small cell lung cancer. J Thorac Oncol. 2006;1:611–21.
21. Burdett S, Rydzewska LH, Tierney JF, Pignon JP. Pre-operative chemotherapy improves survival and reduces recurrence in operable non-small cell lung cancer: preliminary results of a systematic review and meta-analysis of individual patient data from 13 randomised trials. J Thor Oncol. 2011;6(Suppl 2):374–375.
22. Hutchins LF, Unger JM, Crowley JJ, et al. Underrepresentation of patients 65 years of age or older in cancer-treatment trials. N Engl J Med. 1999;341:2061–7.
23. Iacobelli S, Irtelli L, Martino MT. Neoadjuvant chemotherapy for surgically staged IIIAN2 Non-Small Cell Lung Cancer (NSCLC) in the elderly. Proc Am Soc Clin Oncol 20: 2001 (abstr 2725).
24. D´Angelillo RM, Trodella L, Ramella S, et al. Neoadjuvant chemoradiotherapy followed by surgery in elderly patients with locally advanced non-small cell lung cancer: analysis of feasibility, toxicity and factors predicting surgical resection and survival. J Clin Oncol 2004 ASCO Annual Meeting Proceedings (Post-Meeting Edition). Vol 22, No 14S (July 15 Supplement), 2004: 7167.
25. Janssen-Heijnen MLG, Schipper RM, Razenberg PPA, et al. Prevalence of co-morbidity in lung cancer patients and its relationship with treatment: a population-based study. Lung Cancer. 1998;21:105–13.
26. Christensen K, Doblhammer G, Rau R, Vaupel JW. Ageing populations: the challenges ahead. Lancet. 2009;374:1196–208.
27. Tammemagi CM, Nulurd-Dudos C, Simoff L, et al. Impact of comorbidity on lung cancer survival. Int J Cancer. 2003;103:792–802.
28. Pal SK, Katheria V, Hurria A. Evaluating the older patient with cancer: understanding frailty and the geriatric assessment. CA Cancer J Clin. 2010;60:120–32.

29. Davidoff AJ, Tang M, Seal B, et al. Chemotherapy and survival benefit in elderly patients with advanced non-small cell lung cancer. J Clin Oncol. 2010;28:2191–7.
30. Gridelli C, Maione P, Rossi A, et al. Treatment of advanced non-small cell lung cancer in the elderly. Lung Cancer. 2009;66:282–6.
31. Elderly Lung Cancer Vinorelbine Italian Study (ELVIS) Group. Effects of vinorelbine on quality of life and survival of elderly patients with advanced non-small-cell lung cancer. J Natl Cancer Inst. 1999;91:66–72.
32. Gridelli C, Cigolari S, Gallo C, et al. Activity and toxicity of gemcitabine and gemcitabine - vinorelbine in advanced non-small-cell lung cancer elderly patients. Phase II data from the Multicenter Italian Lung Cancer in the Elderly Study (MILES) randomized trial. Lung Cancer. 2001;31:277–84.
33. Fidias P, Supko JG, Martins R, et al. A phase II study of weekly paclitaxel in elderly patients with advanced non-small cell lung cancer. Clin Cancer Res. 2001;7:3942–9.
34. Kudoh S, Takeda K, Nakagawa K, et al. Phase III study of docetaxel compared with vinorelbine in elderly patients with advanced non-small cell lung cancer: results of the West Japan Thoracic Oncology Group Trial (WJTOG 9904). J Clin Oncol. 2006;24:3657–63.
35. Gridelli C, Perrone F, Gallo C, et al. Chemotherapy for elderly patients with advanced non-small-cell lung cancer: the Multicenter Italian Lung cancer in the Elderly Study (MILES) phase III randomized trial. J Natl Cancer Inst. 2003;95:362–72.
36. Feliu J, Martin G, Madronal C, et al. Combination of low-dose cisplatin and gemcitabine for treatment of elderly patients with advanced non-small cell lung cancer. Cancer Chemother Pharmacol. 2003;52:247–52.
37. Ohe Y, Niho S, Kakinuma R, et al. A phase II study of cisplatin and docetaxel administered as three consecutive weekly infusions for advanced non-small-cell lung cancer in elderly patients. Ann Oncol. 2004;15:45–50.
38. Gridelli C, Maione P, Illiano A, et al. Cisplatin plus gemcitabine or vinorelbine for elderly patients with advanced non small-cell lung cancer: the MILES-2P studies. J Clin Oncol. 2007;25:4663–9.
39. Crino L, Cappuzzo F, Zatloukal P, et al. Gefitinib versus vinorelbine in chemotherapy-naive elderly patients with advanced non-small-cell lung cancer (INVITE): a randomized, phase II study. J Clin Oncol. 2008;26:4253–60.
40. Gridelli C, Morabito A, Gebbia V, et al. Cetuximab and gemcitabine in elderly or adult PS2 patients with advanced non-small-cell lung cancer: The cetuximab in advanced lung cancer (CALC1-E and CALC1-PS2) randomised phase II trials. Lung Cancer 67: 86–92.
41. Gridelli C, Rossi A, Mongillo F, et al. A randomized phase II study of sorafenib/gemcitabine or sorafenib/erlotinib for advanced non-small-cell lung cancer in elderly patients or patients with a performance status of 2: treatment rationale and protocol dynamics. Clin Lung Cancer. 2007;8:396–8.
42. Ramalingam S, Perry MC, La Rocca RV, et al. Comparison of outcomes for elderly patients treated with weekly paclitaxel in combination with carboplatin versus the standard 3-weekly paclitaxel and carboplatin for advanced non-small cell lung cancer. Cancer. 2008;113:542–6.
43. Quoix E, Zalcman G, Oster JP, et al. Carboplatin and weekly paclitaxel doublet chemotherapy compared with monotherapy in elderly patients with advanced non-small-cell lung cancer: IFCT-0501 randomised, phase 3 trial. Lancet. 2011;378:1079–88.
44. Azzoli CG, Temin S, Aliff T, et al. Focused update of 2009 American Society of Clinical Oncology Clinical Practice Guideline update on chemotherapy for stage IV non-small-cell lung cancer. J Clin Oncol. 2011;29:3825–31.
45. Felip E, Gridelli C, Baas P, et al. Metastatic non-small-cell lung cancer: consensus on pathology and molecular tests, first-line, second-line, and third-line therapy: 1st ESMO Consensus Conference in Lung Cancer; Lugano 2010. Ann Oncol. 2011;22:1507–19.
46. Rivera MP, Detterbeck F, Socinski M, et al. Impact of preoperative chemotherapy on pulmonary function tests in resectable early-stage non-small cell lung cancer. Chest. 2009;135:1588–95.
47. Rivera C, Jougon J, Dahan M, et al. Are postoperative consequences of neoadjuvant chemotherapy for non-small cell lung cancer more severe in elderly patients? Lung Cancer. 2012;76(2):216–21.

Chapter 11
Curative Radiotherapy in Patients Inoperable for Medical Reasons

Naomi E. Verstegen and Suresh Senan

Abstract Due to changing demographics, increasing numbers of elderly patients are being diagnosed with an early-stage non-small cell lung cancer. These patients may be difficult to treat due to coexistent illnesses and poor performance. Stereotactic radiotherapy is a new and promising treatment option, particularly in the frail elderly. However, the high local control rates and favorable toxicity profile make it also an increasingly attractive treatment for patients who are at increased risk for operative mortality.

Keywords Curative radiotherapy in the elderly • Radiotherapy in the elderly • Radiotherapy in inoperable patients

Epidemiology

Lung cancer is a leading cause of cancer-related death in both men and women in Western countries [1]. Although incidence rates are stable or falling in many Western countries, the growing proportion of the elderly in the population has resulted in an overall increase in the number of elderly lung cancer patients [2]. In the USA, for example, more than two thirds of all patients diagnosed with lung cancer are older than 65 years, with the median age at diagnosis exceeding 70 years [3].

Approximately 80 % of lung cancers can be classified as non-small cell lung subtype, and about 20 % of elderly patients diagnosed with NSCLC present with early-stage disease (stages I–II) [4, 5]. Between 25 and 40 % of elderly patients with stage I and II disease do not undergo a curative treatment [4, 6, 7]. Reasons for the latter include the fact that nearly 70 % of elderly patients diagnosed with lung cancer have significant comorbidities, and concerns about comorbidity, frailty, or

N.E. Verstegen, BSc (✉) • S. Senan, PhD, FRCR, MRCP
Department of Radiation Oncology, VU University Medical Center, Amsterdam, The Netherlands
e-mail: n.verstegen@vumc.nl

C. Gridelli, R.A. Audisio (eds.), *Management of Lung Cancer in Older People*,
DOI 10.1007/978-0-85729-793-8_11, © Springer-Verlag London 2013

efficacy result in the elderly being less likely to receive protocol-specified treatment [2, 4, 8–10]. A lack of evidence-based decision making in elderly patients is also due to the fact that they are less likely participate in clinical trials [11, 12].

Current guidelines recommend surgical resection as standard treatment in early-stage NSCLC [13–15]. When guidelines assessing a patient's fitness to undergo surgery are applied, up to 20 % of patients with early-stage NSCLC are considered medically inoperable [4, 16]. Common reasons for inoperability include a poor lung function, cardiovascular comorbidity as assessed by the American College of Cardiology guidelines, low American Society of Anesthesiologists score, and low general performance as assessed, for example, by using the WHO performance score [13, 15]. As untreated early-stage NSCLC has a 5-year survival of 2 %, alternative curative treatments should be considered in patients who are ineligible for surgery or refuse it [17].

Conventional Radiotherapy

Until recently, conventional radiotherapy has been considered as treatment of choice only for patients either who are medically inoperable or who had refused surgery [14]. Modest improvements in survival are achieved using conventional radiotherapy, when compared with patients who receive no treatment [18]. An analysis of 6,065 patients with histologically confirmed unresected stage I–II NSCLC diagnosed between 1992 and 2002 revealed a median overall survival after radiotherapy of 13 months (95 % confidence interval (CI) of 13–14 months) versus 7 months (95 % CI 6–8 months) in untreated patients [19]. No differences in either acute or late radiation toxicity were observed between patients aged older or younger than 70 years [20]. However, delivery of high radiation doses using conventional techniques may carry the risk of more severe side effects [21].

Stereotactic Radiotherapy

In recent years, stereotactic ablative radiotherapy (SABR or SBRT) has emerged as a highly effective new treatment modality for patients who are unfit for surgery or who refuse surgery. Modern lung SABR is characterized by 4D imaging to account for individual tumor motion, accurate image-guided setup prior to and during each treatment fraction, and treatment delivery times of 10 min or less, depending on equipment used [22] (Fig. 11.1). No randomized clinical trials comparing conventional radiotherapy and SABR have yet been reported. However, a meta-analysis of studies in early-stage NSCLC reported significantly higher 5-year overall survivals after SABR, compared with conventional radiotherapy (42 % vs. 20 % respectively). Disease-specific survival 2 years after treatment was 67 % for conventional radiotherapy versus 83 % for SABR [23]. The lower overall survival in nonsurgically

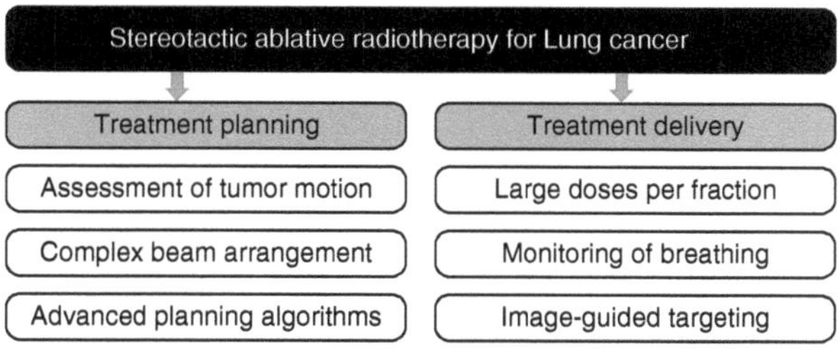

Fig. 11.1 Features of SABR (Courtesy of David Palma, MD, PhD, London, Ontario, Canada)

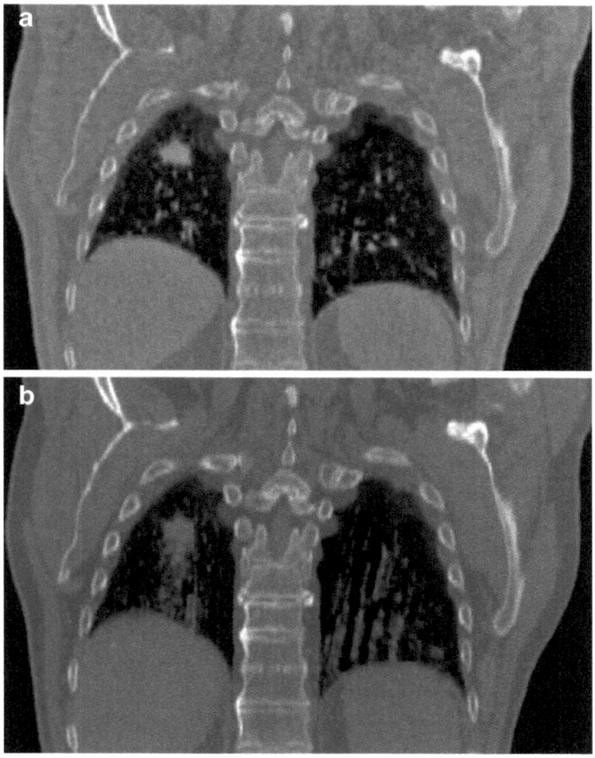

Fig. 11.2 (**a**) 4D CT scan study showing the position of a tumor in the *right upper* lobe in a single phase of the respiratory cycle. (**b**) The corresponding reconstructed image showing tumor position in all positions of the respiratory cycle illustrated in a maximum intensity projection

treated patients reflects the fact that non-cancer-related deaths are very common in such patients [16].

The total doses used in lung SABR are typically between 50 and 60 Gy, and treatment is delivered in 3–8 fractions [22, 24]. Planning target volumes are currently derived using 4-dimensional CT scans [25] (Fig. 11.2). In order to ensure treatment accuracy, patients are comfortably positioned and monitored during SABR. At some centers, techniques to manage tumor motion, such as abdominal compression, respiratory gating, breath holding, or tumor tracking systems, are also applied. However, there is no evidence to suggest that patient fixation or active management of tumor motion leads to improved tumor control. Sophisticated image devices, either present in the treatment room or mounted on-board modern linear

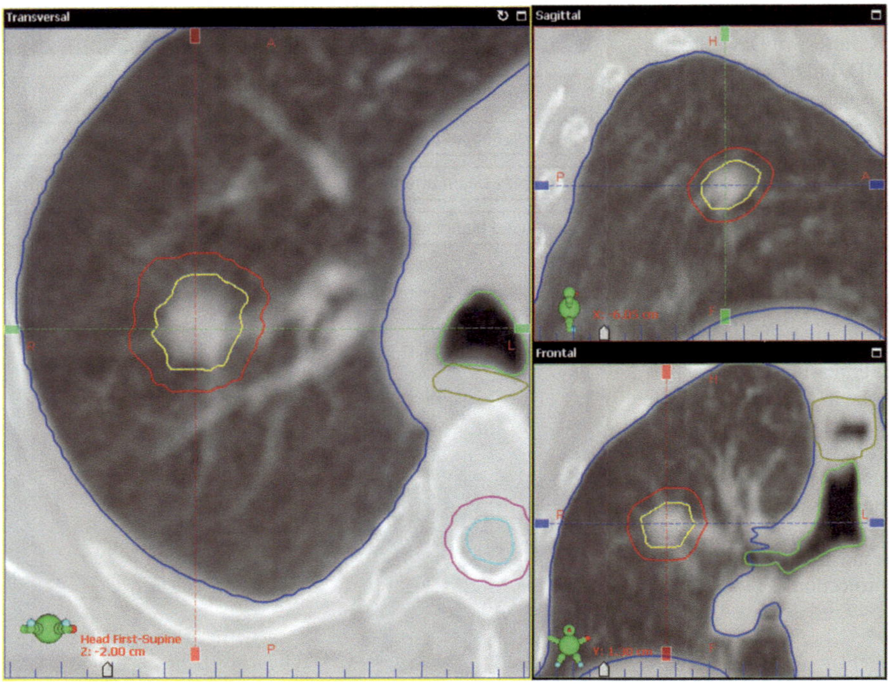

Fig. 11.3 Images of a small lung tumor as seen in all three axes of a planning CT scan. The yellow contour represents tumor position in all phases of the respiratory cycle and the red contour a planning target volume that incorporates an additional "safety" margin of 5 mm

accelerators, allow verification of the tumor position prior to daily treatment [22, 26]. At present, cone-beam computed tomography scans that are acquired just before SABR delivery are a widely used approach for ensuring accurate delivery (Figs. 11.3 and 11.4).

A drawback of some techniques used for SABR delivery is the long treatment durations of up to 1.5 h [27]. Elderly patients, in particular, might better tolerate delivery using volumetric-intensity-modulated arc therapy, which takes less than 7 min at present [28].

The dose fractionation schedules used can vary depending on tumor size and location, and a minimal biologically effective dose (BED) of 100 Gy is considered necessary for optimal local control [22, 24, 29]. Commonly, a more fractionated scheme is used for tumors in close proximity to critical structures such as the mediastinum, chest wall, hilus, or heart. Limiting the volume of irradiation to adjacent normal structures reduces the risk of toxicity. For example, limiting volumes of the chest wall receiving 30 Gy or more can decrease the risk of rib fractures posttreatment [30]. Other critical organs include the bronchial plexus and esophagus, and dose constraints have been recommended for such structures [31].

Local control at 3 years after SABR ranges from 80 to 95 % [29, 32–34], control rates which are much higher than generally reported after conventional

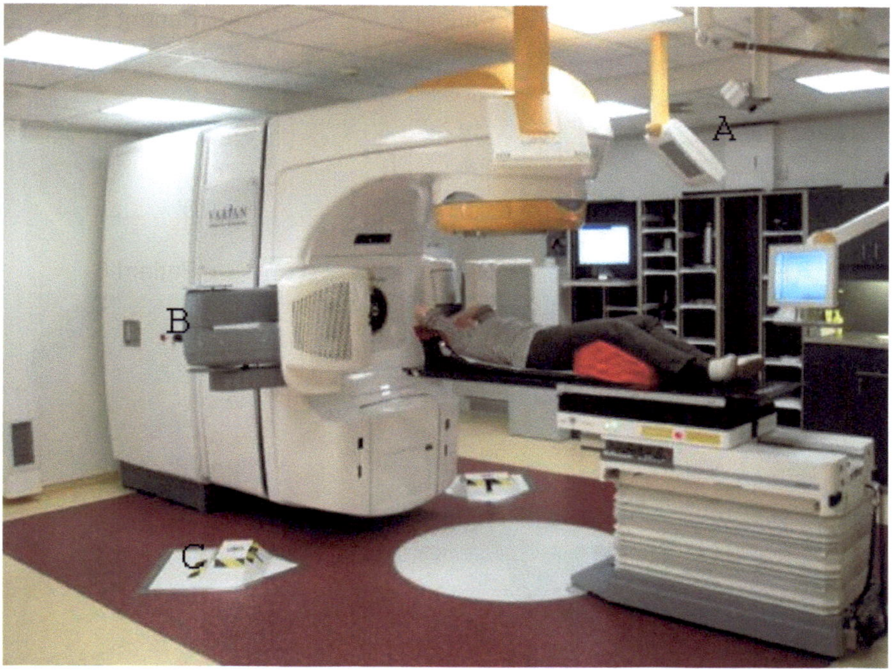

Fig. 11.4 Patient positioned at a linear accelerator (or treatment unit). Adjustable armrests, neck cushion, and mattress ensure patient comfort. Imaging detector panels mounted on the ceiling (*A*) and X-rays sources in the floor (*B*) allow for real-time kilovoltage imaging. A retractable cone-beam CT scan (*C*) allows for volumetric images to be acquired

radiotherapy. These local control rates are also similar to those reported after surgery [35–37]. However, despite high local control rates, patients do remain at risk of recurrence due to systemic relapse. As has been reported in the surgical literature, distant metastases are the main site of recurrences after SABR, occurring in approximately 20 % of patients [29, 32, 33, 38]. Regional recurrences following SABR are observed in less than 10 % of patients [29, 32, 38–40].

Acute and Late Toxicity

Acute toxicity in SABR is usually mild, with the majority of patients not experiencing any adverse effects. Common complaints after SABR are chest wall pain, skin reactions, esophagitis, and general malaise, such as fatigue or dyspnea [24, 29]. Late toxicity usually arises 3–6 months after treatment. Common manifestations include radiation pneumonitis, chest pain, and rib fractures. Severe (grade ≥3 CTCAE) toxicity is uncommon and seldom seen in more than 10 % of treated patients [24, 29]. These low rates of toxicity are similar in both younger and elderly patients [41].

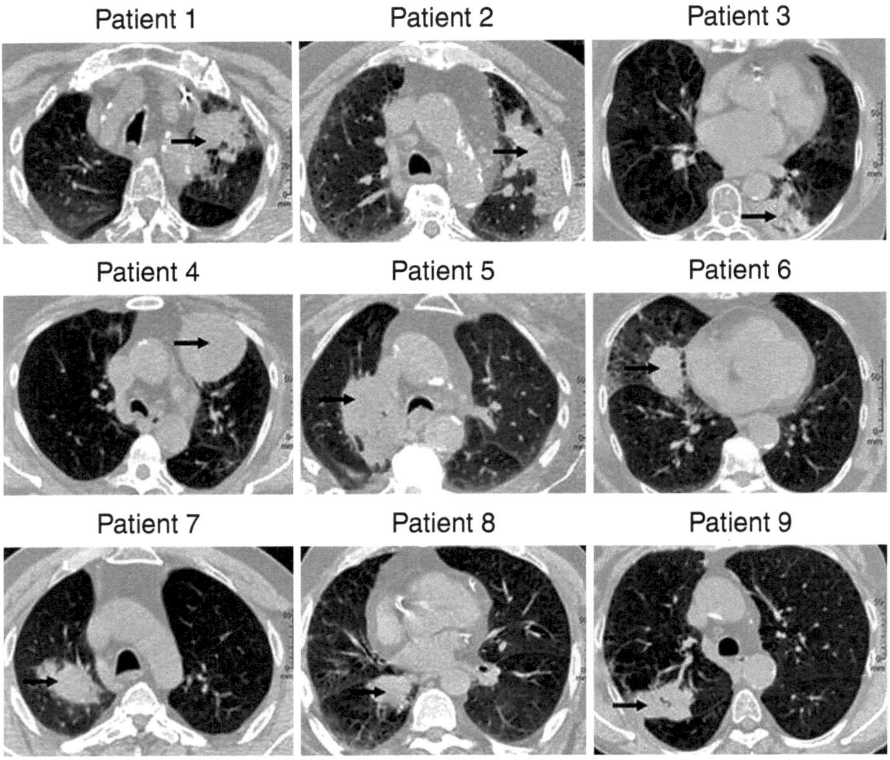

Fig. 11.5 Examples of central lung tumors that are currently being treated outside study protocols using a risk-adapted SABR fractionation scheme delivered in 8 fractions of 7.5 Gy (From Ong et al. [50]. With permission of Elsevier)

SABR is a safe and effective treatment alternative for patients with severe COPD and even in elderly patients with severe COPD [41, 42]. In patients with poor lung function, a systematic review of the literature revealed SABR to have comparable outcomes to surgery [43]. Cause-specific survival after SABR ranges between 67 and 88 % at 3 years posttreatment [32, 33, 39, 44, 45]. However, SABR is commonly performed in patients who are medically inoperable due to extensive comorbidities, and many patients die from other causes than lung cancer. Consequently, overall survival rates usually range between 36 and 70 %, but it can be as high as 90 % [32, 38, 44–46]. An early study on SABR for centrally located tumors, which used high fraction doses typically administered to peripheral lesions, reported high incidences of severe treatment-related toxicity [47]. However, other authors have performed SABR for central lesions using lower doses per fraction, and results indicate this to be a safe and effective approach [48, 49] (Fig. 11.5).

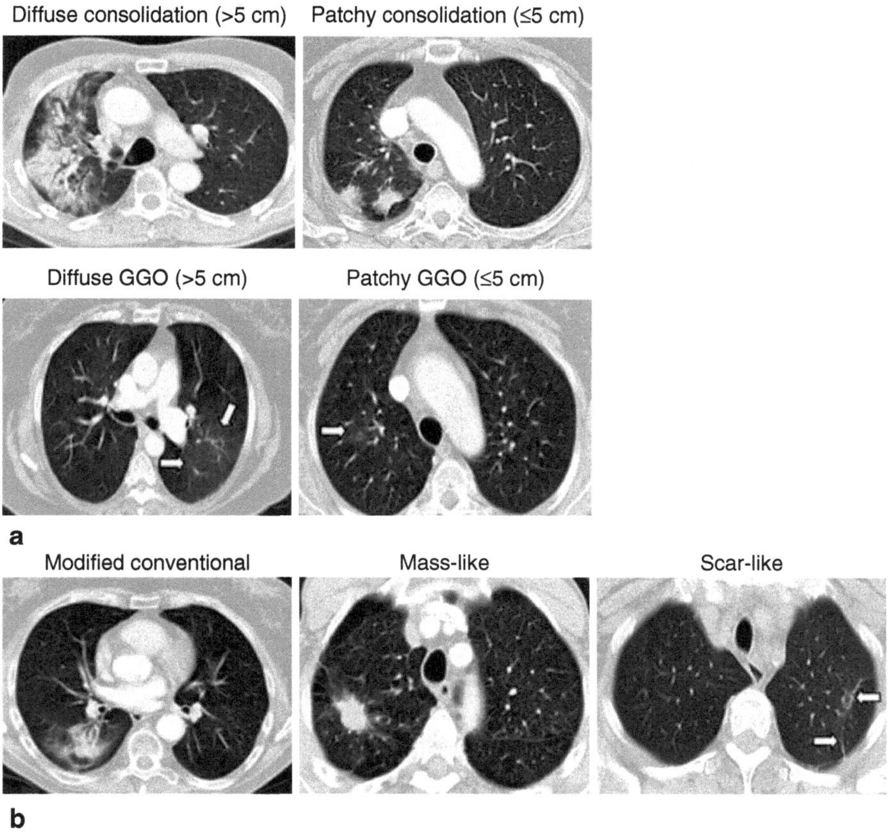

Fig. 11.6 Classification of radiological changes after SABR. (**a**) Acute radiological pneumonitis within 6 months of treatment. (**b**) Late radiological fibrosis after more than 6 months from the time of treatment (From Dahele et al. [52]. With permission Wolters Kluwer)

Care should be paid to restricting doses to critical adjacent structures [48, 51], and optimal SABR schemes for use in central tumors remain under investigation (RTOG 0813 NCT013170560).

Radiation-induced changes in lung parenchyma are common, making it important to distinguish benign fibrosis from disease progression, in order to minimize the risk of invasive diagnostic procedures or inappropriate salvage therapy [52] (Fig. 11.6). Response evaluation using the RECIST criteria may be inappropriate after SABR due to the frequent presence of extensive fibrosis in the high-dose area [53]. Furthermore, moderate to intense FDG uptake observed shortly after SABR is also not a good indicator of residual tumor [54]. Consequently, the evaluation of such radiological findings can be challenging and needs to be addressed in a multidisciplinary team with experience in interpreting post-SABR finding.

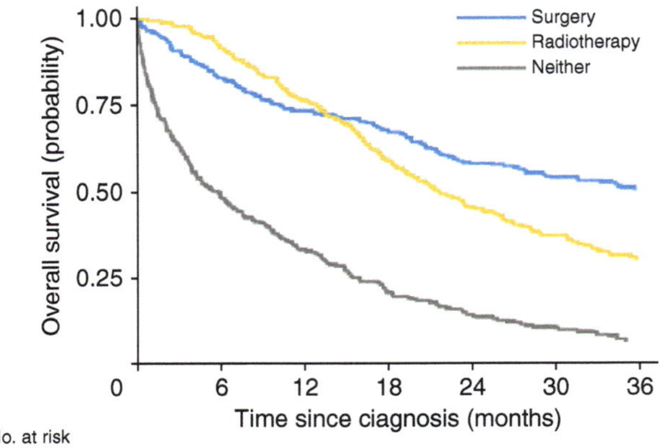

No. at risk							
Surgery	299	248	220	194	154	131	113
Radiotherapy	299	276	229	165	119	86	58
Neither	277	138	93	56	37	25	15

Fig. 11.7 Overall survival in patients aged 75 years or older, who were diagnosed with early-stage NSCLC in a Dutch hospital. Outcomes in untreated patients were poor, and the significant increase in survival after radiotherapy was observed following the introduction of SABR in 2003 (From Palma et al. [7]. With permission of the American Society of Clinical Oncology)

Population Impact of Introducing SABR

The recent introduction of SABR has impacted the survival of elderly patients with early-stage lung cancer, with studies showing an increased use of radiotherapy in elderly patients [7, 55]. A large population-based study performed in the Netherlands explored outcomes in three time periods: one in which SABR was not available, one in which SABR availability was limited, and finally when SABR became fully available. During the study period, the introduction of SABR was associated with a decrease in the proportion of untreated patients and a corresponding increase in the proportion of patients treated with radiotherapy. This increase in treated patients has led to a significant improvement of overall survival in the entire population, a finding that reached statistical significance only for patients who underwent radiotherapy [7] (Fig. 11.7).

Role of SABR in Medically Operable Patients

The high local control rates obtained by using SABR in patients who were medically inoperable, as well as the low toxicity profile, have increased interest in SABR as an alternative to surgical resection in medically fit patients [56]. Recently an increase has been observed in referrals for SABR in the Netherlands for patients in whom no absolute contraindication to surgery was present [57]. Two single-arm phase II trials of SBRT in patients who are fit to undergo surgery have been completed, and the mature results of JCOG 0403 (NCT00238875) and RTOG 0618 (NCT00551369) are awaited.

Several observational studies have reported on the outcomes of SABR for patients who were medically fit but who declined to undergo surgery. The results of these studies reveal that survival comparable with that after surgery can be achieved [39, 57, 58] (Fig. 11.8). A study using Markov modeling indicated that outcomes after either SABR or surgical resection are likely to be similar, with any advantage

Fig. 11.8 Overall survival following SABR in both potentially operable and inoperable patients who underwent SABR for stage I NSCLC. The overall survival observed in potentially operable patients is similar to that reported after surgery

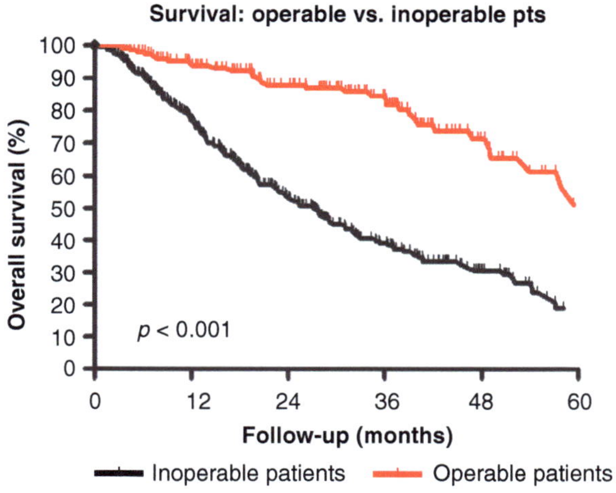

of surgery being lost as soon as the risk of operative mortality exceeds 4 % [42]. These results are especially important for elderly patients who, even after careful selection, experience more postoperative mortality and morbidity compared to younger patients [22, 59].

Recent reports suggest that salvage surgical resections are feasible after SABR, in patients who were fit for surgery but chose instead to undergo SABR. If surgical salvage becomes an established treatment option, it may increase the preference of elderly patients to consider SABR as their preferred treatment option.

In conclusion, due to changing demographics, increasing numbers of elderly patients are being diagnosed with an early-stage non-small cell lung cancer. These patients may be difficult to treat due to coexistent illnesses and poor performance. Stereotactic radiotherapy is a new and promising treatment option, particularly in the frail elderly. However, the high local control rates and favorable toxicity profile make it also an increasingly attractive treatment for patients who are at increased risk for operative mortality.

References

1. Jemal A, Bray F, Center MM, Ferlay J, Ward E, Forman D. Global cancer statistics. CA Cancer J Clin. 2011;61:69–90.
2. Sigel K, Bonomi M, Packer S, Wisnivesky J. Effect of age on survival of clinical stage I non-small-cell lung cancer. Ann Surg Oncol. 2009;16:1912–7.
3. National Cancer Institute. SEER cancer statistics. Available at: http://seer.cancer.gov/statistics. Accessed 11th Nov 2001.
4. Owonikoko TK, Ragin CC, Belani CP, et al. Lung cancer in elderly patients: an analysis of the surveillance, epidemiology, and end results database. J Clin Oncol. 2007;25:5570–7.
5. Edwards BK, Howe HL, Ries LAG, et al. Annual report to the nation on the status of cancer, 1973–1999, featuring implications of age and aging on U.S. cancer burden. Cancer. 2002;94: 2766–92.

6. Bach PB, Cramer LD, Warren JL, Begg CB. Racial differences in the treatment of early-stage lung cancer. N Engl J Med. 1999;341:1198–205.
7. Palma D, Visser O, Lagerwaard FJ, Belderbos J, Slotman BJ, Senan S. Impact of introducing stereotactic lung radiotherapy for elderly patients with stage I non-small-cell lung cancer: a population-based time-trend analysis. J Clin Oncol. 2010;28:5153–9.
8. Janssen-Heijnen ML, Schipper RM, Razenberg PP, Crommelin MA, Coebergh JW. Prevalence of co-morbidity in lung cancer patients and its relationship with treatment: a population-based study. Lung Cancer. 1998;21:105–13.
9. Battafarano RJ, Piccirillo JF, Meyers BF, et al. Impact of comorbidity on survival after surgical resection in patients with stage I non-small cell lung cancer. J Thorac Cardiovasc Surg. 2002;123:280–7.
10. Audisio RA, Zbar AP, Jaklitsch MT. Surgical management of oncogeriatric patients. J Clin Oncol. 2007;25:1924–9.
11. Hutchins LF, Unger JM, Crowley JJ, Coltman CA, Albain KS. Underrepresentation of patients 65 years of age or older in cancer-treatment trials. N Engl J Med. 1999;341:2061–7.
12. Murthy VH, Krumholz HM, Gross CP. Participation in cancer clinical trials: race-, sex-, and age-based disparities. JAMA. 2004;291:2720–6.
13. Scott WJ, Howington J, Feigenberg S, Movsas B, Pisters K. Treatment of non-small cell lung cancer stage I and stage II: ACCP evidence-based clinical practice guidelines (2nd edition). Chest. 2007;132:242.
14. Ettinger DS, Akerley W, Bepler G, et al. Non-small cell lung cancer. J Natl Compr Canc Netw. 2010;8:740–801.
15. Lim E, Baldwin D, Beckles M, et al. Guidelines on the radical management of patients with lung cancer. Thorax. 2010;65 Suppl 3:1–27.
16. Rowell NP, Williams CJ. Radical radiotherapy for stage I/II non-small cell lung cancer in patients not sufficiently fit for or declining surgery (medically inoperable): a systematic review. Thorax. 2001;56:628–38.
17. Detterbeck FC, Gibson CJ. Turning gray: the natural history of lung cancer over time. J Thorac Oncol. 2008;3:781–92.
18. Smith SL, Palma D, Parhar T, Alexander CS, Wai ES. Inoperable early stage non-small cell lung cancer: comorbidity, patterns of care and survival. Lung Cancer. 2011;72:39–44.
19. Wisnivesky JP, Halm E, Bonomi M, Powell C, Bagiella E. Effectiveness of radiation therapy for elderly patients with unresected stage I and II non-small cell lung cancer. Am J Respir Crit Care Med. 2010;181:264–9.
20. Gauden S, Ramsay J, Tripcony L. The curative treatment by radiotherapy alone of stage I non-small cell carcinoma of the lung. Chest. 1995;108:1278–82.
21. Zimmermann FB, Bamberg M, Molls M, Jeremic B. Radiation therapy alone in early stage non-small cell lung cancer. Semin Surg Oncol. 2003;21:91–7.
22. Palma D, Senan S. Stereotactic radiation therapy: changing treatment paradigms for stage I nonsmall cell lung cancer. Curr Opin Oncol. 2011;23:133–9.
23. Grutters JPC, Kessels AGH, Pijls-Johannesma M, De Ruysscher D, Joore MA, Lambin P. Comparison of the effectiveness of radiotherapy with photons, protons and carbon-ions for non-small cell lung cancer: a meta-analysis. Radiother Oncol. 2010;95:32–40.
24. Chi A, Liao Z, Nguyen NP, Xu J, Stea B, Komaki R. Systemic review of the patterns of failure following stereotactic body radiation therapy in early-stage non-small-cell lung cancer: clinical implications. Radiother Oncol. 2010;94:1–11.
25. Underberg RWM, Lagerwaard FJ, Cuijpers JP, Slotman BJ, van Sornsen de Koste J, Senan S. Four-dimensional CT scans for treatment planning in stereotactic radiotherapy for stage I lung cancer. Int J Radiat Oncol Biol Phys. 2004;60:1283–90.
26. Spoelstra FOB, Senan S. Novel tools in radiotherapy. Ann Oncol. 2008;19 Suppl 7:294–9.
27. van der Voort van Zyp N, Prevost JB, Hoogeman MS, et al. Stereotactic radiotherapy with real-time tumor tracking for non-small cell lung cancer: clinical outcome. Radiother Oncol. 2009;91:296–300.

28. Ong CL, Verbakel WFAR, Cuijpers JP, Slotman BJ, Lagerwaard FJ, Senan S. Stereotactic radiotherapy for peripheral lung tumors: a comparison of volumetric modulated arc therapy with 3 other delivery techniques. Radiother Oncol. 2010;97:437–42.
29. Lagerwaard FJ, Haasbeek CJA, Smit EF, Slotman BJ, Senan S. Outcomes of risk-adapted fractionated stereotactic radiotherapy for stage I non-small-cell lung cancer. Int J Radiat Oncol Biol Phys. 2008;70:685–92.
30. Bongers EM, Haasbeek CJA, Lagerwaard FJ, Slotman BJ, Senan S. Incidence and risk factors for chest wall toxicity after risk-adapted stereotactic radiotherapy for early-stage lung cancer. J Thorac Oncol. 2011;6:2052–7.
31. Hurkmans CW, Cuijpers JP, Lagerwaard FJ, et al. Recommendations for implementing stereotactic radiotherapy in peripheral stage IA non-small cell lung cancer: report from the Quality Assurance Working Party of the randomised phase III ROSEL study. Radiat Oncol. 2009;4:1.
32. Onishi H, Shirato H, Nagata Y, et al. Hypofractionated stereotactic radiotherapy (HypoFXSRT) for stage I non-small cell lung cancer: updated results of 257 patients in a Japanese multi-institutional study. J Thorac Oncol. 2007;2:94–9100.
33. Baumann P, Nyman J, Hoyer M, et al. Outcome in a prospective phase II trial of medically inoperable stage I non-small-cell lung cancer patients treated with stereotactic body radiotherapy. J Clin Oncol. 2009;27:3290–6.
34. Nagata Y, Takayama K, Matsuo Y, et al. Clinical outcomes of a phase I/II study of 48 Gy of stereotactic body radiotherapy in 4 fractions for primary lung cancer using a stereotactic body frame. Int J Radiat Oncol Biol Phys. 2005;63:1427–31.
35. Schuchert MJ, Pettiford BL, Pennathur A, et al. Anatomic segmentectomy for stage I non-small-cell lung cancer: comparison of video-assisted thoracic surgery versus open approach. J Thorac Cardiovasc Surg. 2009;138:1318–25.
36. Okada M, Koike T, Higashiyama M, Yamato Y, Kodama K, Tsubota N. Radical sublobar resection for small-sized non-small cell lung cancer: a multicenter study. J Thorac Cardiovasc Surg. 2006;132:769–75.
37. Boyd JA, Hubbs JL, Kim DW, Hollis D, Marks LB, Kelsey CR. Timing of local and distant failure in resected lung cancer: implications for reported rates of local failure. J Thorac Oncol. 2010;5:211–4.
38. Takeda A, Sanuki N, Kunieda E, et al. Stereotactic body radiotherapy for primary lung cancer at a dose of 50 Gy total in five fractions to the periphery of the planning target volume calculated using a superposition algorithm. Int J Radiat Oncol Biol Phys. 2009;73:442–8.
39. Uematsu M, Shioda A, Suda A, et al. Computed tomography-guided frameless stereotactic radiotherapy for stage I non-small cell lung cancer: a 5-year experience. Int J Radiat Oncol Biol Phys. 2001;51:666–70.
40. Fakiris AJ, McGarry RC, Yiannoutsos CT, et al. Stereotactic body radiation therapy for early-stage non-small-cell lung carcinoma: four-year results of a prospective phase II study. Int J Radiat Oncol Biol Phys. 2009;75:677–82.
41. Haasbeek CJA, Lagerwaard FJ, Antonisse ME, Slotman BJ, Senan S. Stage I nonsmall cell lung cancer in patients aged > or =75 years: outcomes after stereotactic radiotherapy. Cancer. 2010;116:406–14.
42. Louie AV, Rodrigues G, Hannouf M, et al. Withholding stereotactic radiotherapy in elderly patients with stage I non-small cell lung cancer and co-existing COPD is not justified: outcomes of a Markov model analysis. Radiother Oncol. 2011;99:161–5.
43. Palma D, Lagerwaard F, Rodrigues G, Haasbeek C, Senan S. Curative treatment of stage I non-small-cell lung cancer in patients with severe COPD: stereotactic radiotherapy outcomes and systematic review. Int J Radiat Oncol Biol Phys. 2011;82:1149–56.
44. Nyman J, Johansson KA, Hulten U. Stereotactic hypofractionated radiotherapy for stage I non-small cell lung cancer–mature results for medically inoperable patients. Lung Cancer. 2006;51:97–9103.
45. Koto M, Takai Y, Ogawa Y, et al. A phase II study on stereotactic body radiotherapy for stage I non-small cell lung cancer. Radiother Oncol. 2007;85:429–34.

46. Kopek N, Paludan M, Petersen J, Hansen AT, Grau C, Hoyer M. Co-morbidity index predicts for mortality after stereotactic body radiotherapy for medically inoperable early-stage non-small cell lung cancer. Radiother Oncol. 2009;93:402–7.
47. Timmerman R, McGarry R, Yiannoutsos C, et al. Excessive toxicity when treating central tumors in a phase II study of stereotactic body radiation therapy for medically inoperable early-stage lung cancer. J Clin Oncol. 2006;24:4833–9.
48. Haasbeek CJA, Lagerwaard FJ, Slotman BJ, Senan S. Outcomes of stereotactic ablative radiotherapy for centrally located early-stage lung cancer. J Thorac Oncol. 2011;6:2036–43.
49. Xia T, Li H, Sun Q, et al. Promising clinical outcome of stereotactic body radiation therapy for patients with inoperable Stage I/II non-small-cell lung cancer. Int J Radiat Oncol Biol Phys. 2006;66:117–25.
50. Ong CL, Palma D, Verbakel WF, et al. Treatment of large stage I-II lung tumors using stereotactic body radiotherapy (SBRT): planning considerations and early toxicity. Radiother Oncol. 2010;97:431–6.
51. Song SY, Choi W, Shin SS, et al. Fractionated stereotactic body radiation therapy for medically inoperable stage I lung cancer adjacent to central large bronchus. Lung Cancer. 2009;66: 89–93.
52. Dahele M, Palma D, Lagerwaard F, Slotman B, Senan S. Radiological changes after stereotactic radiotherapy for stage I lung cancer. J Thorac Oncol. 2011;6:1221–8.
53. Eisenhauer EA, Therasse P, Bogaerts J, et al. New response evaluation criteria in solid tumours: revised RECIST guideline (version 1.1). Eur J Cancer. 2009;45:228–47.
54. Matsuo Y, Nakamoto Y, Nagata Y, et al. Characterization of FDG-PET images after stereotactic body radiation therapy for lung cancer. Radiother Oncol. 2010;97:200–4.
55. Koning CCE, Aarts MJ, Struikmans H, et al. Mapping use of radiotherapy for patients with non-small cell lung cancer in the Netherlands between 1997 and 2008. Clin Oncol (R Coll Radiol). 2011;24:e46–53.
56. Haasbeek CJA, Senan S, Smit EF, Paul MA, Slotman BJ, Lagerwaard FJ. Critical review of nonsurgical treatment options for stage I non-small cell lung cancer. Oncologist. 2008;13: 309–19.
57. Lagerwaard FJ, Verstegen NE, Haasbeek CJA, et al. Outcomes of stereotactic ablative radiotherapy in patients with potentially operable stage I non-small-cell lung cancer. Int J Radiat Oncol Biol Phys. 2011;81:348–53.
58. Onishi H, Shirato H, Nagata Y, et al. Stereotactic body radiotherapy (SBRT) for operable stage I non-small-cell lung cancer: can SBRT be comparable to surgery? Int J Radiat Oncol Biol Phys. 2011;81:1352–8.
59. Wouters MWJM, Siesling S, Jansen-Landheer ML, et al. Variation in treatment and outcome in patients with non-small cell lung cancer by region, hospital type and volume in the Netherlands. Eur J Surg Oncol. 2010;36 Suppl 1:83–92.

Part V
Non Small-Cell Lung Cancer: Treatment of Locally Advanced Disease

Chapter 12
Adjuvant Chemotherapy: Feasibility in the Elderly and Patient Selection

Alejandro Navarro and Enriqueta Felip

Abstract Although adjuvant chemotherapy is considered standard of care for completely resected NSCLC patients with pathologic stage II–III, elderly patients are clearly underrepresented in the adjuvant randomized trials. Furthermore, the positive adjuvant chemotherapy trials employed cisplatin, which is considered a toxic drug in the elderly population. Another consideration is that recovery from surgery can take longer in elderly patients for age-related reasons, and a slow recovery from surgery is also a relevant factor when we consider adjuvant treatment. Subset analyses of NCIC-BR10 and LACE suggest that elderly patients benefit from adjuvant chemotherapy without increased toxicity although almost no information in patients aged ≥80 years was seen because of the extremely low proportion of patients ≥80 years included. Due to the lack of prospective data regarding the use of adjuvant chemotherapy in elderly patients, no general recommendations can be made, and the best approach is to individualize treatment for each patient taking into consideration, factors such as comorbidities, ECOG PS, previous surgical procedure, and, more importantly, patient preference.

Keywords Adjuvant chemotherapy in elderly lung cancer patients • Chemotherapy in elderly lung cancer patients • Elderly patients and chemotherapy • Treatment of elderly lung cancer patients • Chemotherapy toxicity in the elderly

Lung cancer remains the leading cause of cancer-related mortality worldwide, with an estimated 1,600,000 new cases and 1,380,000 deaths in 2008 [1]. More than 80 % of all newly diagnosed cases of lung cancer are non-small cell lung cancer (NSCLC). For patients with early-stage disease, from clinical stage IA through IIB, surgical resection represents the standard of care. However, those patients represent only one third

---

A. Navarro, MD • E. Felip, MD, PhD (✉)
Oncology Department, Vall d'Hebron University Hospital,
119-129, Barcelona 08035, Spain
e-mail: efelip@vhebron.net

C. Gridelli, R.A. Audisio (eds.), *Management of Lung Cancer in Older People*,
DOI 10.1007/978-0-85729-793-8_12, © Springer-Verlag London 2013

of all newly diagnosed cases, and even if they undergo complete resection, approximately 50 % of patients will relapse and die of recurrent disease within 5 years [2].

In order to improve survival in patients with early-stage NSCLC, efforts have been focused on the use of chemotherapy before or after surgery with the aim of reducing the risk of relapse. At present, the benefit of adjuvant chemotherapy is widely accepted and that it should be offered to patients with resected stage II–IIIA NSCLC [3, 4]. However, some aspects still require elucidation; among them the role and feasibility of adjuvant chemotherapy in the elderly population.

Adjuvant Randomized Trials in the General Population

Adjuvant chemotherapy treatment has long been used in dealing with certain types of tumors, and it is considered to be a reasonable option in order to improve the outcome of NSCLC patients who have undergone surgical resection. In 1995, a meta-analysis of 52 studies conducted between 1965 and 1991 which included data from 9,387 patients was published [5]. Eight cisplatin-based studies ($n=1{,}394$) were examined, and the results showed an absolute survival benefit of 5 % at 5 years with the use of adjuvant chemotherapy, although these findings were not statistically significant (HR = 0.87, $p=0.08$). Conversely, adjuvant chemotherapy with older alkylating agents had a detrimental impact on survival. Analyses of five studies ($n=2{,}145$) using alkylating agents showed an absolute decrease in survival of 5 % at 5 years (HR = 1.15, $p=0.005$). Results from this meta-analysis generated optimism and prompted additional evaluation of platinum-based regimens in resectable NSCLC resulting in further prospective randomized phase III trials.

The North American Intergroup Trial ECOG 3590 evaluated the efficacy of four cycles of postoperative cisplatin-etoposide plus concomitant radiotherapy versus postoperative radiotherapy alone in resected stage II and IIIA NSCLC [6]. A total of 463 patients were included and no significant differences in survival between the study arms were found. Radiation toxicity caused by the concomitant administration of chemotherapy may explain the lack of efficacy.

The ALPI-EORTC trial evaluated the efficacy of three cycles of mitomycin, vindesine, and cisplatin versus observation in resected stage I, II, and IIIA NSCLC [7]. A total of 1,209 patients were included and randomly assigned to the two arms with no significant difference in survival being observed. Subgroup analysis showed a 10 % survival advantage at 5 years for chemotherapy-treated stage II patients, although without statistical significance.

The Big Lung Trial (BLT) also evaluated the efficacy of three cycles of cisplatin-based chemotherapy versus observation in resected stage I, II, and III NSCLC [8]. A total of 381 patients were enrolled with no survival differences between arms, although this study may well have been underpowered to detect any survival benefit.

The International Adjuvant Lung Cancer Trial (IALT) was published in 2004 and was the first relevant study to show statistically significant benefit from the use of adjuvant chemotherapy in both disease-free survival (DFS) and overall survival (OS) [9]. A total of 1,867 completely resected stage I, II, and III NSCLC patients were randomized to receive chemotherapy with cisplatin in combination with vinblastine or vinorelbine or etoposide versus observation. Overall survival was longer for patients in the chemotherapy group (HR = 0.86, CI 0.76–0.98, $p < 0.03$). Median DFS was 40.2 versus 30.5 months and median OS was 50.8 versus 44.4 months for the chemotherapy arm and the control arm, respectively. Results of IALT were updated with long-term follow-up in 2008, reporting that the survival benefit from adjuvant chemotherapy was non-significant after a median follow-up of 7.5 years [10].

The Adjuvant Navelbine International Trial Association (ANITA) evaluated the efficacy of cisplatin and vinorelbine versus observation in resected stage IB, II, and III NSCLC patients [11]. A total of 840 patients were included: 36 % stage IB, 25 % stage II, and 39 % stage III. After a median follow-up of 76 months, median survival was significantly longer in the chemotherapy arm, 65.7 months, in comparison with the observation arm, 43.7 months. When subgroup analysis was performed, the benefit appeared to be limited to stage II and III patients. A descriptive analysis suggested that radiotherapy could play a positive role in stage III [12].

The National Cancer Institute of Canada Clinical Trials Group designed a similar trial, known as NCIC-BR10, but limited it to stage IB and II (excluding T3N0) NSCLC [13]. A total of 482 patients were enrolled and randomized to cisplatin and vinorelbine versus observation. PORT was not given in this study. OS was significantly longer (HR = 0.69, $p = 0.04$) in the chemotherapy group, 94 months, in comparison with the observation group, 73 months. There was an absolute gain of 15 % in 5-year survival rate, from 54 to 69 %. Subgroup analyses showed that benefit was limited to stage II patients. The results of this study were updated with long-term follow-up (median follow-up 9.3 years) and the improvement in survival obtained with adjuvant chemotherapy was maintained [14].

The Cancer and Leukemia Group B (CALGB) designed a randomized trial known as CALGB 9633, including only resected stage IB NSCLC patients [15]. This study was closed early based on a positive interim analysis with a total of 344 patients randomized. Although a significant survival benefit was shown at 4 years, it was not confirmed at 6-year follow-up. In an unplanned analysis, patients with tumors of at least 4 cm in size obtained a survival benefit from chemotherapy (HR = 0.66, $p < 0.04$) in contrast with patients with smaller tumors (HR = 1.02, $p = 0.51$). Table 12.1 summarizes a number of randomized trials addressing the role of adjuvant platinum-based chemotherapy in resected NSCLC patients.

The Lung Adjuvant Cisplatin Evaluation (LACE) pooled individual data of 4,854 patients from five randomized adjuvant trials using adjuvant cisplatin combinations, ALPI, ANITA, BLT, IALT, and NCIC-BR10 [16]. Adjuvant chemotherapy was associated with an improvement in OS with an 11 % relative reduction in the risk of death (HR = 0.89, CI 0.82–0.96, $p = 0.04$). However, the degree of benefit varied depending on stage. In stages II and III, OS benefit was 5.3 % at 5 years (HR = 0.83, CI 0.73–0.95 and HR = 0.83, CI 0.72–0.94, respectively), whereas a small but not statistically significant benefit was observed in stage IB (HR = 0.93, CI 0.78–1.10) and a detrimental effect in stage IA (HR = 1.40, CI 0.95–2.06).

Table 12.1 Summary of adjuvant platinum-based chemotherapy trials

Study	Number of patients	Stage	Treatment	OS (HR, 95 % CI) *p* value	Port use per arm experimental/ control (%)	Absolute improvement in 5-year survival (%)
ECOG 3590 (1991–1997)	488	II–IIIA	Cisplatin plus etoposide and concurrent radiotherapy	0.93 (0.74–1.18) $p=0.56$	Yes	
ALPI-EORTC (1994–1999)	1,209	I–IIIA	Mitomycin C, vindesine, and cisplatin	0.96 (0.81–1.13) $p=0.589$	64/70	1.0
ANITA (1994–2000)	840	IB–IIIA	Cisplatin plus vinorelbine	0.80 (0.66–0.96) $p=0.017$	21/33	8.6
JBR.10 (1994–2001)	482	IB–II	Cisplatin and vinorelbine	0.69 (0.52–0.91) $p=0.04$	0/0	15.0
BLT (1995–2001)	381	I–IV	Cisplatin doublet with vindesine, vinorelbine or mitomycin, or triplet vinblastine and mitomycin	1.02 (0.77–1.35) $p=0.9$	NS	−2
IALT (1995–2000)	1,867	IA–IIIB	Cisplatin doublet with vindesine, vinorelbine, vinblastine, or etoposide	0.86 (0.76–0.98) $p<0.03$	64/70	4.1
CALGB 9633 (1996–2003)	344	IB	Carboplatin and paclitaxel	0.83 (0.64–1.08) $p=0.12$	0/0	3

The NSCLC Meta-analyses Collaborative Group recently undertook two systematic reviews and meta-analyses to establish the effect of adding chemotherapy to surgery or to surgery plus radiotherapy [17]. The first meta-analysis of surgery plus chemotherapy versus surgery alone was based on 34 trials and 8,447 patients (3,323 deaths). They reported a benefit of adding chemotherapy after surgery (HR = 0.86, CI 0.81–0.92, $p < 0.0001$), with an absolute increase in survival of 4 % at 5 years. The second meta-analysis of surgery plus radiotherapy and chemotherapy versus surgery plus radiotherapy was based on 13 trials and 2,660 patients (1,909 deaths). They reported a benefit of adding chemotherapy to surgery plus radiotherapy (HR = 0.88, CI 0.81–0.97, $p = 0.009$), representing an absolute improvement in survival of 4 % at 5 years.

A number of studies addressed the role of uracil-tegafur (UFT) in the adjuvant setting. A large trial evaluated the efficacy of adjuvant UFT in NSCLC [18]. A total of 979 patients with completely resected stage I adenocarcinoma were randomized to UFT or observation. There was an increase in OS in the UFT arm (HR = 0.71, CI 0.52–0.98), limited to T2N0 subgroup. UFT is thought to have a particular sensitivity in Japanese populations. No study addressing the role of adjuvant UFT has been performed outside Japan, which is a clear limitation for its use in the clinical practice.

As a result of the several randomized trials mentioned above, the majority of guidelines recommend the use of cisplatin-based chemotherapy in the adjuvant treatment of patients with pathologic stages II–III and complete resection.

Adjuvant Chemotherapy in Elderly Patients

The median age for developing lung cancer is 70 years, with more than 60 % of this population aged >65 years. Adjuvant chemotherapy is still considered an experimental modality of treatment in elderly NSCLC patients mainly because randomized trials, including those mentioned above, rarely include elderly patients. In current practice, the elderly are often deliberately excluded from participation in clinical trials in general and particularly from adjuvant trials. The underrepresentation of the elderly population is relevant because treatment recommendations for lung cancer are obtained from clinical trials. Clinical data obtained in a younger population cannot be automatically extrapolated to the great majority of nonselected elderly patients. One relevant point in this research area is lack of consensus about the definition of "elderly"; some studies define the elderly population as those patients ≥65 years and others as ≥70 years. There are no randomized phase III trials addressing the role of adjuvant chemotherapy in the elderly population and what we have are subset analyses according to age from randomized trials.

In the NCIC-BR10 study, a retrospective analysis was made to evaluate the impact of age on survival, chemotherapy compliance, and toxicity [19]. In this analysis, patients aged <65 years were classified as "young" and those aged ≥65 years as "elderly." Data from 327 young and 155 elderly patients (65 years or older) were analyzed. Younger patients had a major prevalence of adenocarcinoma and had better performance status. Elderly patients received significantly fewer doses of chemotherapy with no significant differences in toxicities when compared with the younger study population. It is important to mention that OS in elderly patients was significantly better in those treated with chemotherapy than in the observation group (HR=0.61, $p=0.04$), but in the few patients older than 75 years ($n=23$) survival was shorter than in those aged 65–75. The conclusion of the authors was that although elderly patients tend to receive lower chemotherapy doses, adjuvant chemotherapy with cisplatin/vinorelbine improves survival in patients older than 65 years with acceptable toxicity and that adjuvant chemotherapy should not be withheld from elderly patients.

In the LACE meta-analysis, the authors determined the efficacy and toxicity of adjuvant cisplatin-based chemotherapy in elderly NSCLC patients. In this report, "elderly" was defined as ≥70 years old [20]. Interestingly, in this meta-analysis, only 9 % of the patients included were ≥70 years old. Elderly patients received a significantly lower total dose of cisplatin and fewer cycles of chemotherapy. Elderly patients enjoyed survival benefits similar to those of the younger cohort. Again the authors concluded that adjuvant cisplatin-based chemotherapy should not be withheld from elderly patients with NSCLC purely on the basis of age. However, caution is required when considering adjuvant cisplatin-based chemotherapy for those patients ≥75 years of age. In the LACE meta-analysis, only 1.3 % of the patients were ≥75 years.

At the 2011 ASCO meeting, two studies dealing with adjuvant chemotherapy in the elderly population were presented. Cuffe et al. analyzed the patients registered in the population-based Ontario Cancer Registry who underwent surgery between 2001 and 2006 [21]. A total of 6,304 patients were registered, 44 % aged ≥70 years. When they analyzed the elderly group defined as those patients aged ≥70 years, they showed that the uptake of adjuvant chemotherapy increased in the 2004–2006 period (in which 16 % of the elderly patients received adjuvant chemotherapy) when compared with the 2001–2003 period (in which only 3 % of the patients received adjuvant chemotherapy). In this registry, cisplatin was less used in patients ≥70 years when compared with those patients <70 years. Interestingly, similar severe toxicity with chemotherapy was observed in the two groups of patients (<70 years and ≥70 years). In this study, the 4-year survival in the elderly group increased in the 2004–2006 period when compared with the 2001–2003 period; one possible explanation for that is the greater proportion of patients receiving adjuvant chemotherapy in the second period. In the study presented by Gu et al., 3,324 resected NSCLC patients with stages II–IIIA and ≥65 years were identified in the SEER-Medicare database between 1992 and 2005 [22]. In these elderly patients, adjuvant carboplatin (79 %) was most often used than cisplatin (16 %) with comparable survival benefit for those patients receiving adjuvant cisplatin and adjuvant carboplatin treatment. Although both studies had some methodological limitations, the results suggest that in the elderly population, there is a benefit from adjuvant chemotherapy (without data for patients ≥80 years) and that although there is no prospective validation, carboplatin may be an alternative to cisplatin.

Summary

Although adjuvant chemotherapy is considered standard of care for completely resected NSCLC patients with pathologic stages II–III, elderly patients are clearly underrepresented in the adjuvant randomized trials. Furthermore, the positive adjuvant chemotherapy trials employed cisplatin, which is considered a toxic drug in the elderly population. Another consideration is that recovery from surgery can take longer in elderly patients for age-related reasons, and a slow recovery from surgery is also a relevant factor when we consider adjuvant treatment. Subset analyses of NCIC-BR10 and LACE suggest that elderly patients benefit from adjuvant chemotherapy without increased toxicity although almost no information in patients aged ≥80 years was seen because of the extremely low proportion of patients ≥80 years included. Due to the lack of prospective data regarding the use of adjuvant chemotherapy in elderly patients, no general recommendations can be made and the best approach is to individualize treatment for each patient taking into consideration factors such as comorbidities, ECOG PS, previous surgical procedure, and, more importantly, patient preference.

References

1. Jemal A, Bray F, Center MM, et al. Global cancer statistics. CA Cancer J Clin. 2011; 61(2):69.
2. Nesbitt JC, Putnam Jr JB, Walsh GL, et al. Survival in early-stage non-small cell lung cancer. Ann Thorac Surg. 1995;60:466–72.
3. Crinò L, Weder W, van Meerbeeck J, et al. Early stage and locally advanced (non-metastatic) non-small-cell lung cancer: ESMO Clinical Practice Guidelines for diagnosis, treatment and follow-up. Ann Oncol. 2010;21 Suppl 5:v103–15.
4. Pisters KM, Evans WK, Azzoli CG, et al. Cancer Care Ontario and American Society of Clinical Oncology adjuvant chemotherapy and adjuvant radiation therapy for stages I-IIIA resectable non small-cell lung cancer guideline. J Clin Oncol. 2007;25:5506–18.
5. Non-small Cell Lung Cancer Collaborative Group. Chemotherapy in non-small cell lung cancer: a meta-analysis using updated data on individual patients from 52 randomised clinical trials. BMJ. 1995;311:899–909.
6. Keller SM, Adak S, Wagner H, et al. A randomized trial of postoperative adjuvant therapy in patients with completely resected stage II or IIIA non-small-cell lung cancer. Eastern Cooperative Oncology Group. N Engl J Med. 2000;343:1217–22.
7. Scagliotti GV, Fossati R, Torri V, et al. Randomized study of adjuvant chemotherapy for completely resected stage I, II, or IIIA non-small-cell lung cancer. J Natl Cancer Inst. 2003;95: 1453–61.
8. Waller D, Peake MD, Stephens RJ, et al. Chemotherapy for patients with nonsmall cell lung cancer: the surgical setting of the Big Lung Trial. Eur J Cardiothorac Surg. 2004;26: 173–1782.
9. Arriagada R, Bergman B, Dunant A, et al. Cisplatin-based adjuvant chemotherapy in patients with completely resected non-small-cell lung cancer. N Engl J Med. 2004;350:351–60.
10. Arriagada R, Dunant A, Pignon JP, et al. Long-term results of the international adjuvant lung cancer trial evaluating adjuvant Cisplatin-based chemotherapy in resected lung cancer. J Clin Oncol. 2010;28:35–42.

11. Douillard JY, Rosell R, De Lena M, et al. Adjuvant vinorelbine plus cisplatin vs. observation in patients with completely resected stage IB-IIIA non-small-cell lung cancer (Adjuvant Navelbine International Trialist Association [ANITA]): a randomised controlled trial. Lancet Oncol. 2006;7:719–27.
12. Douillard JY, Rosell R, De Lena M, et al. Impact of postoperative radiation therapy on survival in patients with complete resection and stage I, II, or IIIA non-small-cell lung cancer treated with adjuvant chemotherapy: the adjuvant Navelbine International Trialist A(ANITA) Randomized Trial. Int J Radiat Oncol Biol Phys. 2008;72:695–701.
13. Winton T, Livingston R, Johnson D, et al. Vinorelbine plus cisplatin vs. observation in resected non-small-cell lung cancer. N Engl J Med. 2005;352:2589–97.
14. Butts CA, Ding K, Seymour L, et al. Randomized phase III trial of vinorelbine plus cisplatin compared with observation in completely resected stage IB and II non-small-cell lung cancer: updated survival analysis of JBR-10. J Clin Oncol. 2010;28:29–34.
15. Strauss GM, Herndon JE, Maddaus MA, et al. Adjuvant paclitaxel plus carboplatin compared with observation in stage IB non-small-cell lung cancer: CALGB 9633 with the Cancer and Leukemia Group B, Radiation Therapy Oncology Group, and North Central Cancer Treatment Group Study Groups. J Clin Oncol. 2008;26:5043–51.
16. Pignon JP, Tribodet H, Scagliotti GV, et al. Lung adjuvant cisplatin evaluation: a pooled analysis by the LACE Collaborative Group. J Clin Oncol. 2008;26:3552–9.
17. NSCLC Meta-analyses Collaborative Group, Arriagada R, Auperin A, Burdett S, et al. Adjuvant chemotherapy, with or without postoperative radiotherapy, in operable non-small-cell lung cancer: two meta-analyses of individual patient data. Lancet. 2010;375:1267–77.
18. Kato H, Ichinose Y, Ohta M, et al. A randomized trial of adjuvant chemotherapy with uracil-tegafur for adenocarcinoma of the lung. N Engl J Med. 2004;350:1713–21.
19. Pepe C, Hassan B, Winton T, et al. Adjuvant vinorelbine and cisplatin in elderly patients: National Cancer Institute of Canada and Intergroup Study JBR.10. J Clin Oncol. 2007;25: 1553–61.
20. Früh M, Rolland E, Pignon JP, et al. Pooled analysis of the effect of age on adjuvant cisplatin-based chemotherapy for completely resected non-small-cell lung cancer. J Clin Oncol. 2008;26:3573–81.
21. Cuffe S, Booth CM, Peng Y, et al. Adjuvant chemotherapy for non-small cell lung cancer in the elderly: A population-based study in Ontario, Canada. J Clin Oncol. 2012;30(15): 1813–21.
22. Gu F, Strauss GM, Wisnivesky JP. Platinum-based adjuvant chemotherapy (ACT) in elderly patients with non-small cell lung cancer (NSCLC) in the SEER-Medicare database: Comparison between carboplatin- and cisplatin-based regimens. ASCO Meeting Abstracts. 2011;29:7014.

Chapter 13
Locally Advanced Non-Small Cell Lung Cancer in the Elderly: What Combination of Therapy Is Best?

Steven E. Schild

Abstract Elderly patients (≥70 years) currently make up about one half of all lung cancer patients in the USA. The normal aging process combined most often with years of smoking leads to physiologic limitations which make aggressive multimodality therapy more challenging. Large modern studies which employed aggressive chemotherapy plus radiotherapy (RT) found that fit elderly patients experienced more myelosuppression and specific non-hematologic toxicities than younger individuals. Despite some degree of increased toxicity from combined modality therapy, it appeared that the fit elderly patients had similar disease control and survival rates as younger patients. Additionally, studies have shown that elderly patients had better survival with the more aggressive regimens of concurrent chemotherapy and radiotherapy rather than sequential therapy or RT alone. These findings suggest that fit elderly patients with locally advanced NSCLC should be encouraged to receive combined modality therapy. Recent clinical trials have been performed specifically for elderly patients. These studies should help clinicians optimize future treatment for the elderly. Research should focus on decreasing treatment toxicity in all patients but especially in the elderly. Treatment-related toxicity may be lessened with the use of newer radiation delivery techniques and novel targeted therapy. Additionally, more studies are needed for elderly patients and those with limited performance status who are grossly underrepresented in current clinical trials.

Keywords Non-small cell lung cancer in the elderly • Lung cancer therapy in the elderly • Chemotherapy for lung cancer in the elderly • Radiotherapy for lung cancer in the elderly • Toxicity from chemotherapy in elderly patients

---

S.E. Schild, MD
Department of Radiation Oncology, Mayo Clinic,
13400 E. Shea Blvd., Scottsdale, AZ 85259, USA
e-mail: sschild@mayo.edu

C. Gridelli, R.A. Audisio (eds.), *Management of Lung Cancer in Older People*,
DOI 10.1007/978-0-85729-793-8_13,

Until recently, radiotherapy (RT) alone was standard therapy for patients with locally advanced medically inoperable or surgically unresectable lung cancer. Conventional RT (60 Gy in 30 daily (QD) fractions) alone resulted in a median survival of 10 months and 5-year survival rate of 5 % [1]. However, during the past 20 years, randomized prospective studies have demonstrated a significant survival advantage for patients who receive chemotherapy in addition to RT for locally advanced NSCLC [2–6]. Additionally, concurrent chemotherapy plus RT results in better survival than sequential therapy [7, 8]. Currently, the treatment strategy associated with the best survival is concurrent thoracic radiotherapy and chemotherapy.

Based on recent SEER data, the median age of patients diagnosed with lung cancer is 70 years [9]. Because half of lung cancer patients are 70 years or older, it is important to understand the effects of modern combined modality therapy in the elderly.

There are two main obstacles which limit enthusiasm for combined modality therapy in elderly lung cancer patients. The first is the notion that aggressive treatment is futile and the second is that therapy is excessively toxic. Therefore, some physicians have advocated the use of single-agent palliative chemotherapy alone, RT alone, or no treatment. While this may be appropriate for frail individuals, there is an expanding cohort of elderly patients who are reasonably fit and desire the chance for cure.

Discussion: The Use of Standard Therapies in the Elderly (Radiotherapy and Chemotherapy)

The dilemma of how to best treat elderly patients has led investigators at the Radiation Therapy Oncology Group (RTOG), Cancer and Leukemia Group B (CALGB), and North Central Cancer Treatment Group (NCCTG) to retrospectively review their experiences [10–13]. The results of combined modality therapy in both elderly and younger individuals were evaluated. This was done to compare tolerance, toxicity, and survival of both age groups to assess the applicability of aggressive therapy to elderly patients.

The RTOG experience has been reported by Langer et al. [10, 11]. In an early report, they reevaluated 3 trials from the late 1980s and early 1990s which included various treatment combinations of chemotherapy and RT. The median survival time of patients age 70 and greater was 11.4 months with daily (QD) RT alone, 9.3 months with twice-daily (BID) RT alone, 11.0 months with induction chemotherapy followed by QD RT, 14.2 months with induction chemotherapy followed by concurrent chemotherapy plus RT, and 11.1 months with concurrent chemotherapy plus BID RT. There was no significant difference in survival based on treatment arm ($p=0.32$). Concurrent chemotherapy and RT resulted in significantly more grade 3 and 4 toxicity, but no improvement in survival compared to less aggressive therapy. Therefore, they concluded that elderly patients did not necessarily appear to benefit from chemotherapy plus RT as opposed to RT alone.

However, in a later study, Langer et al. found that fit elderly patients appeared to benefit from concurrent chemotherapy and QD RT. They evaluated patients 70 years or older who were enrolled in RTOG protocol 94–10. Patients eligible for this study had stage III NSCLC, good performance status, and little weight loss. RTOG 94–10 was a phase III randomized study in which patients received either sequential chemotherapy (cisplatin and vinblastine) then 60 Gy of daily (QD) RT (seq-QD RT), concurrent chemotherapy (cisplatin and vinblastine) plus 60 Gy of QD RT (con-QD RT), or concurrent chemotherapy (cisplatin and etoposide) and 69.6 Gy of twice a day RT (con-BID RT). Of the 595 patients analyzed on this study, 104 were 70 years or older. Grade 3+ (≥3) neutropenia and maximum toxicity were more pronounced in elderly patients. Of those patients who received concurrent therapy, grade 3+ esophagitis was significantly more common in the elderly patients. The median survival in the elderly patients was more favorable with concurrent therapy: 22.4 months with con-QD RT, 16.4 months with con-BID RT, and 10.8 months for seq-QD RT ($p=0.069$). Acute toxicity was judged to be acceptable but was more pronounced in elderly patients. There was no difference in long-term toxicity. Langer et al. concluded that fit elderly patients with stage III NSCLC were candidates for combined modality therapy, although he acknowledged that selection bias was likely to be more pronounced in the elderly.

Rocha Lima et al. evaluated the effect of age on the outcome in two randomized prospective studies performed by the CALGB [12]. CALGB 9130 evaluated the use of combined modality therapy (chemotherapy plus RT) for patients with stage III NSCLC. Eligible patients with good performance status were randomized to receive either cisplatin plus vinblastine followed by QD RT (60 Gy in 30 fractions) or cisplatin plus vinblastine followed by concurrent cisplatin plus QD RT (60 Gy). Elderly patients had significantly more grade 3+ neutropenia ($p=0.04$) and renal toxicity ($p=0.0025$). The renal toxicity was further evaluated based on patient age. There was no severe renal toxicity in patients who were less than 60 years old compared to 6 % of patients age 60–69 and 11 % of patients age 70–79 years. Age was not a factor in survival ($p=0.8$) nor response rate ($p=0.3$).

Schild et al. analyzed the NCCTG experience with elderly patients who received combined modality therapy on NCCTG 94-24-52 [13]. Eligible patients had stage III NSCLC, good performance status (Eastern Cooperative Oncology Group (ECOG) PS=0-1), and adequate organ function. Treatment included the delivery of concurrent etoposide and cisplatin during RT. Patients were randomly assigned to receive either standard QD RT (60 Gy in 30 daily fractions) or BID RT (60 Gy in 40 fractions) [14]. Of the 244 evaluable patients, 181 (74 %) were less than 70 years old and 63 (26 %) were 70 years or older ("elderly"). While grade 3 or greater (grade 3+) toxicity was not more common in elderly patients, grade 4 or greater (grade 4+) toxicity occurred significantly more frequently in the elderly (Table 13.1).

The severity of hematologic toxicity was evaluated for the two age groups. While there was not a significant difference in the occurrence of grade 3+ hematologic toxicity, there was significantly more grade 4+ hematologic toxicity in elderly patients. The severity of non-hematologic toxicity was evaluated for the two age

Table 13.1 Toxicity for patients treated with EP+ either BID RT or QD RT based on age group

	Age <70 (*N*=181)				Age ≥70 (*N*=63)				*P*-value	
	Grade 3+		Grade 4+		Grade 3+		Grade 4+			
Type of toxicity	*N*	%	*N*	%	*N*	%	*N*	%	Grade 3+	Grade4+
All toxicity	155	86	113	62	58	92	51	81	0.18	0.007
Non-hematologic toxicity	104	57	31	17	34	54	12	19	0.63	0.73
Hematologic toxicity	139	77	102	56	55	87	49	78	0.08	0.003
Leukopenia	131	72	56	31	53	84	35	56	0.06	0.0005
Thrombocytopenia	35	19	1	1	21	33	3	5	0.02	0.05 (F)
Anemia	4	2	4	2	2	3	1	2	0.65 (F)	1.00 (F)
Nausea	45	25	0	0	9	14	0	0	0.08	N/A
Vomiting	33	18	23	13	8	13	6	10	0.31	0.50
Esophagitis	31	17	1	1	12	19	1	2	0.73	0.45 (F)
Pneumonitis	22	12	1	1	8	13	4	6	0.91	0.02 (F)

Grades were based on common toxicity criteria version 1
(*F*) Fisher's exact test *p*-value
EP etoposide + cisplatin, *BID RT* twice-daily radiotherapy, *QD RT* daily radiotherapy

groups. Of the non-hematologic toxicities, only grade 4+ pneumonitis (respiratory insufficiency which requires ventilation or continuous oxygen) was more common in elderly patients. This was a relatively uncommon toxicity occurring in 1 % of those younger than 70 years old compared to 6 % of elderly patients ($p=0.02$). Three of the 181 (2 %) patients less than age 70 died of toxicity attributed to treatment compared to 2 of the 63 (3 %) elderly patients ($p=$NS).

There were no significant differences in survival ($p=0.37$) or disease progression ($p=0.2$) rates based on age. The 2-year and 5-year survival rates were 39 and 18 % in the younger patients compared to 36 and 13 % in the elderly (Fig. 13.1).

In a later NCCTG analysis, Schild et al. provided evidence supporting the hypothesis that chemoradiotherapy provided a better outcome than did RT alone for elderly stage III NSCLC patients [15]. This study was performed to assess the value of combined modality therapy in elderly patients by comparing the differences in outcome between patients who received radiotherapy (RT) alone and patients who received RT plus chemotherapy for stage III NSCLC. NCCTG performed 2 recent phase III trials for stage III NSCLC. The first trial, NCCTG 90-24-51, included 3 arms: once-daily RT (QD RT) alone, twice-daily RT (BID RT) alone, and concurrent chemotherapy plus BID RT. The second trial, NCCTG 94-24-52, included 2 arms and compared concurrent chemotherapy with either QD RT or BID RT. The chemotherapy arms of both trials included etoposide and cisplatin administered concurrently with RT. Only the patients aged ≥65 years (elderly) who participated in those trials were included in this analysis. Of the 166 elderly patients included in this analysis, 37 patients received RT alone, and 129 patients received concurrent chemotherapy plus RT. All patients had ECOG performance scores ranging from 0 to 2. The median and 5-year survival rates were 10.5 months and 5.4 % for the RT alone group compared with 13.7 months and

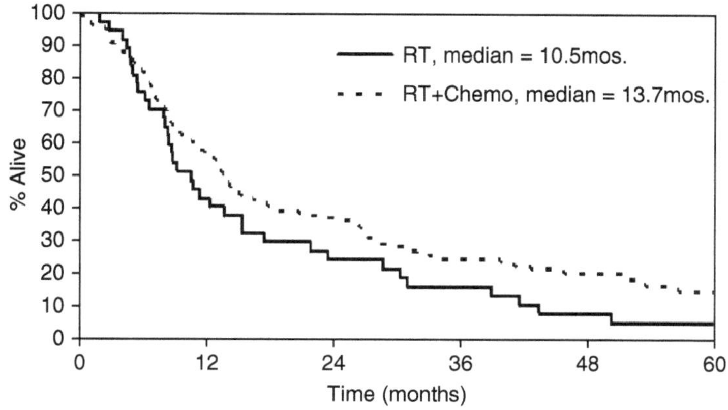

Fig. 13.1 Overall survival by age group (<70 vs. ≥70) ($p = 0.374$) (Data from NCCTG 94-24-52, Schild et al.)

14.7 % for the RT plus chemotherapy group (log-rank $p = 0.05$). Patients who received RT plus chemotherapy experienced significantly greater severe toxicity (grade 3+) compared with patients who received RT alone (89.9 % vs. 32.4 %; $P < 0.01$). They concluded that the elderly patients who participated in these trials appeared to gain a survival advantage from RT and chemotherapy compared with RT alone. As is the case with younger patients, this benefit came at the cost of additional toxicity.

Agati et al. reported a phase II trial examining the feasibility of concurrent thoracic radiotherapy (TRT) and daily low-dose carboplatin (CBDCA) in elderly patients with NSCLC [16]. Forty patients with pathologically documented unresectable stage IIIA or IIIB or medically inoperable stage I or II NSCLC were included. Carboplatin (CBDCA) 30 mg/m^2 was given on days 1–5 in weeks 1–4 concurrently with TRT, mainly as a radiosensitizing agent. TRT was started 1 h after the CBDCA (30-min infusion) was given. TRT was given in 2 Gy/fraction QD, 5 days a week for a total of 50–60 Gy. The main toxicities were hematological toxicity with grade 3 or greater leukopenia and anemia occurring in 27 (68 %) and 13 (32.5 %) of patients, respectively. Other toxicities were grade 2 esophagitis in one (2.5 %) patient, grade 3 nausea/vomiting in one (2.5 %), and grade 4 pulmonary toxicity in two (5 %). There was one treatment-related death due to pulmonary toxicity. For stage IIIA + IIIB patients, the median survival time was 15.1 months and 1- and 2-year actuarial survival rates were 52.6 and 20.5 %, respectively. For stage I + II patients, 1- and 3-year actuarial survival rates were 90.9 and 69.3 %, respectively. They concluded that TRT with daily low-dose CBDCA in elderly patients is effective and feasible because of its low toxicity and reasonable survival.

The JCOG performed a phase III trial (JCOG 0301) in which elderly patients (>70 years) with unresectable stage III NSCLC were randomly assigned to chemoradiotherapy (60 Gy/30 fractions plus concurrent low-dose carboplatin

[30 mg/m^2 per day, 5 days a week for 20 days]) or TRT alone [17]. Patients were stratified for ECOG performance status (0 vs. 1 vs. 2), stage (IIIA vs. IIIB), and institution. The primary end point was survival and there were 100 patients in each of the two arms. The median survival for the chemoradiotherapy and TRT alone groups were 22.4 months and 16.9 months, respectively (hazard ratio 0.68, log-rank, one-sided p-value=0.0179). More patients had grade 3–4 hematological toxic effects in the chemoradiotherapy group than in the radiotherapy alone group, including leukopenia (61 [63.5 %] vs. none), neutropenia ([57.3 %] vs. none), and thrombocytopenia ([29.2 %] vs. [2.0 %]). Grade 3 infection was more common with chemoradiotherapy (12 patients [12.5 %]) than with TRT (four patients [4.1 %]). Incidences of grade 3–4 pneumonitis and late lung toxicity were similar between groups. There were seven treatment-related deaths: three of 100 patients (3.0 %) in the chemoradiotherapy group and four of 100 (4.0 %) in the radiotherapy group. They concluded that for a select group of elderly patients with locally advanced NSCLC, combination chemoradiotherapy provides a clinically significant benefit over radiotherapy alone.

The survival data appears consistent with the results of other trials which included patients of all age groups and which demonstrated better survival with chemotherapy plus RT than RT alone [12, 18, 19].

Jeremic et al. performed a phase II trial of low-dose BID RT (51 Gy/34 fractions) plus concurrent carboplatin and etoposide in 58 elderly (>70 years) patients with stage III NSCLC [20]. The median survival was 10 months, and the 1-, 2-, and 5-year survival rates were 45, 24, and 9.1 %, respectively. Hematological, esophageal, and bronchopulmonary acute grade 3+ (3 or greater) toxicities were observed in 22, 7, and 4 % of the patients, respectively. There was no grade 5 toxicity or late grade >3 toxicity. They concluded that the toxicity was relatively low, and the survival results appeared to be comparable to those obtained in younger patients with treated by standard RT alone.

Coate et al. analyzed the Princess Margaret Hospital experience treating 740 elderly patients with stage III NSCLC [21]. Patients were classified by treatment plan: palliative (palliative chemotherapy or radiation [≤ 40 Gy]), nonsurgical multimodality (>40 Gy radiation ± chemotherapy), or surgical multimodality (chemotherapy, radiation, and surgery). Elderly patients (>65 years) were more likely to have poor performance status ($p<0.0001$), multiple comorbidities ($p<0.0001$), and to receive palliative therapy only ($p<0.0001$). Patients treated with curative intent with nonsurgical bimodality therapy or trimodality therapy (including surgery) had similar rates of grade 3/4 toxicity by age group (0–65 years, 39 %; 66–75 years, 43 %; 76+ years, 5 %; $p=0.18$) and toxic death (0–65 years, 4 %; 66–75 years, 4 %; 76+ years, 0 %; $p=0.76$). Survival was worse with increasing age ($p<0.0001$). The authors attributed this to greater use of palliative treatment in the elderly. When survival was analyzed for patients treated with curative intent, there was no difference between age groups for nonsurgical ($p=0.32$) or surgical ($p=0.53$) therapy. They concluded that in fit elderly patients, combined modality therapy is tolerable and associated with survival similar to that of younger patients.

Attempts to Decrease Toxicity by Using Targeted Agents and RT in High-Risk Patients (Primarily the Elderly)

Jatoi et al. [22] performed a prospective trial (NCCTG N0422) which included cetuximab+radiation for elderly and/or poor performance status patients with locally advanced NSCLC. Those eligible included older patients [≥65 years with an Eastern Cooperative Oncology Group performance status (ECOG PS) of 0–2] or younger patients with an ECOG PS of 2. All patients received cetuximab 400 mg/m^2 IV on day 1 followed by weekly cetuximab 250 mg/m^2 IV with concomitant radiation of 6,000 cGy in 30 daily fractions. The primary end point was survival. This 57 patient cohort had a median age of 77 years (range: 60–87), and 12 (21 %) patients had a performance status of 2. The median survival was 15.1 months and the median time to cancer progression was 7.2 months. No treatment-related deaths occurred, but 31 (54 %) patients experienced grade 3+ adverse events, most commonly fatigue, anorexia, dyspnea, rash, and dysphagia, each of which occurred in <10 % of patients. The authors concluded that this combination merits further study in this group of patients.

Jensen et al. performed a similar phase II trial which included intensity-modulated radiation (IMRT) and cetuximab in stage III NSCLC patients considered unfit for chemoradiation [23]. Treatment consisted of IMRT (66 Gy/33 fractions) and weekly cetuximab followed by a 13-week maintenance period. Thirty patients (median age, 71 years) were treated on this protocol. The median survival was 19.5 months, with an estimated 1- and 2-year survival of 66.7 and 34.9 %, respectively. Stage (IIIA vs. IIIB) and histologic subtype did not have a significant impact on survival. Treatment was tolerated well with only mild toxicity (grade 3 pneumonitis: 3.3 %, any grade 3 acute toxicity: 36.7 %). They concluded that IMRT with cetuximab was safe and feasible, especially in elderly patients with multiple comorbidities.

Proton Beam RT and Implications for Elderly Patients

Sejpal et al. hypothesized that proton beam therapy for patients with NSCLC could permit higher tumor doses with less toxicity than photon RT delivered with 3-dimensional conformal RT (3D-CRT) or intensity-modulated RT (IMRT) [24]. This is possible because a proton beam peaks in energy deposition (dose delivered) within a body at the Bragg peak. At this point the protons are stopped because of mass to mass interactions and there is no significant radiation delivered beyond this point. The Bragg peak can be adjusted in position within the patient to overlay a tumor by altering the energy of the beam. In contrast, photons (X-rays) have little or no mass and travel straight through the patient delivering dose both during the entrance and exit of the beam through the patient.

These investigators compared the toxicity of proton therapy plus concurrent chemotherapy in 62 patients with NSCLC (treatment period 2006–2008) with patients with similar disease given 3D-CRT plus chemotherapy ($n=74$; treatment period 2001–2003) or IMRT + chemotherapy ($n=66$; treatment period 2003–2005). Proton therapy to the gross tumor volume was given with weekly IV paclitaxel (50 mg/m^2) and carboplatin (area under the curve 2 mg/mL/min). The primary end point was toxicity. The median total radiation dose was 74 Gy (RBE) for the proton group and 63 Gy for the other groups. Rates of severe (grade 3+) pneumonitis and esophagitis in the proton group (2 and 5 %) were lower than the other groups (3D-CRT, 30 and 18 %; IMRT, 9 and 44 %; $P<0.001$ for all) despite the higher radiation dose. They concluded that higher doses of proton radiation could be delivered to lung tumors with a lower risk of esophagitis and pneumonitis. A randomized comparison of chemotherapy plus either IMRT or proton therapy is being performed to provide better evidence of a possible advantage to proton therapy. Proton therapy would likely be safer than photon therapy when used for any patient with stage III NSCLC. This could be especially attractive for use in the elderly as they do suffer a high risk of serious toxicity from conventional therapy. The improved beam profile within the tissue traversed by the beam during entrance coupled with the lack of a beam exit translates to a better dose distribution which appears to result in greater safety.

Comorbidity and Prognosis

Semrau et al. evaluated the value of concurrent chemoradiotherapy (CRT) for treatment of locally advanced non-small cell lung cancer (NSCLC) in elderly [25]. They specifically investigated the correlation between impaired organ function, age, tumor-associated symptoms, social factors with acute toxicity, and survival following CRT. Retrospective data collection and analysis were performed on the variables age and functional parameters: forced expiratory volume in 1 s (FEV1), vital capacity (VC), diffusion capacity (DLCO), left ventricular ejection volume (LVEF), creatinine clearance, age, several categories of comorbidity, WHO performance status, alcohol and nicotine habits, toxicity according CTC-criteria, and survival of all patients ($n=66$) with inoperable NSCLC suffering substantial comorbidities or advanced age (>70 years). Patients were treated with chemoradiotherapy (CRT) consisting of two cycles cisplatin or carboplatin plus vinorelbine and a conventionally fractionated radiotherapy up to 63 Gy. The median survival of all patients was 13 months. Univariate analyses showed significantly poorer survival (12 months vs. 15 months) in patients with LVEF <50 % compared with LVEF ≥50 % ($P=0.022$, in log-rank test). The other variables did not exhibit a significant correlation to survival. Multivariate analyses revealed significantly inferior survival in patients suffering from cardiac or pulmonary dysfunction ($P=0.039$, hazard ratio [HR]: 2.18). Elderly patients (>70 years) had a higher prevalence of hematotoxicity of higher degree than younger patients (≤70 years) but without significant impact on the feasibility of both treatment modalities. They concluded that cardiac and pulmonary dysfunction may be associated with a reduced survival in elderly or poor-risk patients with inoperable NSCLC after CRT.

In a later retrospective analysis, Semrau et al. evaluated of the effects of tumor- and patient-related factors (cardiopulmonary and heart function) on the toxicity, and prognosis [26]. Cardiopulmonary function had no effect on the toxicity or feasibility of treatment; effects on survival were observed in the univariate analysis. Median survival varied as follows: cardiac function: 13.0 months for left ventricular ejection fraction (LVEF) >50 % vs. 10.0 months for LVEF ≤50 % ($p=0.003$); pulmonary function: 16.0 months for no lung function deficits (vital capacity [VC] ≥ 60 %, forced expiratory volume in 1 s ≥80 %, and diffusing capacity of the lung for carbon monoxide (DLCO) ≥60 %) vs. 14.0 months for one or two function deficits vs. 8.0 months for three lung function deficits ($p=0.001$); T stage: 19.0 months for rcT0/cT1/cT2 vs. 12.0 months for cT3/cT4 ($p=0.039$); and age: 11.0 months for <60 years vs. 18.0 months for 60–69 years vs. 12.0 months for ≥70 years ($p=0.008$). Prognostic factors identified in the multivariate analysis were LVEF ≤50 % ($p=0.043$; hazard ratio [HR], 1.74), reduced pulmonary function ($p=0.001$; HR, 1.71 or 5.05), and T stage ($p=0.026$; HR: 1.71). They concluded that in addition to T stage, cardiac and pulmonary function variables affected the survival of NSCLC patients after chemoradiotherapy.

Conclusions

The results of the above-mentioned studies are reasonably consistent. The studies found that elderly patients experienced more myelosuppression than younger patients [12, 13, 27]. Elderly patients also experienced greater non-hematologic toxicity as a result of the treatment. Elderly patients in NCCTG 94-24-52 had more pneumonitis, those in RTOG 94–10 had more esophagitis, and those in CALGB 9130 had more renal toxicity. Elderly patients may experience greater toxicity because of coexisting morbidities, decreased clearance of the chemotherapy, and decreased marrow reserve. Therefore, physicians should be more cautious when monitoring the effects of therapy in elderly patients.

Despite increased toxicity from combined modality therapy, these studies strongly suggest that fit elderly patients have similar disease control and survival rates as younger patients. Additionally, the JCOG (0301), RTOG (94–10), and NCCTG (90-24-51 and 94-24-52) investigators found that elderly patients had better survival with the more aggressive regimens incorporating concurrent therapy rather than sequential therapy or RT alone. The study by Jeremic et al. also illustrates a very important lesson: lower than standard RT doses in elderly patients appear to produce a bit less optimal results.

The Agati et al. studies revealed that concurrent chemotherapy (carboplatin) and radiotherapy were feasible in elderly patients. The results of their phase II trial were promising enough to perform a phase III trial of RT vs. RT+carboplatin. Agati reported a significant 5.5-month advantage in median survival with chemoradiotherapy compared to TRT alone. More patients had grade 3–4 hematological toxic effects and grade 3 infections in the chemoradiotherapy group.

The results of RT+chemotherapy appear for the most part similar to those obtained with combinations of the targeted therapy, cetuximab with RT. Jatoi et al. (NCCTG N0422) and the trial of Jensen et al. reported median survival durations of 15 and 19.5 months in spite of the inclusion of both elderly and poor PS patients. These trials also reported a bit more modest toxicity.

The prognosis of elderly patients with NSCLC appears dependent on both pulmonary and cardiac function. This makes sense in that both lung and heart functions are needed to withstand the stress of tumor, chemotherapy, and radiotherapy. These two organ systems are also affected by both advanced age and smoking which frequently coexist in NSCLC patients.

These findings suggest that fit elderly patients with locally advanced NSCLC should be encouraged to receive combined modality therapy, preferably on clinical trials. Future research should focus on decreasing treatment toxicity especially in the elderly. Toxicity may potentially be lessened with the use of targeted agents, certain chemotherapy agents, and proton therapy. Additional elderly-specific trials in locally advanced NSCLC will help delineate the optimal approach to therapy for these patients.

References

1. Perez CA. Non-small cell carcinoma of the lung: dose-time parameters. Cancer Treat Symp. 1985;2:131–42.
2. Dillman RO, Herndon J, Seagren SL, et al. Improved survival in stage III non-small-cell lung cancer: seven-year follow-up of cancer and leukemia group B (CALGB) 8433 trial. J Natl Cancer Inst. 1996;88:1210–5.
3. Komaki R, Seiferheld W, Curran W, et al. Sequential vs. concurrent chemotherapy and radiation therapy for inoperable non-small cell lung cancer (NSCLC): analysis of failures in a phase III study (RTOG 9410)(abstract). Int J Radiat Oncol Biol Phys. 2000;48:113.
4. Le Chevalier T, Arriagada R, Quoix E, et al. Radiotherapy alone versus combined chemotherapy and radiotherapy in unresectable non-small cell lung carcinoma. Lung Cancer. 1994;10 Suppl 1:S239–244.
5. Chemotherapy in non-small cell lung cancer: a meta-analysis using updated data on individual patients from 52 randomised clinical trials. Non-small Cell Lung Cancer Collaborative Group. BMJ. 1995;311:899–909.
6. Sause WT, Scott C, Taylor S, et al. Radiation Therapy Oncology Group (RTOG) 88–08 and Eastern Cooperative Oncology Group (ECOG) 4588: preliminary results of a phase III trial in regionally advanced, unresectable non-small-cell lung cancer. J Natl Cancer Inst. 1995;87: 198–205.
7. Furse KFM, Kawahara M, Nishikawa H, Takada Y, Kudoh S, et al. Phase III study of concurrent versus sequential thoracic radiotherapy in combination with mitomycin, vindesine, and cisplatin in unresectable stage III non-small cell lung cancer. J Clin Oncol. 1999;17:2692–9.
8. Komaki RSW, Curran W, et al. Sequential vs. concurrent chemotherapy and radiation therapy for inoperable non-small cell lung cancer (NSCLC): analysis of failures in a phase III study (RTOG 9410) (abstract). Int J Radiat Oncol Biol Phys. 2004;48:113.
9. Jemal A, Murray T, Ward E, et al. Cancer statistics, 2005. CA Cancer J Clin. 2005;55:10–30.

10. Langer CJ, Hsu J, Curran WJ, et al. Elderly patients with locally advanced non-small cell lung cancer (LA NSCLC) benefit from combined modality therapy, secondary analysis of radiation therapy oncology group (RTOG) 94–10. Proc ASCO. 2002;21:299a.
11. Langer CJ, Scott C, Byhardt RW. Effect of advanced age on outcome in radiation therapy oncology group studies of locally advanced NSCLC (LA-NSCLC). Lung Cancer. 2000;29:104.
12. Rocha Lima CM, Herndon 2nd JE, Kosty M, et al. Therapy choices among older patients with lung carcinoma: an evaluation of two trials of the Cancer and Leukemia Group B. Cancer. 2002;94:181–7.
13. Schild SE, Stella PJ, Geyer SM, et al. The outcome of combined-modality therapy for stage III non-small-cell lung cancer in the elderly. J Clin Oncol. 2003;21:3201–6.
14. Schild SE, Stella PJ, Geyer SM, et al. Phase III trial comparing chemotherapy plus once-daily or twice-daily radiotherapy in Stage III non-small-cell lung cancer. Int J Radiat Oncol Biol Phys. 2002;54:370–8.
15. Schild SE, Mandrekar SJ, Jatoi A, et al. The value of combined-modality therapy in elderly patients with stage III nonsmall cell lung cancer. Cancer. 2007;110:363–8.
16. Atagi S, Kawahara M, Ogawara M, et al. Phase II trial of daily low-dose carboplatin and thoracic radiotherapy in elderly patients with locally advanced non-small cell lung cancer. Jpn J Clin Oncol. 2000;30:59–64.
17. Atagi S, Kawahara M, Yokoyama A, et al. Thoracic radiotherapy with or without daily low-dose carboplatin in elderly patients with non-small-cell lung cancer: a randomised, controlled, phase 3 trial by the Japan Clinical Oncology Group (JCOG0301). Lancet Oncol. 2012;13:671–8.
18. Videtic G, Vokes E, Turrisi A, et al. The survival of patients treated for stage III non-small cell lung cancer in North America has increased during the past 25 years. (Abstract 2557). The 39th annual meeting of the American Society of Clinical Oncology. 2003; Chicago: ASCO. p. 291.
19. Langer CJ, Hsu C, Curran WJ, et al. Elderly patients (pts) with locally advanced non-small cell lung cancer (LA-NSCLC) benefit from combined modality therapy: secondary analysis of Radiation Therapy Oncology Group (RTOG) 94–10. In: Proceedings of the American Society of Clinical Oncology. Vol 21. Lippincott Williams & Wilkins; Philadelphia, PA, 2002. p. 299a.
20. Jeremic B, Shibamoto Y, Milicic B, et al. A phase II study of concurrent accelerated hyperfractionated radiotherapy and carboplatin/oral etoposide for elderly patients with stage III non-small-cell lung cancer. Int J Radiat Oncol Biol Phys. 1999;44:343–8.
21. Coate LE, Massey C, Hope A, et al. Treatment of the elderly when cure is the goal: the influence of age on treatment selection and efficacy for stage III non-small cell lung cancer. J Thorac Oncol. 2011;6:537–44.
22. Jatoi A, Schild SE, Foster N, et al. A phase II study of cetuximab and radiation in elderly and/or poor performance status patients with locally advanced non-small-cell lung cancer (N0422). Ann Oncol. 2010;21:2040–4.
23. Jensen AD, Munter MW, Bischoff HG, et al. Combined treatment of nonsmall cell lung cancer NSCLC stage III with intensity-modulated RT radiotherapy and cetuximab: the NEAR trial. Cancer. 2011;117:2986–94.
24. Sejpal S, Komaki R, Tsao A, et al. Early findings on toxicity of proton beam therapy with concurrent chemotherapy for nonsmall cell lung cancer. Cancer. 2011;117:3004–13.
25. Semrau S, Klautke G, Virchow JC, et al. Impact of comorbidity and age on the outcome of patients with inoperable NSCLC treated with concurrent chemoradiotherapy. Respir Med. 2008;102:210–8.
26. Semrau S, Klautke G, Fietkau R. Baseline cardiopulmonary function as an independent prognostic factor for survival of inoperable non-small-cell lung cancer after concurrent chemoradiotherapy: a single-center analysis of 161 cases. Int J Radiat Oncol Biol Phys. 2011;79:96–104.
27. Langer CJ, Hsu C, Curran WJ, et al. Elderly patients with locally advanced non-small cell lung cancer (LA NSCLC) benefit from combined modality therapy, secondary analysis of radiation therapy oncology group (RTOG) 94–10. Proc Am Soc Clin Oncol. 2002;21:299a (abstract 1193).

Part VI
Non Small-Cell Lung Cancer: Treatment of Advanced Disease

Chapter 14
First-Line Treatment and the New Paradigm of Histology-Based Treatment

Cesare Gridelli, Antonio Rossi, and Paolo Maione

Abstract Today, no data are available concerning the histological NSCLC subtypes and treatment in elderly population in which the relationship between histology and therapy can be extrapolated from that of general population. Thus, pemetrexed and bevacizumab can be used in non-squamous histology due to a better efficacy or for safety concerns, respectively. Squamous cell carcinoma could benefit from third-generation-based treatment due to the lack of biological agents resulting active in this histology. The diagnosis of NSCLC NOS is still frequent, but the new immunohistochemical techniques, better defining the histotype, are reducing the incidence of this histology.

Keywords First-line treatment for lung cancer • Histology-based treatment of lung cancer in the elderly • Non-small cell lung cancer in the elderly • Retrospective analyses in NSCLC

In the past, there were two main histological lung cancer subtypes differing for prognosis and treatment approach: non-small cell lung cancer (NSCLC) and small cell lung cancer. In the last few years, there is an emerging role of histology for the decision-making treatment of advanced NSCLC. To date, the advances in biologic knowledge of NSCLC and the development of drugs active in specific histological subtypes are changing the diagnostic and therapeutic approach for this disease with the histology of NSCLC being essential in the choice of first-line treatment. Three subtypes can be included in the NSCLC histology: squamous cell carcinoma,

C. Gridelli, MD (✉)
Department of Oncology/Hematology, S.G. Moscati Hospital, Avellino, Italy
e-mail: cgridelli@libero.it

A. Rossi, MD • P. Maione, MD
Division of Medical Oncology, S.G. Moscati Hospital, Avellino, Italy

C. Gridelli, R.A. Audisio (eds.), *Management of Lung Cancer in Older People*,
DOI 10.1007/978-0-85729-793-8_14,

NSCLC not otherwise specified (NOS), non-squamous cell carcinoma comprising adenocarcinoma and undifferentiated large cell carcinoma. The incidence of these histological subtypes has changed worldwide in the last few decades, now being marked by a growing of adenocarcinoma diagnosis and a concurrent decline in the incidence of squamous cell carcinoma [1]. A possible explanation of this different distribution may be due to the changes in cigarette designing (lower tar and nicotine), which have changed the anatomic location (more peripheral lesions) and histologic subtype (more adenocarcinoma) [2].

The availability of pemetrexed for the treatment of advanced NSCLC patients has shown that histology represents an important variable in decision making. In fact, pemetrexed resulted more active in non-squamous NSCLC histology, in which it is currently registered, and the possible explanation may relate to the baseline thymidylate synthase expression levels, an enzyme inhibited by pemetrexed, which are significantly higher in squamous cell carcinoma compared with adenocarcinoma [3]. These recent evidences led to investigate if previous trials involving older agents had pointed out an association between histology and efficacy outcomes. However, despite NSCLC histological subtypes are always reported for patients enrolled in clinical trials, their relationship with the therapy outcomes and consequently their possible predictive and/or prognostic role has never been explored. A literature review of the last 25 years identified 408 publications reporting an association between advanced NSCLC histology, patient prognosis, and the efficacy of specific chemotherapeutic agents. Eleven trials only reported a prognostic association between histology and clinical outcomes, showing a better survival in patients affected by adenocarcinoma or other type of carcinoma rather than squamous. Seven studies suggested that histologic subtype was a predictive factor in patients treated with specific cytotoxic regimens [4]. A phase III trial comparing cisplatin-docetaxel to docetaxel-gemcitabine showed a significantly higher response rate with the non-platinum regimen among patients with adenocarcinoma, while patients with a non-adenocarcinoma subtype demonstrated a significantly higher response rate with the platinum-based chemotherapy. However, no significant differences in progression-free or overall survival were reported [5]. Another retrospective analysis investigated the survival and time to progression data from a phase III trial comparing paclitaxel plus carboplatin, gemcitabine plus cisplatin, and vinorelbine plus cisplatin administered to 607 advanced NSCLC patients. A survival advantage for squamous cell carcinoma over adenocarcinoma ($p=0.0021$) independently from the schedule was reported [6]. A randomized phase III trial comparing cisplatin plus vinorelbine and cisplatin plus docetaxel in 390 advanced NSCLC patients showed a better median survival for adenocarcinoma with both regimens (11.73 and 11.60 months, respectively) than squamous cell carcinoma (8.87 and 9.92 months, respectively) [7]. Overall, none of these data can be considered reliable, because all these studies were not aimed to assess the role of histology.

The issue of histology has been addressed for NSCLC patients regardless of age, but this is also an important topic for elderly patients. Unfortunately, no studies investigating the relationship between therapy and histology specifically in elderly patients are available.

Retrospective Analyses

The impact on the elderly population of both chemotherapy and new targeted agents has been investigated through retrospective analyses. Regrettably, no correlation data have been reported concerning the different histological NSCLC subgroups and outcomes of treatments.

Chemotherapy

Platinum-based chemotherapy is considered the standard first-line treatment for advanced NSCLC [8–10]. In spite of several concerns in the use of platinum-based chemotherapy in elderly patients, the American Society of Clinical Oncology (ASCO) recommends the use of this regimen regardless the age [8]. The issue of platinum-based therapy for elderly patients with advanced NSCLC has been firstly addressed by retrospective analyses of large randomized trials which had no age limit for enrolling patients. Overall, these analyses showed that the treatment outcomes were similar between patients younger and older than 70 years but with a small increase in toxicity in the elderly group, suggesting that advanced age alone should not preclude this subset of patients to platinum-based chemotherapy [11–15]. All these retrospective analyses did not evaluate the role of histology. Nevertheless, the elderly patients enrolled in these trials are not representative of the real elderly population but rather of a small subgroup considered by investigators to be eligible for aggressive treatments [16].

The activity of pemetrexed in combination with cisplatin versus cisplatin and gemcitabine in chemotherapy-naive patients was retrospectively considered. In this study, 32.7 % of the 1,252 non-squamous patients were ≥65 and 12.8 % were ≥70 years old. Patients treated with pemetrexed plus cisplatin had significantly longer survival compared with those treated with gemcitabine plus cisplatin with hazard ratio (HR) values, favoring pemetrexed, of 0.89 (95 % confidence interval [CI] 0.76–1.05), 0.75 (95 % CI 0.59–0.94), 0.83 (95 % CI 0.72–0.95), and 0.85 (95 % CI 0.59–1.22) for the <65, ≥65, <70, and ≥70 age groups, respectively. Dose intensity delivered and toxicities observed for patients treated with pemetrexed were manageable and similar between the older and younger age groups [17].

The maintenance therapy, generally defined as the continuation of treatment in patients not progressing to four cycles of platinum-based induction treatment, has been investigated in several large randomized phase III trials. A retrospective analysis addressed the role of maintenance therapy in elderly patients. A phase III randomized trial enrolled 539 non-progressing non-squamous NSCLC patients, after four cycles of chemotherapy induction with cisplatin plus pemetrexed, to receive maintenance pemetrexed 500 mg/m^2 day 1 every 3 weeks or placebo until progression or unacceptable toxicity. The primary end point was progression-free survival which statistically improved by maintenance pemetrexed. Subgroup analyses were done for patients aged <70 years and those aged ≥70 years. A total of 92 patients, 52 in pemetrexed arm and 40 in placebo group, were aged ≥70 years. Maintenance pemetrexed reduced the risk of progression by 65 % (HR 0.35, 95 % CI 0.20–0.63; $p=0.00041$), with a median progression-free survival of 6.4 months for the pemetrexed arm and 3.0 months for placebo group. More elderly patients experienced drug-related grade 3–4 anemia and neutropenia, potentially due to greater number of cycles received and worse PS than younger patients [18]. These data confirm the activity and efficacy of maintenance pemetrexed in non-squamous NSCLC histology with a good safety profile also in elderly patients.

Targeted Therapy

Retrospective analysis has been used also to evaluate the impact of new agents in the elderly population because to date, prospective data are still lacking. Bevacizumab is a monoclonal antibody inhibitor of vascular endothelial growth factor (VEGF) currently registered in combination with chemotherapy for first-line treatment of advanced non-squamous NSCLC patients due to a higher incidence of pulmonary hemorrhage reported in squamous histology. Thus, for bevacizumab therapy the choice to treat only non-squamous histology is based simply on safety concern and not on specific biomarkers. In the randomized phase III ECOG 4599 trial, the combination of carboplatin, at the dose of area under curve (AUC) 6, plus paclitaxel, at the dose 200 mg/m^2, was compared with the same regimen plus bevacizumab, at the dose of 15 mg/kg, all drugs given on day 1 every 3 weeks. A subgroup analysis of the older patients ($n=224$ ≥70 years) yielded a trend toward higher response rate (29 % versus 17 %; $p=0.067$) and higher progression-free survival (5.9 versus 4.9 months; $p=0.063$) in favor of the bevacizumab arm and no difference in median survival (11.3 versus 12.1 months; $p=0.4$). However, the older patients enrolled in the bevacizumab arm experienced significant grade ≥3 toxicities compared to their younger counterparts. Seven treatment-related deaths were observed among elderly patients treated with the three-drug combination compared with only two deaths in the chemotherapy alone arm [19]. The AVAiL (AVAstin in Lung) was another phase III randomized trial addressed to non-squamous advanced NSCLC patients in which the combination of cisplatin, 80 mg/m^2 on day 1, plus gemcitabine, 1,250 mg/m^2 on day 1 and 8, every 3 weeks was administered alone or in combination with two different doses of bevacizumab, 7.5 or 15 mg/kg, on day 1, all regimens recycled every 3 weeks. An exploratory not-planned retrospective analysis of the 304 patients older than 65 years was performed also for the AVAiL study. Patients who received bevacizumab derived a clinically relevant improvement in progression-free survival compared with placebo (7.5 mg/kg bevacizumab: HR 0.71; $p=0.023$; 15 mg/kg bevacizumab: HR 0.84; $p=0.25$). Response rates were 40, 29, and 30 % in the 7.5, 15 mg/kg bevacizumab, and placebo arms, respectively. Median survival was similar for each bevacizumab arm versus placebo (7.5 mg/kg bevacizumab: HR 0.84; $p=0.31$; 15 mg/kg bevacizumab: HR 0.88; $p=0.44$). Only grade ≥3 thrombocytopenia occurred more frequently with bevacizumab compared with placebo in patients

Table 14.1 Main retrospective data analyses from randomized phase III trials of elderly patients affected by advanced non-squamous non-small cell lung cancer and enrolled in phase III trials with bevacizumab-based chemotherapy

Author	Age	Treatment	No. pts	ORR (%)	OS (months)
Ramalingam et al. [19]	≥70	CBDCA+PAC+BEV 15[a] vs	111	29	11.3
		CBDCA+PAC	113	27	12.1
Leighl et al. [20]	≥65	CDDP+GEM+BEV 7.5[a] or	89	40	HR 0.84
		CDDP+GEM+BEV 15[a]	103	29	HR 0.88
		vs CDDP+GEM	112	30	–

No. pts number of patients, *ORR* objective response rate, *OS* overall survival, *CBDCA* carboplatin, *PAC* paclitaxel, *BEV* bevacizumab, *CDDP* cisplatin, *GEM* gemcitabine, *HR* hazard ratio
[a]mg/kg

aged ≥65 years (13 % higher in the 7.5 mg/kg arm and 11 % in the 15 mg/kg arm) than those aged <65 years. The incidence of other grade ≥3 adverse events with bevacizumab was similar in older and younger patients (Table 14.1) [20]. The safety of bevacizumab combined with various type of chemotherapy was assessed retrospectively in older patients (≥65 years; $n=361$) enrolled within an open-label study showing no difference in the incidence of serious adverse events between older and younger patients, reporting the same outcome results [21]. Contrasting results about the potential role of bevacizumab in elderly patients are reported, particularly about safety profile. The last two retrospective analyses did not advice any safety concerns for the use of bevacizumab in the elderly, yet in both analyses the cutoff age used to consider a patient elderly was 65 years.

Overall, retrospective analyses should generate hypotheses to verify in prospective trials. Thus, due to the reported results, platinum-based regimens have been prospectively investigated in elderly patients. Also bevacizumab is under investigation in strictly selected elderly patients aged ≥70 years with advanced non-squamous NSCLC.

Prospective Studies

Both chemotherapy and targeted agents have been investigated prospectively in studies addressed specifically to elderly patients. Also in these trials no correlation between histology and outcomes has been investigated.

Chemotherapy

Seven randomized phase III trials have been performed as first-line treatment of advanced NSCLC elderly patients [22–28]. Four trials investigated the role of third-generation drugs administered as single agent or combined in non-platinum-based

Table 14.2 Results from prospective randomized phase III trials with non-platinum-based chemotherapy in patients aged ≥70 years with advanced non-small cell lung cancer regardless of histological subtypes

Author	Treatment	No. pts	ORR (%)	OS (months)
ELVIS [22]	VNR vs BSC	76	20	6.5
		78	NA	4.8
Kudoh et al. [23]	VNR vs TXT	91	9.9	9.9
		88	22.7	14.3
Frasci et al. [24]	VNR vs VNR+GEM	60	15	4.2
		60	22	6.7
Gridelli et al. [25]	VNR or GEM vs VNR+GEM	233	18	8.3
		233	16	6.5
		232	21	6.9

No. pts number of patients, *ORR* objective response rate, *OS* overall survival, *ELVIS* Elderly Lung cancer Vinorelbine Italian Study, *VNR* vinorelbine, *BSC* best supportive care, *NA* not applicable, *TXT* docetaxel, *GEM* gemcitabine

doublet (Table 14.2). The first randomized phase III study ever performed in elderly patients was the ELVIS (Elderly Lung cancer Vinorelbine Italian Study) trial in which 191 patients aged ≥70 years, with an Eastern Cooperative Oncology Group (ECOG) performance status (PS) ≤2, were randomized to single-agent vinorelbine ($n=76$), at the dose of 30 mg/m^2 day 1 and 8 every 3 weeks, plus best supportive care (BSC) or BSC alone ($N=78$). Quality of life (QoL) was the primary end point of the study which resulted improved in vinorelbine-treated patients. Vinorelbine improved median overall survival which was 27 versus 21 weeks reported by BSC alone ($p=0.04$). The relative HR for death for vinorelbine-treated patients was 0.65 (95 % CI 0.45–0.93) [22]. Another randomized phase III trial compared 182 patients, aged ≥70 years and with a PS ≤2 vinorelbine ($n=91$), at the dose of 25 mg/m^2 day 1 and 8, versus docetaxel ($n=88$), administered at 60 mg/m^2 day 1, recycled every 3 weeks. Docetaxel reported a better median survival (14.3 versus 9.9 months, respectively; HR 0.780; 95 % CI 0.561–1.085; $p=0.138$), improved progression-free survival (5.5 versus 3.1 months; HR 0.606, 95 % CI 0.450–0.816; $p<0.001$), and response rate (22.7 % versus 9.9 %; $p=0.019$) than vinorelbine. However, docetaxel was associated with more grade 3–4 neutropenia (82.9 % versus 69.2 %; $p=0.031$). No significant difference, in terms of QoL, was observed between the two arms (odds ratio [OR] 1.30; 95 % CI 0.80–2.11) [23].

Two randomized phase III trials addressed the issue of non-platinum-based doublet. In both trials the doublet investigated was the combination of gemcitabine and vinorelbine [24, 25]. Gemcitabine 1,200 mg/m^2 plus vinorelbine 30 mg/m^2 versus vinorelbine 30 mg/m^2, given on day 1 and 8, recycled every 3 weeks were administered to 120 patients, 60 per each arm aged ≥70 years and with a PS ≤2. The primary end point was OS. This trial was closed early due to an interim analysis showing a survival advantage for the doublet over the single agent (OS: 29 versus 18 weeks, respectively; $p<0.01$). The 1-year survival was 30 and 18 %, respectively, with a HR for death of 0.48 (95 % CI 0.29–0.79). The response rate was 22 % versus 15 %,

Table 14.3 Results from prospective randomized phase III trials with platinum-based chemotherapy in patients aged ≥70 with advanced non-small cell lung cancer regardless of histological subtypes

Author	Treatment	No. pts	ORR (%)	OS (months)
Quoix et al. [26]	VNR or GEM vs CBDCA+PAC	226	10.2	6.2
		225	27.1	10.3
Abe et al. [27]	TXT vs CDDP+TXT	137	24.6	14.8
		139	34.4	13.3
Biesma et al. [28]	CBDCA+GEM vs CBDCA+PAC	90	27	8.6
		91	19	6.9

No. pts number of patients, *ORR* objective response rate, *OS* overall survival, *ELVIS* Elderly Lung cancer Vinorelbine Italian Study, *VNR* vinorelbine, *GEM* gemcitabine, *TXT* docetaxel, *CBDCA* carboplatin, *CDDP* cisplatin, *PAC* paclitaxel

respectively. Grade 3 or 4 neutropenia and thrombocytopenia occurred in 38 and 13 % of patients in the doublet arm and in 28 and 8 % of those in the vinorelbine group, respectively [24]. The largest randomized phase III trial ever performed in the elderly NSCLC patients, named MILES (Multicenter Italian Lung Cancer in the Elderly Study), accrued 698 patients aged ≥70 years and with PS ≤2. This trial showed that the combination of vinorelbine (25 mg/m^2) plus gemcitabine (1,000 mg/m^2) was no more effective than single-agent vinorelbine (30 mg/m^2) or gemcitabine (1,200 mg/m^2) given on day 1 and 8, recycled every 3 weeks. The primary end point was median survival between each single agent and doublet and it was 36, 28, and 30 weeks, and the probability of being alive at 1 year of 38, 28, and 30 %, for vinorelbine, gemcitabine, or their combination, respectively. The HR for death was 1.17 (95 % CI 0.95–1.44) for the combination treatment versus vinorelbine and 1.06 (95 % CI 0.86–1.29) for the combining regimen versus gemcitabine. Although QoL was similar across the three treatment arms, the combination treatment was slightly more toxic than the two drugs given singly. In fact, combination chemotherapy resulted in higher thrombocytopenia and hepatic toxicity compared to single-agent vinorelbine and higher neutropenia, vomiting, fatigue, cardiac toxicity, and constipation compared to single-agent gemcitabine [25].

Three studies investigated the role of platinum-based doublets in the treatment of elderly patients (Table 14.3) [26–28]. Single-agent gemcitabine, at the dose of 1,150 mg/m^2, or vinorelbine, at the dose 8 of 30 mg/m^2, given on day 1 and 8, every 3 weeks versus carboplatin, at the dose of AUC 6 on day 1, plus paclitaxel, at the dose of 90 mg/m^2 on day 1, 8, and 15, every 4 weeks. A total of 451 patients aged from 70 to 89 years, with PS 0–2, were randomized. The median survival, primary end point, was significantly longer for patients treated with combination chemotherapy (10.4 versus 6.2 months; HR 0.639, 95 % CI 0.515–0.792; $p<0.0001$). The 1-year survival was 45.1 % for the doublet and 26.9 % for the single agent with a median progression-free survival of 6.1 versus 3.0 months, respectively. Response rate was 29 % versus 10.9 %, respectively. However, grade 3–4 hematologic toxicities and treatment-related deaths were significantly more frequent in patients treated with carboplatin and paclitaxel as compared to single-agent therapy [26]. A total of

276 elderly patients aged ≥70 years with PS ≤1 were randomized to receive 3-weekly docetaxel at the dose of 60 mg/m² or cisplatin, at the dose of 25 mg/m², plus docetaxel, at the dose of 20 mg/m², both given on day 1, 8, and 15, recycled every 4 weeks. At the first interim analysis, median survival, the primary end point, was 17.3 months for the docetaxel and 13.3 months for the doublet (HR 1.557, 99.99 % CI 0.624–3.884; *p* 0.969). The predictive probability that the doublet could be superior to docetaxel at the final analysis was 0.996 %, so the study was stopped. The updated median survival was 13.3 months for the doublet and 14.8 for the single agent (HR 1.183, 95 % CI 0.830–1.687; $p=0.824$), progression-free survival was 4.7 and 4.4 months (HR 0.924, 95 % CI 0.714–1.197; $p=0.303$) and response rate was 34.4 and 24.6 % ($p=0.101$), respectively. Hematologic toxicities were higher in 3-weekly docetaxel, with grade 4 neutropenia reported in 68 % of patients versus doublet (1 %), and grade 3–4 febrile neutropenia 15 % versus 0 %, respectively. On the contrary non-hematologic toxicities were higher for the doublet arm in which three treatment-related deaths were observed. A subset analysis evaluated the survival of the patients aged <75 years ($n=62$) with 24.1 months for docetaxel and 17.3 months for doublet (HR 1.474, 95 % CI 0.621–3.501) and of those aged ≥75 years ($n=210$) with 15.4 and 13.3 months, respectively (HR 1.131, 95 % CI 0.767–1.669). Thus, no differences between the two arms of each group were reported, but a higher median survival was showed by the patients younger than 75 years [27].

There is only one trial comparing two platinum-based doublets. A total of 181 patients, aged ≥70 years and with PS ≤2, were randomized to receive carboplatin at the dose of AUC 5 on day 1, plus gemcitabine, given at 1,250 mg/m² on day 1 and 8, or paclitaxel, at the dose of 175 mg/m² on day 1, recycled every 3 weeks for a maximum of four cycles. The main end point was QoL. Mean global QoL score at baseline did not differ between both arms without any statistical difference at 18 weeks analysis. The number of QoL responders (12 and 5 % in carboplatin plus gemcitabine or paclitaxel, respectively) was not significantly different. A comprehensive geriatric assessment (CGA) was also carried out with 38 and 25 % of patients enrolled in gemcitabine-based arm and paclitaxel-based arm reporting ≥2 comorbidities, respectively. Almost half of patients had limitations in instrumental activities of daily living (IADL), and more than a quarter had abnormal depression scores. There were no significant interactions between CGA scores and treatment. Overall, grade 3–4 toxicity occurred in 75 and 60 % of patients treated with carboplatin plus gemcitabine or paclitaxel, respectively. The confirmed response rate was 27 and 19 % with a median progression-free survival of 4.7 and 4.5 months and a median survival of 8.6 and 6.9 months, respectively [28].

It is important to consider that the doses and schedules employed in these trials were similar to the ones generally administered in younger patients. In spite of the data seem to favor the platinum-based combinations, the toxicities reported by the elderly should be strongly considered before standardizing this approach to the whole elderly population. Several phase II studies investigated innovative third-generation platinum-based doublets modified with attenuated platinum doses or weekly schedules that would be more suitable in the elderly. Overall, these trials showed that these regimens could maintain the efficacy without increasing toxicity [29]. Among these studies, the MILES-2P, a phase I/II randomized trial, evaluated the feasibility of cisplatin at attenuated doses combined with gemcitabine or vinorelbine in patients aged ≥70 years and with PS 0–1. Cisplatin was feasible and active at 60 mg/m^2 on day 1, with gemcitabine at the fixed dose of 1,000 mg/m^2 on day 1 and 8, and at 40 mg/m^2 on day 1, with vinorelbine given at the fixed dose of 25 mg/m^2 on day 1 and 8, recycled every 3 weeks. With the former combination, 83.3 % of patients were treated without unacceptable toxicity, response rate was 43.5 % (95 % CI 30.6–56.8), median progression-free survival was 25.3 weeks, and median survival of 43.6 weeks. With the latter combination, 82 % of patients were treated without unacceptable toxicity, response rate was 36.1 % (95 % CI 24.2–49.4), and median progression-free survival and survival were 21.1 and 33.1 weeks, respectively [30]. Based on the results coming from MILES-2P study, a randomized phase III trial, named MILES-3, comparing, in patients aged ≥70 years with PS 0–1, cisplatin plus gemcitabine versus gemcitabine alone, is ongoing. A further randomized phase III trial addressed to non-squamous elderly patients, named MILES-4, is going to compare in a factorial design cisplatin plus pemetrexed versus pemetrexed alone versus cisplatin plus gemcitabine versus gemcitabine alone addressing two question: the role of combination platinum-based chemotherapy versus single agent and pemetrexed-based versus gemcitabine-based chemotherapy.

Targeted Therapy

A lot of cellular pathways are involved in the lung cancer development and several of them have been deeply studied. Among these the epidermal growth factor receptor (EGFR) pathway was one of the first against which targeted drugs had been developed and investigated. Gefitinib and erlotinib are two small molecules, given orally, and EGFR tyrosine kinase inhibitors (TKIs) which were investigated firstly, alone or in combination with chemotherapy, in the treatment of unselected patients and then, as single agent, in patients selected for clinical and biological factors [31]. Retrospective analyses of several studies reported a higher benefit obtained in some patient subgroups, such as females, never smokers, Asians, and patients with adenocarcinoma histology. Although clinical characteristics may identify candidates for EGFR-TKIs therapy, the ideal patient selection should mostly rely on biological tumor features, and, in particular, EGFR gene mutations. These represent the most important factor for selecting NSCLC patients who might benefit from EGFR-TKIs therapy and are more frequently correlated with the above mentioned clinical features [32]. Four randomized phase III trials investigated both gefitinib and erlotinib as first-line treatment of advanced NSCLC patients versus chemotherapy. The main end point of each trial was progression-free survival which was statistically improved by EGFR-TKIs therapy [33–36]. Thus, gefitinib is registered for the treatment of advanced NSCLC EGFR mutated patients in any line of therapy. Erlotinib is still waiting for the approval in this setting. All the trials were not addressed specifically to elderly patients; however, in two trials there was the limit age at 75 years and in other two no age limit to enroll patients. Obviously, the most histological NSCLC subtypes included were adenocarcinoma due to the higher incidence of EGFR mutations in this histology. Overall, in presence of an advanced NSCLC harboring an EGFR mutation, the standard of care is gefitinib regardless of the age. In fact, a small phase II study investigated gefitinib in 31 chemotherapy-naïve patients of 75 years of age or older and with PS 0–1 affected by advanced NSCLC harboring EGFR mutations. Almost all of them ($n=30$) were affected by adenocarcinoma. Overall response rate was 74 % with a disease control rate of 90 %. The median progression-free survival was 13.6 months with a 1-year survival rate of 77.4 %. One treatment-related death by interstitial lung disease was observed [37].

A phase II randomized trial compared gefitinib, at the daily dose of 250 mg orally ($n=97$), to vinorelbine, at the dose of 30 mg/m^2 day 1 and 8, every 3 weeks ($n=99$) as first-line treatment of patients aged ≥70 years and with PS ≤2. The primary end point was progression-free survival. The HRs for gefitinib versus vinorelbine were 1.19 (95 % CI 0.85–1.65) for progression-free survival and 0.98 (95 % CI 0.66–1.47) for overall survival. The response and disease control rates were 3.1 and 43.3 %, for gefitinib, and 5.1 and 53.5 %, for vinorelbine, respectively. Overall QoL and pulmonary symptoms improvement rates were 24.3 and 36.6 %, for gefitinib, and 10.9 and 31 %, for vinorelbine, respectively. Gefitinib was better tolerated with fewer treatment-related grade 3–5 adverse events (12.8 %) than with vinorelbine (41.7 %) [38].

Erlotinib, at the daily dose of 150 mg orally, was investigated in 80 unselected elderly patients (≥70 years) with previously untreated advanced NSCLC reporting a response rate of 10 % with a stable disease of 41 %. There was an overall survival of 10.9 months. Rash and diarrhea, the most common toxicities, occurred in 81 and 69 % of the patients, respectively [39].

A phase II randomized trial investigated prospectively two bevacizumab-based regimen as first-line therapy of patients aged ≥70 years with PS 0–1 affected by non-squamous NSCLC. Patients were randomized to pemetrexed, at the dose of 500 mg/m^2, plus gemcitabine, at the dose of 1,500 mg/m^2, plus bevacizumab, given at 10 mg/kg, days 1 and 15 of 28–day cycles, or pemetrexed, at the same dose, plus carboplatin, at AUC 5, plus bevacizumab given at 15 mg/kg, day 1 of 21–day cycles. Patients not progressing after six cycles continued maintenance bevacizumab until disease progression. A total of 110 patients were randomized reporting a time to progression, primary end point, of 4.7 and 10.2 months in non-platinum-based regimen and platinum-based regimen, respectively; with median survival of 7.5 and 14.8 months, respectively, the response rate was 35 % in both arms. Three and two treatment-related deaths occurred, respectively. Thus, the combination of pemetrexed plus carboplatin plus bevacizumab was associated with improved outcomes in this elderly population leading to a further evaluation (Table 14.4) [40]. Targeted therapies, with the exception of gefitinib, are still under investigation properly in the older population due to the lack of large prospective studies.

Table 14.4 Results from prospective trials with new biological agents in patients aged ≥70 years with advanced non-small cell lung cancer regardless of histological subtypes

Author	Type of study	Treatment	No. pts	ORR (%)	OS (months)
Crinò et al. [38]	II randomized	Gefitinib vs Vinorelbine	97	3.1	5.9
			99	5.1	8.0
Jackman et al. [39]	II	Erlotinib	80	10	10.9
Spigel et al. [40][a]	II randomized	PEM+GEM+BEV 10[b] vs	55	35	7.5
		PEM+CBDCA+BEV 15[b]	55	35	14.8

No. pts number of patients, *ORR* objective response rate, *OS* overall survival, *PEM* pemetrexed, *GEM* gemcitabine, *CBDCA* carboplatin, *BEV* bevacizumab
[a]Only in non-squamous histology
[b]mg/kg

Conclusions

Still today, no data are available concerning the histological NSCLC subtypes and treatment in elderly population in which the relationship between histology and therapy can be extrapolated from that of general population. Thus, pemetrexed and bevacizumab can be used in non-squamous histology due to a better efficacy or for safety concerns, respectively. Squamous cell carcinoma could benefit from third-generation-based treatment due to the lack of biological agents resulting active in this histology. The diagnosis of NSCLC NOS is still frequent, but the new immunohistochemical techniques, better defining the histotype, are reducing the incidence of this histology.

These considerations underline an important topic: the need of an adequate amount of cancer tissue to perform the diagnosis of the type of NSCLC histology and the biomolecular analyses, in order to better address the treatment. Elderly patients affected by NSCLC harboring EGFR mutations should receive gefitinib. Elderly patients with PS 0–1, no major comorbidities, should receive a third-generation platinum-based regimen, but schedules investigated specifically in old population are preferred. In the general elderly population, a third-generation single-agent drug is a valid option. In conclusion, although several data have been already produced, further trials need to better address first-line chemotherapy and/or targeted therapy in elderly NSCLC patients.

References

1. Gabrielson E. Worldwide trends in lung cancer pathology. Respirology. 2006;11:533–8.
2. Strauss GM, Jemal A, McKenna MB, et al. The epidemic of smoking-related adenocarcinoma of the lung: the role of the tobacco industry and filtered and low-tar cigarettes. J Thorac Oncol. 2007;2 Suppl 4:S305 (abstr. PRS-01).
3. Scagliotti G, Hanna N, Fossella F, et al. The differential efficacy of pemetrexed according to NSCLC histology: a review of two Phase III studies. Oncologist. 2009;14:253–63.

4. Hirsch FR, Spreafico A, Novello S, et al. The prognostic and predictive role of histology in advanced non-small cell lung cancer: a literature review. J Thorac Oncol. 2008;3:1468–81.
5. Georgoulias V, Papadakis E, Alexopoulos A, et al. Platinum-based and non-platinum-based chemotherapy in advanced non-small-cell lung cancer: a randomised multicentre trial. Lancet. 2001;357:1478–84.
6. Scagliotti GV, de Marinis F, Rinaldi M, et al. The role of histology with common first-line regimens for advanced non-small cell lung cancer: a brief report of the retrospective analysis of a three-arm randomized trial. J Thorac Oncol. 2009;4:1568–71.
7. Tan EH, Rolski J, Grodzki T, et al. Global Lung Oncology Branch trial 3 (GLOB3): final results of a randomised multinational phase III study alternating oral and i.v. vinorelbine plus cisplatin versus docetaxel plus cisplatin as first-line treatment of advanced non-small-cell lung cancer. Ann Oncol. 2009;20:1249–56.
8. Azzoli CG, Baker Jr S, Temin S, et al. American Society of Clinical Oncology Clinical Practice Guideline update on chemotherapy for stage IV non-small-cell lung cancer. J Clin Oncol. 2009;27:6251–66.
9. Felip E, Gridelli C, Baas P, et al. Metastatic non-small-cell lung cancer: consensus on pathology and molecular tests, first-line, second-line, and third-line therapy: 1st ESMO Consensus Conference in Lung Cancer; Lugano 2010. Ann Oncol. 2011;22:1507–19.
10. de Marinis F, Rossi A, Di Maio M, et al. Treatment of advanced non-small-cell lung cancer: Italian Association of Thoracic Oncology (AIOT) clinical practice guidelines. Lung Cancer. 2011;73:1–10.
11. Langer CJ, Vangel M, Schiller J, et al. Age-specific subanalysis of ECOG 1594: fit elderly patients (70–80 yrs) with NSCLC do as well as younger pts (<70). Proc Am Soc Clin Oncol. 2003;22:639 (abstr. 2571).
12. Hensing TA, Peterman AH, Schell MJ, et al. The impact of age on toxicity, response rate, quality of life, and survival in patients with advanced, stage IIIB or IV nonsmall cell lung carcinoma treated with carboplatin and paclitaxel. Cancer. 2003;98:779–88.
13. Belani CP, Fossella F. Elderly subgroup analysis of a randomized phase III study of docetaxel plus platinum combinations versus vinorelbine plus cisplatin for first-line treatment of advanced nonsmall cell lung carcinoma (TAX 326). Cancer. 2005;104:2766–74.
14. Ramalingam S, Perry MC, La Rocca RV, et al. Comparison of outcomes for elderly patients treated with weekly paclitaxel in combination with carboplatin versus the standard 3-weekly paclitaxel and carboplatin for advanced nonsmall cell lung cancer. Cancer. 2008;113:542–6.
15. Blanchard EM, Moon J, Hesketh PJ, et al. Comparison of platinum-based chemotherapy in patients older and younger than 70 years: an analysis of Southwest Oncology Group Trials 9308 and 9509. J Thorac Oncol. 2011;6:115–20.
16. Perrone F, Gallo C, Gridelli C. Re: cisplatin-based therapy for elderly patients with advanced non-small-cell lung cancer: implications of Eastern Cooperative Oncology Group 5592, a randomized trial. J Natl Cancer Inst. 2002;94:1029–31.
17. Gridelli C, Brodowicz T, Langer CJ, et al. Pemetrexed therapy in elderly patients with good performance status: analysis of two phase III trials of patients with nonsquamous non-small cell lung cancer. Clin Lung Cancer. 2012;13(5):340–6.
18. Gridelli C, Thomas M, Prabhash K, et al. Pemetrexed (pem) maintenance therapy in elderly patients (pts) with good performance status (PS) – analysis of PARAMOUNT phase III study of pem versus placebo in advanced nonsquamous non-small cell lung cancer (NSCLC). Eur J Cancer. 2011;47 Suppl 1:S613 (abstr. 9072).
19. Ramalingam SS, Dahlberg SE, Langer CJ, et al. Outcomes for elderly, advanced-stage non small-cell lung cancer patients treated with bevacizumab in combination with carboplatin and paclitaxel: analysis of Eastern Cooperative Oncology Group Trial 4599. J Clin Oncol. 2008;26:60–5.
20. Leighl N, Zatloukal P, Mezger J, et al. Efficacy and safety of bevacizumab-based therapy in elderly patients with advanced or recurrent nonsquamous non-small cell lung cancer in the phase III BO17704 study (AVAiL). J Thorac Oncol. 2010;5:1970–6.

21. Griesinger F, Pavlakis N, Garrido P, et al. MO19390 (SAiL): safety and efficacy of first-line bevacizumab plus chemotherapy in elderly patients with advanced or recurrent non-squamous non-small cell lung cancer (NSCLC). J Thorac Oncol. 2009;4 suppl 1:S359 (abstr. C2.6).
22. The Elderly Lung Cancer Vinorelbine Italian Study Group. Effects of vinorelbine on quality of life and survival of elderly patients with advanced non small cell lung cancer. J Natl Cancer Inst. 1999;91:66–72.
23. Kudoh S, Takeda K, Nakagawa K, et al. Phase III study of docetaxel compared with vinorelbine in elderly patients with advanced non-small-cell lung cancer: results of the West Japan Thoracic Oncology Group trial (WJOG 9904). J Clin Oncol. 2006;24:3657–63.
24. Frasci G, Lorusso V, Panza N, et al. Gemcitabine plus vinorelbine versus vinorelbine alone in elderly patients with advanced non-small-cell lung cancer. J Clin Oncol. 2000;18:2529–36.
25. Gridelli C, Perrone F, Gallo C, et al. Chemotherapy for elderly patients with advanced non-small-cell lung cancer: the Multicenter Italian Lung Cancer in the Elderly Study (MILES) phase III randomized trial. J Natl Cancer Inst. 2003;95:362–72.
26. Quoix E, Zalcman G, Oster JP, et al. Carboplatin and weekly paclitaxel doublet chemotherapy compared with monotherapy in elderly patients with advanced non-small-cell lung cancer: IFCT-0501 randomised, phase 3 trial. Lancet. 2011;378:1079–88.
27. Abe T, Yokoyama A, Takeda K, et al. Randomized phase III trial comparing weekly docetaxel (D)-cisplatin (P) combination with triweekly D alone in elderly patients (pts) with advanced non-small cell lung cancer (NSCLC): an intergroup trial of JCOG0803/WJOG4307L. J Clin Oncol. 2011;29:478s (abstr. 7509).
28. Biesma B, Wymenga ANM, Vincent A, et al. Quality of life, geriatric assessment and survival in elderly patients with non-small-cell lung cancer treated with carboplatin-gemcitabine or carboplatin-paclitaxel: NVALT-3 a phase III study. Ann Oncol. 2011;22:1520–7.
29. Gridelli C, Maione P, Rossi A. Therapy for elderly patients with advanced non-small cell lung cancer. In: 47th annual meeting of American Society of Clinical Oncology Educational Book. Alexandria, VA: American Society of Clinical Oncology; 2011. p. 300–4.
30. Gridelli C, Maione P, Illiano A, et al. Cisplatin plus gemcitabine or vinorelbine for elderly patients with advanced non small-cell lung cancer: the MILES-2P studies. J Clin Oncol. 2007;25:4663–9.
31. Rossi A, Galetta D, Gridelli C. Biological prognostic and predictive factors in lung cancer. Oncology. 2009;77 Suppl 1:90–6.
32. Shigematsu H, Gazdar AF. Somatic mutations of epidermal growth factor receptor signalling pathway in lung cancers. Int J Cancer. 2006;118:257–62.
33. Mitsudomi T, Morita S, Yatabe Y, et al. Gefitinib versus cisplatin plus docetaxel in patients with non-small-cell lung cancer harbouring mutations of the epidermal growth factor receptor (WJTOG3405): an open label, randomised phase 3 trial. Lancet Oncol. 2010;11:121–8.
34. Maemondo M, Inoue A, Kobayashi K, et al. Gefitinib or chemotherapy for non-small-cell lung cancer with mutated EGFR. N Engl J Med. 2010;362:2380–8.
35. Zhou C, Wu YL, Chen G, et al. Erlotinib versus chemotherapy as first-line treatment for patients with advanced EGFR mutation-positive non-small-cell lung cancer (OPTIMAL, CTONG-0802): a multicentre, open-label, randomised, phase 3 study. Lancet Oncol. 2011;12: 735–42.
36. Rosell R, Gervais R, Vergnenegre A, et al. Erlotinib vs chemotherapy (CT) in advanced non-small-cell lung cancer (NSCLC) patients (p) with epidermal growth factor receptor (EGFR) activating mutations: Interim results of the European Tarceva vs Chemotherapy (EURTAC) phase III randomized trial. J Clin Oncol. 2011;29(15S):476s (abstr. 7503).
37. Mineshi Y, Maemondo M, Okinaga S, et al. First-line gefitinib therapy for elder advanced non-small cell lung cancer patients with epidermal growth factor receptor mutations: multicenter phase II trial (NEJ 003 study). J Clin Oncol. 2010;28(18S):553s (abstr. 7561).
38. Crinò L, Cappuzzo F, Zatloukal P, et al. Gefitinib versus vinorelbine in chemotherapy-naive elderly patients with advanced non-small-cell lung cancer (INVITE): a randomized, phase II study. J Clin Oncol. 2008;26:4253–60.

39. Jackman DM, Yeap BY, Lindeman NI, et al. Phase II clinical trial of chemotherapy-naïve patients ≥70 years of age treated with erlotinib for advanced non-small-cell lung cancer. J Clin Oncol. 2007;25:760–6.
40. Spigel DR, Hainsworth JD, Shipley DL, et al. A randomized phase II trial of pemetrexed/gemcitabine/bevacizumab or pemetrexed/carboplatin/bevacizumab in the first-line treatment of elderly patients with advanced non-small cell lung cancer. J Thorac Oncol. 2012;7(1):196–202.

Chapter 15
Treatment of Frail Patients and Octogenarians with Advanced NSCLC

Cesare Gridelli, Paolo Maione, and Antonio Rossi

Abstract Octogenarians and frail patients with advanced non-small cell lung cancer (NSCLC) constitute a clinical setting commonly faced by the oncologist as a consequence of the high incidence of lung cancer in the elderly. The selection of the treatment approach in this setting is often difficult because of the extreme paucity of prospective data regarding the safety of standard treatment strategies for advanced NSCLC. However, for fit octogenarian patients with advanced NSCLC, single-agent chemotherapy can be a reasonable treatment choice. On the contrary, frail patients should be treated with supportive care only with the exception of carefully selected cases (i.e., gefitinib or erlotinib in patients with tumor harboring an EGFR-activating mutation). Only specifically designed prospective trials (with separation of fit octogenarians from frail patients), will clarify the optimal systemic treatment for advanced NSCLC in these two peculiar patient populations.

Keywords NSCLC in the elderly • Non-small cell lung cancer in the elderly • Octogenarians with advanced NSCLC • The frail patient with lung cancer • Chemotherapy and targeted therapies in unfit elderly patients

C. Gridelli, MD (✉)
Department of Oncology/Hematology,
S.G. Moscati Hospital,
Avellino, Italy
e-mail: cgridelli@libero.it

P. Maione, MD • A. Rossi, MD
Division of Medical Oncology,
S.G. Moscati Hospital,
Avellino, Italy

C. Gridelli, R.A. Audisio (eds.), *Management of Lung Cancer in Older People*,
DOI 10.1007/978-0-85729-793-8_15, © Springer-Verlag London 2013

Lung cancer in the older individual is an increasingly common problem faced by the oncologist. There are substantial concerns about treating older patients with advanced non-small cell lung cancer (NSCLC). Elderly patients often present with medical and physiologic characteristics that make the selection of their optimal treatment more challenging [1]. In fact, aging causes physiologic changes in functional status, organ function, and drug pharmacokinetics [2]. Furthermore, concomitant diseases, which may significantly affect functional status, general health, and tumor symptoms, are frequently present in this patient population. These comorbidities may also result in a higher prevalence of polypharmacy and related risks. Given these health concerns, it is important to carefully assess the potential benefit of a systemic treatment.

Performance status (PS) 2 patients usually account for a small proportion of patients enrolled in trials of first-line treatment for advanced NSCLC [3] but represent a significantly higher proportion (up to 30–40 %) when population-based surveys are conducted [4]. Thus, unfit older patients represent a significant proportion of advanced NSCLC patients, for whom specific prospective data are very scarce. Consequently, medical treatment of this special population is often empirical and further prospective investigation is absolutely warranted. Unfortunately, among elderly patients only data regarding PS 2 patients, subgroup that can be considered including vulnerable patients, are available and only retrospective evidences exist from clinical trials dedicated to PS 2 patients without age limits or specifically designed for the elderly. The doubts and fears in treating elderly patients with lung cancer increase when the patients are older than 80 years, due to very few data available.

Octogenarians and Lung Cancer

A study using the surveillance, epidemiology and end results (SEER) database from 1988 to 2003 showed that patients aged 80 years or older accounted for 14 % of all patients with lung cancer [5]. Moreover, from actuarial tables of the population at large, the life expectancies of 80-year-old men and women are 87.3 and 89.0 years, respectively. In addition only a minority of these 80 years of age and older and 85 years of age and older have dementia [6, 7].

The increase of octogenarians with lung cancer, and often in good clinical conditions, raises the importance of finding an optimal treatment for these very elderly patients. In fact, there are limited data describing the specific therapies for patients aged 80 years or older because rarely they are included in phase III trials.

A recent study of the SEER database [8] found that lung cancer patients older than the age of 80 had an inferior 5-year survival rate (8.3 %) compared with younger patients (16.2 %, $p \leq 0.0001$), controlling for stage, gender, and race. It also demonstrated that in practice, fewer of these very elderly NSCLC patients receive surgery or radiation treatments compared with younger patients. An earlier analysis of NSCLC patients in the SEER database found that the rate of receiving guideline-recommended therapy was lower among patients aged 80 and older (33 %) than among patients aged 50–59 (66 %) [9].

In conclusion, because patients 80 years of age and older constitute between 10 and 20 % of all lung cancer patients and the median survival of healthy octogenarians is approaching a decade, it is important to consider whether these patients can benefit from chemotherapy.

Frailty and Cancer

The trajectory of aging, which begins in early adulthood, involves progressive decline in the functional reserve of multiple organs and systems. Seemingly, this is due to a combination of factors including predetermined limitation in individual functional reserve, ongoing damage from environmental agents, increased prevalence of chronic diseases, and the emergence of a number of conditions termed geriatric syndromes [10–12]. The loss of functional reserve leads to functional impairment, disability, handicaps, functional dependence, and ultimately death. Loss of functional reserve also increases the susceptibility of older individuals to stress so that acute diseases are more common, more prolonged, more disabling, and more toxic in older individuals. In addition, complications associated with the medical interventions occur more frequently. The evaluation of the older-aged individual explores all dimensions of aging including function (expressed as activities of daily living [ADLs] and instrumental activities of daily living [IADLs]), comorbidity (with special attention to cardiovascular diseases, depression, anemia, and other cancers), social support, cognitive status, and presence of geriatric syndromes. The Comprehensive Geriatric Assessment (CGA) has reduced the rate of hospitalization and institutionalization of older individuals and also might have prolonged their survival. In geriatric oncology, the advantages of a CGA are threefold: it identifies reversible conditions that might interfere with the treatment of older patients, it ascertains an estimate of life expectancy and treatment tolerance, and it establishes a common language in the classification of older individuals in alternative to the use of chronologic age. Patients with dependence in one or more ADLs, with severe comorbidities, and with one or more geriatric syndromes are considered candidates for symptom management only. The underlying assumption is that the functional reserve of these individuals is so limited that they could not tolerate even minimal stress.

Until recently, a consistent definition of frailty remained elusive [13]. However, emerging data are providing a uniform definition of frailty within the geriatric population. A position statement from the American Medical Association defined the term "frailty" as characterizing "the group of patients that presents the most complex and challenging problems to the physician and all health care professionals," because these are the individuals who have a higher susceptibility to adverse outcomes, such as institutionalization or mortality [14–16].

Although frailty models provide important prognostic information for the geriatric population at large, data applicable to oncology patients are lacking. Frailty criteria for older adults with cancer have been proposed, combining elements of existing definitions. For example, the Balducci criteria are derived in part from observations reported in a study by Winograd et al. assessing predictors of mortality and institutionalization among male patients aged 65 years and older at the Palo Alto Veterans Affairs Medical Center [17]. Winograd et al. identified functional impairment, comorbidity, and the presence of geriatric syndromes as predictors. The Balducci frailty criteria supplement these predictors with a criterion of age older than 85 years, given the purported high incidence of functional and cognitive changes in this demographic [18].

In conclusion, several definitions of frailty have been described including empiric criteria as defined by Balducci et al. [18]. The challenge for the oncologist is to incorporate elements from these definitions into a framework optimized for the older adult with cancer. The geriatric assessment may serve as the framework, because this tool includes components with independent prognostic implications for the older cancer patient.

The geriatric assessment has emerged as a useful oncology tool. It adds information to more generalized measures of functional status usually employed in oncology, such as the Karnofsky or ECOG PS. Repetto et al. juxtaposed assessment by ECOG PS and by geriatric assessment in a cohort of 363 patients admitted with a diagnosis of a solid or hematologic malignancy [19]. Elements of the geriatric assessment used in this study included demographic characteristics, physical function, disability, depression, and cognitive status. Components of the geriatric assessment and ECOG PS were found to be strongly associated. For example, the presence of ADL or IADL dependence conferred a fivefold higher risk of poor PS (ECOG PS of 2 or higher). However, no association between comorbidity and PS was observed in this study. Presumably, these data suggest that although some domains of the geriatric assessment (i.e., disability assessment) may serve as a surrogate for PS, other components (such as comorbidity) may offer supplementary information that could augment its prognostic value.

Chemotherapy and Targeted Therapies in Unfit Elderly Patients

Oncologists must choose among several treatment options for elderly patients with advanced NSCLC: best supportive care without chemotherapy, single-agent chemotherapy with a third-generation drug, non-platinum-based combination chemotherapy, platinum-based combination chemotherapy, or new biologic agents. Unfit older patients have been usually excluded from this type of clinical trials dedicated to PS 0–1 subgroup, and the feasibility of platin-based chemotherapy in this special population is absolutely not proven and should be avoided. Based on these observations, single-agent chemotherapy should be considered a reasonable treatment choice and the standard for comparison in unselected elderly patients with advanced NSCLC

[20]. Although this assumption is yet debatable for PS 0–1 elderly patients considering the potential role of platin-based regimens, on the contrary should be considered the optimal choice for unfit older patients (or elderly patients with PS 2). The results of a European Experts Panel on the topic indicate that single-agent chemotherapy could be the preferred option in the treatment of PS 2 patients, with carboplatin-based or low-dose cisplatin-based doublets representing alternative options [21]. This suggestion on single-agent chemotherapy as preferred option for PS 2 patients should be considered particularly wise for PS 2 elderly patients. In fact, in the ELVIS trial, the first randomized phase III trial that demonstrated a survival advantage in favor of single-agent chemotherapy with vinorelbine versus best supportive care in the treatment of elderly patients with advanced NSCLC, the percentage of PS 2 patients was 24 %. Also in this subgroup of PS 2 elderly patients, the advantage of vinorelbine versus best supportive care was confirmed [22]. Moreover, in the MILES phase III randomized trial that compared polychemotherapy with gemcitabine + vinorelbine versus single-agent chemotherapy with vinorelbine or gemcitabine, no advantage was found in terms of survival in favor of polichemotherapy versus monochemotherapy, also in the subgroup of PS 2 patients. In addition, polichemotherapy was demonstrated to be more toxic. In this large trial (about 700 patients randomized), the percentage of PS 2 patients was about 20 % [23]. Targeted therapies are an alternative to chemotherapy in the treatment of elderly advanced NSCLC patients, and some of them, because of their favorable safety profile, may be particularly suitable to unfit older patients. In fact, the results reported in phase I, II, and III trials performed with several targeted agents in younger patients indicate that the safety profile of most of these new drugs makes them more suitable than cytotoxic chemotherapy for elderly patients. Erlotinib, an epidermal growth factor receptor tyrosine kinase inhibitor (EGFR-TKI), is characterized by a mild safety profile that makes it particularly suitable to be tested prospectively as single agent in the first-line treatment of elderly patients as an alternative to cytotoxic chemotherapy. Jackman and colleagues have formally tested erlotinib in a phase II study in 80 patients over 70 years of age with previously untreated advanced NSCLC. Erlotinib was well tolerated with encouraging activity [24]. They reported a response rate of 10 % and disease stabilization rate of 41 %. There was a significant improvement of key symptoms (dyspnea, cough, fatigue, pain) and an intriguing median survival of 10.9 months. Rash and diarrhea were the most common toxicities occurring in 81 and 69 % of the patients, respectively. In this trial, also PS 2 patients were enrolled. Thus, these results can be considered also for unfit elderly patients. Crinò et al. have published the results of the INVITE trial [25]. This phase II, open-label, parallel-group study compared gefitinib (another EGFR-TKI) with vinorelbine in chemotherapy- naïve elderly patients with advanced NSCLC. About 200 patients were enrolled. Hazard ratios (HR; gefitinib versus vinorelbine) were 1.19 (95 % CI, 0.85–1.65) for progression-free survival and 0.98 (95 % CI, 0.66–1.47) for overall survival. Response rate and disease control rates were 3.1 % (95 % CI, 0.6–8.8) and 43.3 % (for gefitinib) and 5.1 % (95 % CI, 1.7–11.4) and 53.5 % (for vinorelbine), respectively. There were fewer treatment-related grade 3–5 adverse events with gefitinib (12.8 %) than with vinorelbine (41.7 %).

The authors concluded that there was no statistical difference between gefitinib and vinorelbine in efficacy in chemotherapy-naïve, unselected elderly patients with advanced NSCLC, but there was better tolerability with gefitinib. Considering that also PS 2 patients were enrolled onto this trial, the better safety profile demonstrated by gefitinib compared with vinorelbine must be taken into consideration when selecting treatment for unfit elderly patients. Unfit older patients with lung cancer are at risk of both empirical under-treatment resulting in poor survival and excessive toxicity from standard therapy. Thus, specifically designed prospective studies are mandatory to provide definitive recommendations for the treatment of unfit elderly patients with lung cancer. At the moment, single-agent chemotherapy should be considered the best option for unfit elderly patients. If the EGFR-TKIs erlotinib and gefitinib were approved for use also in the first-line treatment of advanced NSCLC, to date they are approved only for patients with tumors harboring EGFR mutations; they would represent a valid alternative to single-agent chemotherapy for a large proportion of unfit older patients because of their more favorable safety profile. Asami et al. recently performed a phase II study aimed to investigate the efficacy and usefulness of gefitinib therapy as a first-line treatment for elderly patients affected by advanced lung adenocarcinoma with EGFR mutations. They enrolled patients aged 75 years or older. Between April 2008 and November 2009, 17 patients were enrolled. Overall response rate was 59 % (95 % confidence interval [CI]: 33–81 %), with two patients achieving complete response and eight partial response. Stable disease was noted in five patients, and disease control rate was 88 % (95 % CI: 62–98 %). Median progression-free survival was 12.9 months (95 % CI: 2.2–23.6 months), and median overall survival had not yet been reached. Major grade 3 toxicities were skin rash (12 %) and increased levels of aspartate aminotransferase or alanine aminotransferase (18 %). The authors concluded that first-line treatment with gefitinib was effective and well tolerated in elderly patients with EGFR mutations [26]. It is to note that in this trial 17 % of the patients were PS 2 and the median age was 81 (range 75–88 years). Thus, the results of this trial that confirm the good safety profile of gefitinib in the elderly can be considered valid also for octogenarian patients.

For frail elderly patient group with poorer clinical conditions and PS 3–4, to date in absence of data, best supportive care alone is recommended. However, in patients with PS 3–4 whose tumors harbor EGFR mutations, an EGFR-TKI (gefitinib or erlotinib) should be considered as demonstrated by the study by Inoue et al. [27]. In fact these authors performed a phase II study to investigate the efficacy and feasibility of gefitinib for patients with advanced NSCLC harboring *EGFR* mutations without indication for chemotherapy as a result of poor PS. Chemotherapy-naïve patients with poor PS (patients 20–74 years of age with PS 3–4, 75–79 years of age with PS 2–4, and ≥80 years of age with PS 1–4) who had EGFR mutations were enrolled and received gefitinib (250 mg/day) alone. Between February 2006 and May 2007, 30 patients with NSCLC and poor PS, including 22 patients with PS 3–4, were enrolled. The overall response rate was 66 % (90 % CI, 51–80 %), and the disease control rate was 90 %. PS improvement rate was 79 % ($p \leq .00005$); in particular, 68 % of the 22 patients improved from ≥PS 3 at baseline to ≤PS 1. The median progression-free survival, median survival time, and 1-year survival rate were 6.5, 17.8 months, and 63 %, respectively. No treatment-related deaths were observed in this trial. This interesting trial demonstrates that when clinical characteristics suggest that EGFR mutational analysis should be performed, frailty, poor PS, and age ≥80 must not be a limit, because when tumors harbor EGFR mutations, dramatic responses can be achieved also in these peculiar and extreme patient populations [28].

Retrospective Data on Octogenarians with Advanced NSCLC

Few reports have described the distribution of treatment modalities in octogenarians with advanced NSCLC. Chen et al. performed a retrospective study to characterize the treatment modalities and outcomes for octogenarian Taiwanese patients with advanced NSCLC and to investigate the impact of EGFR-TKIs on survival [29]. From January 2000 to December 2006, patients with NSCLC aged 80 years or older with stage IIIB or IV disease at National Taiwan University Hospital were included. The medical records were reviewed and analyzed. A Cox proportional hazard model was used to calculate the hazard ratio and its 95 % confidence interval for gender, performance status, histologic types, disease stages, smoking history, comorbidities, and initial treatment modalities. A total of 203 patients were included. Among the 203 patients, 93 (45.8 %) received supportive care only. Regarding the initial antitumor therapy, 65 patients (32.0 %) received EGFR-TKI therapy, 17 (8.4 %) received chemotherapy, and 28 (13.8 %) received palliative radiotherapy. Sixty-five patients (32.0 %) were treated with EGFR-TKI as the first-line therapy, and all of them were admitted after 2003. After 2003, the proportion of supportive care significantly decreased ($p \leq 0.001$), whereas those of chemotherapy and radiotherapy showed no significant change. There was a trend of an increase in median survival from 2003 (2000: 37 days, 2001: 62 days, 2002: 69 days, 2003: 110 days, 2004: 85 days, 2005: 188 days, and 2006: 195 days). When compared with those who received supportive care only, patients who received EGFR-TKI therapy had a significantly better prognosis (hazard ratio: 0.56, 95 % confidence interval: 0.40–0.80), whereas no significant survival benefit was found in patients who received chemotherapy or radiotherapy. Obviously, these data, although interesting, cannot be generalized because they are collected in Asiatic patients where the impact of EGFR-TKIs is larger. However, these data demonstrate that the safety profile of EGFR-TKIs is particularly suitable to a peculiar patient population as octogenarians or frail patients.

In another retrospective study, all patients with chemotherapy-naive advanced non-small cell lung cancer 80 years of age and older treated at the MD Anderson Cancer Center with one or more follow-ups were identified from the database for the years 1997–2004 [30]. A cohort of patients younger than 80 years old was matched based on treatment year, race, histology, and gender in a 2:1 ratio. Of 13,690 thoracic oncology patients, 496 (3.6 %) were 80 years of age and older, of whom 46 met the criteria. In older and younger patients, respectively, platinum doublets were given in 43 % versus 79 % ($p \leq 0.0001$), the response rate was 41 % versus 47 %, the median progression-free survival was 5.55 versus 3.91 months ($p \leq 0.216$), and the median overall survival was 10.7 versus 9.8 months ($p \leq 0.43$). Hematologic and nonhematologic toxicities were similar. These data indicate that selected patients 80 years of age and older may tolerate and benefit from chemotherapy, and prospective evaluation of these patients is indicated. However, the SEER database has given the percentage of lung cancer patients 80 years of age and older as 17.8 %, but the data registry of MD Anderson Cancer Center showed that these patients constituted only 3.6 % of the MD Anderson Cancer Center lung cancer population. This difference suggests that MD Anderson Cancer Center's elderly population may be highly selected and not representative of the elderly population in the community.

An abstract presented in 2005 at the American Society of Clinical Oncology by Hesketh et al. [31] reported outcomes from two first-line advanced NSCLC trials for patients 70 years of age and older: the Southwest Oncology Group (S0027) (sequential vinorelbine and docetaxel) and an investigator-initiated multicenter trial (LUN 6) (single-agent docetaxel). Between these trials, the 47 patients (21.5 %) who were 80 years of age and older had similar disease control, although the patients with a PS of 0/1 had shorter survival than the younger patients, but the very elderly patients with a PS of 2 had a similar overall survival. They noted that the regimens were well tolerated by the patients 80 years of age and older and concluded that selected patients in this age group may benefit from single-agent chemotherapy. These data encourage to investigate whether patients 80 years of age and older might benefit from standard chemotherapy doublets. However, this was a retrospective study, so there may be selection bias. Thus, patients 80 years of age and older may have a lesser or greater tendency to be treated, resulting in a population of patients who are in a different condition than the younger patients.

Oxnard et al. performed a retrospective chart review of 111 outpatients with NSCLC aged 80 or older [32]. Patient treatment regimens were evaluated for consistency with contemporaneous stage-specific guideline-recommended therapy. Attention was paid to how patient characteristics and attitudes influence therapy decisions. Patient characteristics included median age of 82.6 years (range, 80–92), 30 % stage I–II, 39 % stage IV, 59 % performance status 0–1, and 25 % performance status ≥2 (performance status unavailable for 15 %). Eighty-four percent of the patients received some form of antineoplastic therapy, and 11 % were treated with best supportive care alone. Of 34 patients with localized disease, 53 % underwent tumor resection and 38 % received definitive radiation. Of 70 patients with stage III or IV disease, 36 % received cytotoxic chemotherapy and 27 % received oral-targeted therapy alone. Thirty-two percent of patients received the stage-specific guideline-recommended therapy. Of the patients who did not receive guideline-recommended therapy, 26 % electively refused the offered guideline-recommended therapy and 74 % were not offered guideline-recommended therapy. The authors concluded that in their experience the vast majority of octogenarian patients with NSCLC receive antineoplastic therapy, but only one third of this population receives stage-specific guideline-recommended therapy. In the age-specific subset analysis of trial ECOG 1594 (n =1,139) on platin-based chemotherapy in NSCLC, only nine patients were aged 80 years or older. These patients had a shorter time to progression and survival than that of the patients aged 70–79 years, with only one being able to receive three cycles of chemotherapy [33].

Prospective Data on Octogenarians or Frail Patients with Advanced NSCLC

Only one clinical trial of chemotherapy for advanced NSCLC has been specifically performed in patients aged 80 and older [34]. This was a phase II clinical trial conducted to evaluate the efficacy and toxicity of vinorelbine plus gemcitabine in very old patients with inoperable (stage IIIb or IV) NSCLC. Vinorelbine 20 mg/m^2 and gemcitabine 800 mg/m^2 were given on days 1, 8, and 15 of each 28-day cycle. From March 1998 to December 2001, 20 patients (16 males, 4 females) were enrolled in the study. The median age was 83 years, within the range 80–88 years. The median number of treatment cycles per patient was four. With the exception of one, all patients received at least two cycles of treatment. Thirteen patients achieved a partial response, with an overall response rate of 65 % (95 % confidence interval, 44.1–85.9 %). Median survival was 10 months. The significant (WHO grade 3/4) toxicities were myelosuppression, including leukopenia in five (25 %) patients, neutropenia in eight (40 %), anemia in six (30 %), and thrombocytopenia in three (15 %) patients. Febrile neutropenia occurred in two patients and accounted for one treatment-related death. Nonhematological toxicity was generally mild, except one patient who suffered from grade 3 interstitial pneumonitis. Another patient suffered from a cerebral infarction after three cycles of treatment. The authors concluded that the combination of vinorelbine and gemcitabine in very old patients with advanced NSCLC is a highly active regimen with an acceptable toxicity profile.

Yanagitani et al. performed a phase I study to determine the maximum tolerated dose (MTD) and to evaluate the toxicity of the biweekly paclitaxel and carboplatin combination chemotherapy in frail patients with advanced NSCLC [35]. Seventeen unresectable and previously untreated NSCLC patients participated in this study. Frail patients (>80 years old with PS 0–1 and adequate organ functions or <80 years old with PS 2 or <80 with PS 0–1 and one inadequate organ function of bone marrow, liver, or kidney) of NSCLC were enrolled in this study. Both paclitaxel and carboplatin were administered on day 1 and repeated biweekly. The starting dose of paclitaxel was 120 mg/m^2 and carboplatin was AUC 3 on day 1 every 2 weeks for four to eight cycles. The major hematologic toxicity was neutropenia. Nonhematologic toxicities, including numbness and constipation, were generally mild and reversible. The MTD of paclitaxel were determined as 140 mg/m^2. The recommended phase II study dose of paclitaxel was determined as 120 mg/m^2 and of carboplatin as AUC 3 biweekly. Objective responses were observed in 8 of 17 frail patients (47 %). The authors concluded that combination chemotherapy of biweekly paclitaxel and carboplatin appears to be tolerable and sufficiently effective in frail patients with NSCLC to launch a phase II trial.

Le Caer et al. evaluated the feasibility and activity of weekly docetaxel monotherapy (30 mg/m^2) in frail elderly patients with advanced-stage NSCLC, selected on the basis of their precise age, general condition, and number of comorbid disorders (Charlson score) [36]. Fifty patients were enrolled and 42 were assessable. Five patients (10 % [3.7–22.6]) had objective responses, 14 (28 % [16.9–41.6]) had stable disease, and 23 (46 % [32.6–52.8]) progressed. The main grade 3–4 toxicity was fatigue (30 %). Quality of life remained stable during treatment. The median survival time was 4.3 months, and the 1-year survival rate was 21.8 %. The authors concluded that in frail elderly patients selected on the basis of their age, general condition, and comorbidity, weekly docetaxel monotherapy has acceptable toxicity and does not negatively affect quality of life, although it has only moderate activity.

Conclusions

Frail patients and octogenarians with advanced NSCLC are overlapping populations, but they are not the same. Thus, treatment approaches are sometimes similar and sometimes different. In particular, frail elderly patients should be treated in selected cases with single-agent chemotherapy and in unselected cases with best supportive care only. Frail and octogenarian patients should be treated always with best supportive care. Fit octogenarian patients with advanced NSCLC can be treated with chemotherapy; however, in the absence of large prospective and specific data on the safety of platinum-based chemotherapy in this patient population, single-agent chemotherapy should be considered the standard treatment for fit octogenarian patients with advanced NSCLC. About the EGFR-TKIs erlotinib and gefitinib, they are probably the best drugs to use in frail patients and octogenarians with advanced NSCLC because of their favorable safety profile, but their use in the first-line treatment is limited to patients whose tumors harboring EGFR mutations. Only specifically designed prospective trials (with separation of fit octogenarians from frail patients) will clarify the optimal systemic treatment for advanced NSCLC in these two peculiar patient populations.

References

1. Fentiman IS, Tirelli U, Monfardini S, et al. Cancer in the elderly: why so badly treated? Lancet. 1990;335:1020–2.
2. McLean AJ, Le Couteur DG. Aging biology and geriatric clinical pharmacology. Pharmacol Rev. 2004;56:163–84.
3. Gridelli C, Perrone F, Monfardini S. Lung cancer in the elderly. Eur J Cancer. 1997;33:2313–4.

4. Radzikowska E, Glaz P, Roszkowski K. Lung cancer in women: age, smoking, histology, performance status, stage, initial treatment and survival. Population based study of 20651 cases. Ann Oncol. 2002;13:1087–93.
5. Owonikoko TK, Ragin CC, Belani CP, et al. Lung cancer in elderly patients: an analysis of the surveillance, epidemiology, and end results database. J Clin Oncol. 2007;25:5570–7.
6. Fitzpatrick AL, Kuller LH, Ives DG, et al. Incidence and prevalence of dementia in the cardiovascular health study. J Am Geriatr Soc. 2004;52:195–204.
7. Skoog I, Nilsson L, Palmertz B, et al. A population-based study of dementia in 85-year-olds. N Engl J Med. 1993;328:153–8.
8. Owonikoko TK, Belani C, Cai C, et al. Lung cancer in patients ≥80 years of age: analysis of the national surveillance, epidemiology and end results (SEER) database. J Clin Oncol. 2006;24(Suppl):7156.
9. Potosky AL, Saxman S, Wallace RB, et al. Population variations in the initial treatment of non-small-cell lung cancer. J Clin Oncol. 2004;22:3261–8.
10. Balducci L. Aging, frailty and chemotherapy. Cancer Control. 2007;14(1):7–12.
11. Carreca I, Balducci L, Extermann M. Cancer in the older person. Cancer Treat Rev. 2005;31:380–402.
12. Kinney JM. Nutritional frailty, sarcopenia and falls in the elderly. Curr Opin Clin Nutr Metab Care. 2004;7:15–20.
13. Kumar Pal S, Katheria V, Hurria A. Evaluating the older patient with cancer: understanding frailty and geriatric assessment. CA Cancer J Clin. 2010;60:120–32.
14. [No authors listed]. American Medical Association white paper on elderly health. Report of the Council on Scientific Affairs. Arch Intern Med. 1990;150:2459–72.
15. Fried LP, Tangen CM, Walston J, et al. Frailty in older adults: evidence for a phenotype. J Gerontol A Biol Sci Med Sci. 2001;56:M146–57.
16. Rockwood K, Howlett SE, MacKnight C, et al. Prevalence, attributes, and outcomes of fitness and frailty in community dwelling older adults: report from the Canadian study of health and aging. J Gerontol A Biol Sci Med Sci. 2004;59:1310–7.
17. Winograd CH, Gerety MB, Chung M, et al. Screening for frailty: criteria and predictors of outcomes. J Am Geriatr Soc. 1991;39:778–84.
18. Balducci L, Extermann M. Management of the frail person with advanced cancer. Crit Rev Oncol Hematol. 2000;33:143–8.
19. Repetto L, Fratino L, Audisio RA, et al. Comprehensive geriatric assessment adds information to Eastern Cooperative Oncology Group performance status in elderly cancer patients: an Italian Group for Geriatric Oncology Study. J Clin Oncol. 2002;20:494–502.
20. Gridelli C, Maione P, Rossi A, et al. Management of unfit older patients with advanced NSCLC. Cancer Treat Rev. 2009;35:517–21.
21. Gridelli C, Ardizzoni A, Le Chevalier T. Treatment of advanced non-small-cell lung cancer patients with ECOG performance status 2: results of an European Experts Panel. Ann Oncol. 2004;15:419–26.
22. The Elderly Lung Cancer Vinorelbine Italian Study Group. Effects of vinorelbine on quality of life and survival of elderly patients with advanced non-small cell lung cancer. J Natl Cancer Inst. 1999;91:66–72.
23. Perrone F, Di Maio M, Gallo C, et al. Outcome of patients with a performance status of 2 in the Multicenter Italian Lung Cancer in the Elderly Study (MILES). J Clin Oncol. 2004;22:5018–20.
24. Jackman DM, Yeap BY, Lindeman NI, et al. Phase II clinical trial of chemotherapy-naive patients = or >70 years of age treated with erlotinib for advanced non-small-cell lung cancer. J Clin Oncol. 2007;25:760–6.
25. Crinò L, Cappuzzo F, Zatloukal P, et al. Gefitinib versus vinorelbine in chemotherapy-na elderly patients with advanced non-small-cell lung cancer (INVITE): a randomized, phase II study. J Clin Oncol. 2008;26:4253–60.

26. Kazuhiro A, Koizumi T, Hirai K, et al. Gefitinib as first-line treatment in elderly epidermal growth factor receptor-mutated patients with advanced lung adenocarcinoma: results of a Nagano Lung Cancer Research Study. Clin Lung Cancer. 2011;12:387–92.
27. Inoue A, Kobayashi K, Usui K, et al. First-line gefitinib for patients with advanced non-small-cell lung cancer harboring epidermal growth factor receptor mutations without indication for chemotherapy. J Clin Oncol. 2009;27:1394–400.
28. Langer CJ. The "Lazarus response" in treatment-naïve, poor performance status patients with non-small cell lung cancer and epidermal growth factor receptor mutation. J Clin Oncol. 2009;27:1350–4.
29. Chen KY, Chen JH, Shih JY, et al. Octogenarians with advanced non-small cell lung cancer. Treatment modalities, survival, and prognostic factors. J Thorac Oncol. 2010;5:82–9.
30. Altundag O, Stewart DJ, Fossella FV, et al. Many patients 80 years and older with advanced non-small cell lung cancer (NSCLC) can tolerate chemotherapy. J Thorac Oncol. 2007;2:141–6.
31. Hesketh PJ, Lilenbaum R, Chansky K, et al. Chemotherapy in patients _80 with advanced non small cell lung cancer: combined results from SWOG 0027 and LUN 6. In: Abstracts of the 2005 ASCO annual meeting, Orlando, 13–17 May 2005, abstract no. 7147.
32. Oxnard GR, Fidias P, Muzikansky A, Sequist LV. Non-small cell lung cancer in octogenarians: treatment practices and preferences. J Thorac Oncol. 2007;2:1029–35.
33. Langer CJ, Vangel M, Schiller J, et al. Age-specific subanalysis of ECOG 1594: fit elderly patients (70–80 yrs) with NSCLC do as well as younger pts (≤70) [abstract]. Proc Am Soc Clin Oncol. 2003;22:abstract 2571.
34. Chen YM, Perng RP, Chen MC, Tsai CM, Ming-Liu J, Whang-Peng J. Phase II trial of vinorelbine plus gemcitabine in previously untreated inoperable (stage IIB/IV) non-small cell lung cancer patients aged 80 or older. Lung Cancer. 2003;440:221–6.
35. Yanagitani N, Tsuchiya S, Kaira K, et al. Phase I study of biweekly paclitaxel and carboplatin for frail patients with advanced non-small cell lung cancer. Am J Clin Oncol. 2007;30(5):487–91.
36. Le Caer H, Barlesi F, Robinet G, et al. An open multicenter phase II trial of weekly docetaxel for advanced-stage non-small-cell lung cancer in elderly patients with significant comorbidity and/or poor performance status: the GFPC 02-02b study. Lung Cancer. 2007;57(1):72–8.

Chapter 16
Are Second- and Third-Line Treatments in the Elderly Feasible?

Cesare Gridelli, Antonio Rossi, and Paolo Maione

Abstract Currently, pemetrexed, docetaxel, erlotinib, and gefitinib have to be considered the standard treatment for patients with pretreated advanced NSCLC. Given the similar efficacies of the three currently available agents, patient's preference, comorbidities, and convenience are important issues to consider when selecting a therapeutic agent. Although these considerations come from trials performed in the general population, it is reasonable to use them for the choice of second- and third-line therapy of elderly patients as well. Unfortunately, second-line studies are still lacking in the elderly patients, but the large amount of new agents which are investigating in NSCLC patients may help in increasing the knowledge in this specific setting.

Keywords Treatment for NSCLC in the elderly • Lung cancer in the elderly • Non-small cell lung cancer in the elderly • Second-line therapy in the elderly with lung cancer • Third-line therapy in the elderly with lung cancer

Patients affected by advanced unresectable non-small cell lung cancer (NSCLC) are only suitable for systemic treatment approaches reaching a disease control rate in about two third of them, but all patients ultimately suffer of a progression of disease. At the time of disease progression, many patients still have a good performance

---

C. Gridelli, MD (✉)
Department of Oncology/Hematology,
S.G. Moscati Hospital, Avellino, Italy
e-mail: cgridelli@libero.it

A. Rossi, MD • P. Maione, MD
Division of Medical Oncology,
S.G. Moscati Hospital, Avellino, Italy

C. Gridelli, R.A. Audisio (eds.), *Management of Lung Cancer in Older People*,
DOI 10.1007/978-0-85729-793-8_16,

status (PS) and can be considered for further active treatment. It is estimated that in clinical research studies, between 40 and 50 % of cases go on to receive second-line therapy [1]. This emphasizes the high selection of patients who are suitable of further treatments. In fact, patients who experience disease progression during or after first-line treatment for advanced NSCLC have a limited life expectancy. Quality of life is often compromised by disease-related symptoms, by residual toxicity of previous chemotherapy, and by comorbid diseases. The aims of second-line treatment should be palliation of symptoms, benefit in quality of life, and prolongation of survival. The benefits of treatment should outweigh toxicity and inconvenience to the patient. However, the impact of treatment on the natural history of the disease is modest. In fact, an analysis of 19 phase III trials, in the second-line or later setting, showed that the median objective response rate was 6.8 % and the median overall survival was 6.6 months [2]. Life expectancy of these patients is largely dependent on their clinical condition at the start of second-line treatment. Patients with PS 2, who are considered fit for further treatment, may have a relative benefit from treatment similar to patients with better PS. However, the absolute benefit is small, with most studies reporting a median survival of 3–4 months.

Due to the availability of new drugs, the length of time spent by patients receiving antitumor treatment has been increasing recently. However, most patients with advanced NSCLC who receive second-line treatment are near the end of life. In a retrospective review of patients treated for advanced NSCLC in a community oncology setting, the mean line of chemotherapy in patients who were receiving active treatment at the time of death was second-line [3]. Chemotherapy was given within 1 month and 2 weeks of death to 43 and 20 % of patients, respectively. This can be explained in part by the increased demand for additional treatment by patients and their relatives who are unable to accept the futility of further therapy and the inevitability of death from progressive NSCLC. It may also be due to physicians' inability to correctly predict life expectancy of these patients. This emphasizes the importance of identifying predictive markers of response, survival benefit, and toxicity in pretreated NSCLC patients.

While the prognostic factors associated with improved survival with first-line therapy have been extensively studied, less information exists about the prognostic factors in second-line therapy. For the treating physician, prognostic factors may assist in determining the likelihood of clinical benefit of further therapy. The analysis of prognostic factors in a second-line trial comparing docetaxel with paclitaxel poliglumex in 849 patients was reported. There was no outcome difference between the two treatment arms with the median survival of 6.9 months for both treatments [4]. The following factors were associated with shorter survival: a PS score of 2 versus 0–1 (hazard ratio [HR] 2.19; $p<0.001$), a hemoglobin level of <11 g/dl versus 11 g/dl (HR 1.78; $p<0.001$), an LDH level of <200 U/l versus 200 U/l (HR 1.72; $p<0.001$), a lung cancer symptom score of <18 versus 18 (HR 1.47; $p<0.001$), male gender (HR 1.39; $p=0.005$), extrathoracic metastases (HR 1.45; $p<0.001$), prior radiation therapy (HR 1.40; $p=0.001$), and starting second-line chemotherapy <4 months after the start of first-line chemotherapy (HR 1.37; $p=0.003$) [5]. Unfortunately, specific data concerning the elderly patients are not available but what reported before could be generalized to the entire population affected by advanced NSCLC.

Overall, four drugs are currently approved for the second-line therapy: two cytotoxic chemotherapy agents, docetaxel and pemetrexed, and two epidermal growth factor receptor tyrosine kinase inhibitors (EGFR-TKI), erlotinib and gefitinib. Gefitinib is approved only in patients affected by recurrent NSCLC harboring activating EGFR mutations, and both gefitinib, in the same setting, and erlotinib are approved for third-line therapy. These agents were approved regardless the age and so also elderly patients could benefit from their administration.

Second-Line Therapy

Docetaxel has been the first drug investigated in second-line setting within two phase III randomized trials [6, 7]. In the TAX317 study [6], docetaxel, administered at the dose of 100 mg/m^2 on day 1 recycled every 3 weeks, was compared to the best supportive care. When interim safety data monitoring identified a significantly higher toxic death rate in the chemotherapy arm, the protocol was amended and the dose was reduced to 75 mg/m^2. Docetaxel scored better than the best supportive care in all efficacy outcomes reporting also all quality of life parameters improvement [8]. Febrile neutropenia was the most relevant toxicity reported with docetaxel, but was less frequent with the lower dose. In the TAX320 phase III randomized trial [7], patients were randomized to receive docetaxel (100 or 75 mg/m^2, day 1, every 3 weeks) versus vinorelbine or ifosfamide at the investigator's discretion. All outcome parameters favored docetaxel arm with the exception of median survival which was similar between the two arms although the 1-year survival was significantly greater with docetaxel 75 mg/m^2 than with the control treatment (32 % versus 19 %; $p = 0.025$). Patients assigned to docetaxel had more neutropenia and febrile neutropenia compared to the control arm, but the lower dose of docetaxel was generally well tolerated. Based on the results coming from these studies, docetaxel was licensed for second-line therapy, but myelosuppression resulted extremely frequent and severe with safety concerns properly in elderly patients. Thus, weekly scheduling of docetaxel has been investigated to improve the toxicity profile of the drug in pretreated NSCLC patients. Several randomized trials compared the weekly with the standard 3-week schedule of docetaxel in the second-line treatment of advanced NSCLC. These trials were included in a meta-analysis based on individual patient data with the aim of comparing the efficacy of the two different docetaxel schedules. No significant difference in efficacy outcomes for weekly schedule of docetaxel compared to standard 3-weekly administration as second-line treatment of patients with advanced NSCLC was reported. No relevant differential effect was detected in subgroup analyses including age. A significantly less severe and febrile neutropenia was reported with weekly schedule ($p < 0.00001$ for both), whereas no significant differences were observed for anemia, thrombocytopenia, and non-hematologic toxicity [9]. Based on an advantageous profile of toxicity and no relevant difference in survival, weekly docetaxel represents a valid alternative to 3-weekly administration, particularly in elderly patients.

Pemetrexed, a multi-targeted antifolate agent, at the dose of 500 mg/m^2, day 1 recycled every 3 weeks, was compared to docetaxel 75 mg/m^2, day 1 every 3 weeks, within a phase III randomized trial in 571 recurrent NSCLC patients [10]. The study was originally designed to test for superiority of pemetrexed, but in an amendment to the protocol, a non-inferiority design was adopted. A similar activity but a significant improvement of the safety profile for pemetrexed arm was reported. Pemetrexed works much better in non-squamous histology due to a higher expression of thymidylate synthase, a target enzyme of pemetrexed activity, in squamous NSCLC and lower in adenocarcinomas, leading to lower sensitivity to pemetrexed in the squamous histotype and higher in adenocarcinoma. Data emerged from first- and second-line randomized studies [11]. In current practice pemetrexed is licensed for the treatment of non-squamous NSCLC patients.

Erlotinib plus best supportive care was compared with placebo plus best supportive care in 731 unselected patients with recurrent NSCLC. Patients were required to have received one or two previous line of chemotherapy and not be eligible for further chemotherapy [12]. Patients were randomized in a 2:1 ratio to receive either erlotinib 150 mg orally daily or placebo. This trial revealed statistically significant higher progression-free and overall survival rates with erlotinib treatment (median survival times and 1-year survival rates of 6.7 versus 4.7 months and 31 % versus 22 % for the erlotinib and placebo groups, respectively). Erlotinib was well tolerated and the principal toxicities were rash and diarrhea. An exploratory univariate analysis demonstrated that the survival benefit with erlotinib therapy was similar across multiple subgroups. Treatment with erlotinib also showed significant benefits in quality of life and lung cancer-related symptoms of cough, dyspnea, and pain [13]. Based on the results coming from this trial, erlotinib is currently approved for the second-line treatment of recurrent NSCLC patients not selected for any biological factors, i.e., EGFR mutations.

On the contrary, gefitinib did not demonstrate any survival improvement when compared with placebo in second-line treatment of unselected patients [14], but the significant outcomes advantage reported when compared with chemotherapy in patients affected by advanced NSCLC harboring EGFR mutations, even if as first-line treatment [15–18], led to its registration in this subgroup of patients in any line of treatment.

Unfortunately, to date, few data, prevalently retrospective analyses, are available for second-line therapy of advanced NSCLC elderly patients. A retrospective analysis was performed in 86 elderly (≥70 years) out of a total of 571 patients enrolled in a randomized phase III trial comparing second-line pemetrexed to docetaxel. Elderly patients receiving pemetrexed ($n=47$) or docetaxel ($n=39$) had a median survival of 9.5 and 7.7 months compared with 7.8 and 8.0 months for younger patients receiving pemetrexed ($n=236$) or docetaxel ($n=249$), respectively. Elderly patients treated with pemetrexed had a longer time to progression (4.6 versus 2.9 months) and a longer median survival (9.5 versus 7.7 months) than their counterpart patients treated with docetaxel (not statistically significant). Pemetrexed produced a more favorable toxicity profile with less febrile neutropenia (2.5 % versus 19 %; $p=0.025$)

Table 16.1 Retrospective subgroup analyses of elderly from randomized phase III trials of second-line therapy in non-small cell lung cancer patients

Author	Age	Treatment	No. pts	ORR (%)	PFS (months)	OS (months)
Weiss et al. [19]	≥70	Pemetrexed	47	5.0	4.6[a]	9.5
		vs docetaxel	39	5.6	2.9[a]	7.7
	<70	Pemetrexed	224	9.8	3.0[a]	7.8
		vs docetaxel	238	9.2	3.9[a]	8.0
Wheatley-Price et al. [20]	≥70	Erlotinib	112	7.6	3.0	7.6
		vs placebo	51	NR	2.1	5.0
	<70	Erlotinib	376	9.3	2.1	6.4
		vs placebo	192	NR	1.8	4.7

No. pts number of patients, *ORR* objective response rate, *PFS* progression-free survival, *OS* overall survival, *NR* not reported
[a]Time to progression

than docetaxel and with no toxic deaths (one death as result of toxicity was reported in the docetaxel arm) [19].

Another retrospective analysis evaluated 163 elderly patients (112 on erlotinib, 51 on placebo) out of 731 randomized to erlotinib versus placebo. For elderly patients randomly assigned to erlotinib or placebo, progression-free survival was 3.0 versus 2.1 months ($p=0.009$) and median survival was 7.6 versus 5.0 months ($p=0.67$). Elderly patients, compared with young patients, had significantly more overall and severe (grades 3 and 4) toxicity (35 % versus 18 %; $p<0.001$), were more likely to discontinue treatment as a result of treatment-related toxicity (12 % versus 3 %; $p<0.0001$), and had lower relative dose-intensity (64 % versus 82 % received >90 % planned dose; $p<0.001$). Overall, elderly patients treated with erlotinib gained survival and quality of life benefits similar to younger patients but experienced greater toxicity (Table 16.1) [20].

A prospective phase II trial investigated a modified schedule of docetaxel (37.5 mg/m^2, days 1–8, every 3 weeks) given as second-line therapy to 33 elderly patients who had progressed after 1 line of chemotherapy [21]. The objective response was reached in seven patients (21.2 %), while 12 patients (36.3 %) reported a stable disease. Grade 3 neutropenia and anemia were observed in 9 and 3 % of patients, respectively. The main non-hematologic toxicity consisted of grade 3 nausea/vomiting, diarrhea, and asthenia in 6 % of patients each and grade 3 nail toxicity in 3 % of patients. Unfortunately, to date, these are the only prospective data available in second-line therapy for advanced NSCLC elderly patients.

Third-Line Therapy

No trials addressing the third-line therapy in elderly patients are available. In general, in the phase III randomized trial comparing erlotinib to placebo, patients were required to have received one or two previous line of chemotherapy to be eligible in the study [12]. In fact, based on the results of this trial, erlotinib is licensed worldwide

Table 16.2 Clinical factors influencing the choice of second-line therapy in patients affected by recurrent non-small cell lung cancer

First-line treatment: type of therapy, response, toxicity, progression-free survival
Patient's characteristics: performance status, comorbidities, age, sex, race, smoking, patient's preference
Disease-related characteristics: histology, symptoms, extension of disease
Second-line characteristics: expected toxicity, patient's compliance, costs

for third-line therapy of unselected NSCLC patients. The retrospective analysis performed from this trial and addressed to elderly patients did not evaluate the difference between the second- and third-line impact of erlotinib [20], but we can state that it is a valid option also in this setting.

Factors Affecting the Choice of Second-Line Therapy

The availability of chemotherapeutics and biologic agents for second-line therapy raises the question about what should be the factors driving the choice of the agent to use in this setting. In presence of a patient affected by recurrent NSCLC harboring an activating EGFR mutations, the choice of gefitinib or erlotinib is mandatory. In patients affected by recurrent NSCLC with EGFR wild-type or unknown, the selection of a second-line agent may depend on a number of factors. Gefitinib has been compared with docetaxel in randomized phase II and III trials addressing the second-line therapy in unselected NSCLC patients reporting similar activity but a better safety profile [22–25]. A meta-analysis based on individual patient data, grouping these four randomized trials, confirmed the results favoring gefitinib administration [26]. Erlotinib has been also investigated, in second-line setting, versus chemotherapy, docetaxel, or pemetrexed, reporting the same activity and a good safety profile [27]. However, all these trials did not answer to the question of which therapy should be the best choice in second-line setting. The problem is that several clinical factors should be considered for the choice of the most appropriate agent to use in that specific patient as second-line therapy. Factors related to the tolerance and response to the previous chemotherapy, patient's comorbidities, and patient's preference may impact the selection of second-line therapies (Table 16.2) [28]. These factors coming from the analysis of trials and from the clinical practice of the general population should be considered also for the elderly patients.

Conclusions

Currently, pemetrexed, docetaxel, erlotinib, and gefitinib have to be considered the standard treatment for patients with pretreated advanced NSCLC. Given the similar efficacies of the three currently available agents, patient's preference, comorbidities, and convenience are important issues to consider when selecting a therapeutic agent. Although these considerations come from trials performed in the general population, it is reasonable to use them for the choice of second- and third-line therapy of elderly patients as well. Unfortunately, second-line studies are still lacking in the elderly patients, but the large amount of new agents which are investigating in NSCLC patients may help in increasing the knowledge in this specific setting.

References

1. Cullen M. Second-line treatment options in advanced non-small cell lung cancer: current status. Semin Oncol. 2006;33 Suppl 1:S3–8.
2. Hotta K, Fujiwara Y, Kiura K, et al. Relationship between response and survival in more than 50000 patients with advanced non-small cell lung cancer treated with systemic chemotherapy in 143 phase III trials. J Thorac Oncol. 2007;2:402–7.
3. Murillo JR, Koeller J. Chemotherapy given near the end of life by community oncologists for advanced non-small-cell lung cancer. Oncologist. 2006;11:1095–9.
4. Paz-Ares L, Ross H, O'Brien M, et al. Phase III trial comparing paclitaxel poliglumex vs docetaxel in the second-line treatment of non-small-cell lung cancer. Br J Cancer. 2008;98:1608–13.
5. Bonomi P, Langer C, O'Brien M, et al. Analysis of prognostic factors in patients with advanced relapsed/refractory NSCLC: Cox regression analysis of a randomized phase III trial comparing docetaxel and paclitaxel poliglumex (PPX). J Clin Oncol. 2006;24(S18):374s (abstr. 7040).
6. Shepherd FA, Dancey J, Ramlau R, et al. Prospective randomized trial of docetaxel versus best supportive care in patients with non-small-cell lung cancer previously treated with platinum-based chemotherapy. J Clin Oncol. 2000;18:2095–103.
7. Fossella FV, DeVore R, Kerr RN, et al. Randomized phase III trial of docetaxel versus vinorelbine or ifosfamide in patients with advanced non-small-cell lung cancer previously treated with platinum-containing chemotherapy regimens. The TAX 320 Non-Small Cell Lung Cancer Study Group. J Clin Oncol. 2000;18:2354–62.
8. Dancey J, Shepherd FA, Gralla RJ, et al. Quality of life assessment of second-line docetaxel versus best supportive care in patients with non-small-cell lung cancer previously based with platinum-based chemotherapy: results of a prospective, randomized phase III trial. Lung Cancer. 2004;43:183–94.
9. Di Maio M, Perrone F, Chiodini P, et al. Individual patient data meta-analysis of docetaxel administered once every 3 weeks compared with once every week second-line treatment of advanced non-small-cell lung cancer. J Clin Oncol. 2007;25:1377–82.
10. Hanna N, Shepherd FA, Fossella FV, et al. Randomized phase III trial of pemetrexed versus docetaxel in patients with non-small-cell lung cancer previously treated with chemotherapy. J Clin Oncol. 2004;22:1589–97.
11. Scagliotti G, Hanna N, Fossella F, et al. The differential efficacy of pemetrexed according to NSCLC histology: a review of two phase III studies. Oncologist. 2009;14:253–63.
12. Shepherd FA, Rodrigues Pereira J, Ciuleanu T, et al. Erlotinib in previously treated non-small-cell lung cancer. N Engl J Med. 2005;353:123–32.
13. Bezjak A, Tu D, Seymour L, et al. Symptom improvement in lung cancer patients treated with erlotinib: quality of life analysis of the National Cancer Institute of Canada Clinical Trials Group Study BR.21. J Clin Oncol. 2007;24:3831–7.
14. Thatcher N, Chang A, Parikh P, et al. Gefitinib plus best supportive care in previously treated patients with refractory advanced non-small-cell lung cancer: results from a randomised, placebo-controlled, multicentre study (Iressa Survival Evaluation in Lung Cancer). Lancet. 2005;366:1527–37.

15. Mok TS, Wu YL, Thongprasert S, et al. Gefitinib or carboplatin-paclitaxel in pulmonary adenocarcinoma. N Engl J Med. 2009;361:947–57.
16. Lee JS, Park K, Kim SW, et al. A randomized phase III study of gefitinib (IRESSA) versus standard chemotherapy (gemcitabine plus cisplatin) as a first-line treatment for never-smokers with advanced or metastatic adenocarcinoma of the lung. J Thorac Oncol. 2009;4 Suppl 1:S283–4 (abstr PRS.4).
17. Mitsudomi T, Morita S, Yatabe Y, et al. Gefitinib versus cisplatin plus docetaxel in patients with non-small-cell lung cancer harbouring mutations of the epidermal growth factor receptor (WJTOG3405): an open label, randomised phase 3 trial. Lancet Oncol. 2010;11:121–8.
18. Maemondo M, Inoue A, Kobayashi K, et al. Gefitinib or chemotherapy for non-small-cell lung cancer with mutated EGFR. N Engl J Med. 2010;362:2380–8.
19. Weiss GJ, Langer C, Rosell R, et al. Elderly patients benefit from second-line cytotoxic chemotherapy: a subset analysis of a randomized phase III trial of pemetrexed compared with docetaxel in patients with previously treated advanced non-small-cell lung cancer. J Clin Oncol. 2006;24:4405–11.
20. Wheatley-Price P, Ding K, Seymour L, et al. Erlotinib for advanced non-small-cell lung cancer in the elderly: an analysis of the National Cancer Institute of Canada Clinical Trials Group Study BR.21. J Clin Oncol. 2008;26:2350–7.
21. Tibaldi C, Bernardini I, Chella A, et al. Second-line chemotherapy with a modified schedule of docetaxel in elderly patients with advanced-stage non-small-cell lung cancer. Clin Lung Cancer. 2006;7:401–5.
22. Cufer T, Vrdoljak E, Gaafar R, et al. Phase II, open-label, randomized study (SIGN) of single-agent gefitinib (IRESSA) or docetaxel as second-line therapy in patients with advanced (stage IIIB or IV) non-small-cell lung cancer. Anticancer Drugs. 2006;17:401–9.
23. Kim ES, Hirsch V, Mok T, et al. Gefitinib versus docetaxel in previously treated non-small-cell lung cancer (INTEREST): a randomized phase III trial. Lancet. 2008;372:1809–18.
24. Maruyama R, Nishiwaki Y, Tamura T, et al. Phase III study, V-15-32, of gefitinib versus docetaxel in previously treated Japanese patients with non-small-cell lung cancer. J Clin Oncol. 2008;26:4244–52.
25. Lee DH, Park K, Kim JH, et al. Randomized phase III trial of gefitinib versus docetaxel in non-small cell lung cancer patients who have previously received platinum-based chemotherapy. Clin Cancer Res. 2010;16:1307–14.
26. Shepherd FA, Douillard J, Fukuoka M, et al. Comparison of gefitinib and docetaxel in patients with pretreated advanced non-small cell lung cancer (NSCLC): meta-analysis from four clinical trials. J Clin Oncol. 2009;27(15S):409s (abstr 8011).
27. Ciuleanu T, Stelmakh L, Cicenas S, et al. Erlotinib versus docetaxel or pemetrexed as second-line therapy in patients with advanced non-small cell lung cancer (NSCLC) and poor prognosis: efficacy and safety results from the phase III TITAN study. J Thorac Oncol. 2010;5 Suppl 12:S560–1 (abstr LBOA5).
28. Gridelli C, Ardizzoni A, Bernardo G, et al.: Progetto CHALLENGE. Tarceva highlights: agreement on its role in the second line treatment in non-small cell lung cancer. Tumori. 2010;96:15–24.

Part VII
Small-Cell Lung Cancer: Therapeutics

Chapter 17
Treatment of Limited-Stage Disease in Older Patients: The Role of Thoracic Radiotherapy and Prophylactic Cranial Irradiation

Rovel J. Colaco, Anna P. Britten, Fiona H. Blackhall, and Corinne Faivre-Finn

Abstract Elderly patients should neither be undertreated nor overtreated with RT or CTRT. Treatment selection should not be made on the basis of chronological age and should take into account performance status, stage, comorbidities, nutritional status, and patients' preference. The benefits of concurrent CTRT have to be balanced against the risks of radiation esophagitis and pneumonitis which are more likely to lead to hospitalization, malnutrition, and deterioration of QoL in the elderly compared to their younger counterparts. Future studies in SCLC including elderly patients are urgently needed with emphasis on toxicity, QoL, and efficacy. The use of geriatric assessments may help to define groups of patients more likely to benefit from aggressive treatments such as concurrent CTRT and may also enable more robust stratification of elderly patients in prospective studies. Furthermore, advances in RT planning and delivery, such as omitting elective nodal irradiation, 4-D conformal RT planning, intensity-modulated radiotherapy (IMRT), and image-guided radiotherapy (IGRT), are likely to widen the therapeutic window, and the resulting reduction in toxicity should make future RT more tolerable for elderly patients.

Keywords Lung cancer in the elderly • Limited-stage lung cancer in the elderly • Elderly patients and lung cancer • Thoracic radiotherapy in the elderly • Prophylactic cranial irradiation • Cranial irradiation in the elderly

---

R.J. Colaco, FRCR • A.P. Britten, MRCP • C. Faivre-Finn, MD, PhD(✉)
Department of Clinical Oncology,
The Christie NHS Foundation Trust,
Manchester, UK
e-mail: corinne.finn@christie.nhs.uk

F.H. Blackhall, PhD, FRCP
Department of Medical Oncology,
The Christie NHS Foundation Trust,
Wilmslow Rd, Manchester, M20 4BX, UK

C. Gridelli, R.A. Audisio (eds.), *Management of Lung Cancer in Older People*,
DOI 10.1007/978-0-85729-793-8_17,

Lung cancer is one of the most common types of cancer in Western countries and is increasingly becoming a disease of the elderly. According to Western epidemiological reports, the median age of individuals at diagnosis of lung cancer, of all histological subtypes, is 71 years, with 69 % of patients ≥65 years and 36 % ≥75 years. Over the last decade, the incidence of death from lung cancer has decreased in patients ≤50 years of age, but has increased in those ≥70 years old [1].

For small cell lung cancer (SCLC), data from the Surveillance, Epidemiology and End Results (SEER) database (cohort of 6,271 patients diagnosed from 1983 to 1998) showed that the proportion of patients with limited-stage (LS) SCLC and who are ≥70 years old had increased such that they accounted for almost half of the cohort [2]. A further SEER report also showed that 10 % of patients with SCLC were ≥80 years of age [1]. An increase in life expectancy can explain the proportion of elderly patients diagnosed with SCLC; however, this is balanced with the decline in the overall general incidence of SCLC, which currently accounts for approximately 13 % of all lung cancers [3].

In the last two decades, we have gained a better understanding of the optimal way to combine chemotherapy and radiotherapy (RT) and of the role of prophylactic cranial irradiation (PCI) contributing to improvements in both local control and overall survival [4, 5]. Moreover, recent improvements in RT planning and delivery techniques have reduced the impact of toxicity and have had a positive impact on the outcome of RT treatment in this disease [6].

The most favorable 5-year survival rates in clinical trials have been reported with early concurrent chemoradiotherapy (CTRT) [7–10]. However, these more intensive treatments, while being associated with better outcomes and survival, are also associated with increased toxicity which can render them unsuitable particularly in the context of an elderly population. RT therefore plays an important role in the curative and palliative treatment of SCLC as elderly patients commonly have multiple comorbidities and/or poor performance status [11, 12] that may prohibit the use of chemotherapy as a treatment option. PCI is considered to be standard of care in LS-SCLC, but concerns regarding long-term toxicity have limited its application in elderly patients [13].

Generally, 70 years of age is used as the cutoff for participation in clinical trials as the incidence of age-related comorbidities starts to increase after 70 years [14]. As a result we have a paucity of data from the available literature on the best management of elderly patients with LS-SCLC.

Thoracic Radiotherapy in the Elderly

Thoracic RT has played an important role in the management of SCLC since the 1980s and has led to significant reductions in the rate of intrathoracic failure when added to chemotherapy. A meta-analysis examining the role of thoracic RT in LS-SCLC showed a 3-year survival advantage of 5.4 %, but a subgroup analysis showed a trend toward a larger reduction in mortality among younger patients. The relative risk of death with combined therapy compared to chemotherapy alone ranged from 0.72 for patients ≤55 years (95 % confidence interval, 0.56–0.93) to 1.07 (0.70–1.64) for patients ≥70 years [15]. However, it should be noted that the studies included in the meta-analysis used dated RT techniques (2D RT, large volume of irradiation) possibly associated with increased morbidity/mortality in elderly patients. Evidence addressing the impact of age as an independent prognostic variable in LS-SCLC is conflicting. A pooled SWOG/CALGB analysis [16] suggests age is an important prognostic factor in LS-SCLC, but this has been refuted in other studies [17–19].

The SEER data showed that there was an increase in the proportion of younger patients treated with RT, such an increase was not reported for patients aged ≥70. The study also showed that patients who were diagnosed from 1993 to 1998 and received RT had improved survival compared to patients in the earlier study period (HR = 0.53; CI 0.47–0.58; $p < 0.0001$), whose survival was better than patients from the same time era who did not receive RT (HR = 0.77; CI 0.69–0.85; $p < 0.0001$). A subset analysis based on the patient age (≤59, 60–69, and ≥70 years old) confirmed that the mortality hazard ratio for RT use appeared consistent in each age group. A further analysis of the SEER database shows that very elderly patients, aged 80 years or older, with lung cancer were less likely to receive RT than younger patients. The analysis did not report the separate figures for patients with SCLC and non-small cell lung cancer (NSCLC) [1].

The role of palliative thoracic RT in lung cancers is based on a limited number of trials involving only a small proportion of patients ≥60 years [20]. The only known prospective study of palliative thoracic RT in elderly patients with NSCLC and SCLC compared a cohort of 83 patients with a median age of 78 with 49 patients with a median age of 60 years [21]. Symptom palliation rates, in particular hemoptysis and chest pain, were similar in both groups. Similarly, acute toxicity rates, were comparable.

Chemoradiotherapy in the Elderly

Although it is well recognized that the standard of care for good performance status LS-SCLC is early concurrent CTRT [4, 22], elderly patients are less likely to receive this treatment regimen compared to their younger counterparts. A retrospective review performed on 174 patients with LS-SCLC referred to the British Columbia Cancer Agency from 1991 to 1999 showed that combined modality CTRT was given in 86, 66, and 40 % of patients ages ≤65, 65–74, and ≥75 years, respectively ($p < 0.0001$) [23]. Age was not found to be significantly associated with survival in a multivariate analysis, and treatment toxicity was similar among the three age cohorts.

These findings were echoed in a population-based study from the nationwide Netherlands Cancer Registry from 1997 to 2007 which showed that among patients with LS-SCLC ($n = 4{,}701$), the proportion receiving CTRT increased from 35 % to almost 60 % for those aged 60–69, from 28 to 48 % in age group 70–74, from 17 to 33 % in age group 75–79, but remained <10 % for those aged ≥80 [24]. As a result survival has only improved for patients <80 years during the study period.

Evidence on the impact of age on the compliance, toxicity, and efficacy of CTRT in the elderly comes from retrospective analysis of randomized controlled trials. It should be emphasized that these patients with good performance status and low burden of comorbidities are not representative of the general elderly population.

The landmark study by Turrisi et al. compared once-daily (OD) RT (45 Gy in 25 fractions) versus twice-daily (BD) RT (45 Gy in 30 fractions) concurrently with cisplatin and etoposide (EP) [10]. In this study, 40 % of the 206 patients in the ODRT group and 31 % of the 211 patients in the BDRT group were age ≥65. The oldest patient included was 82 years with only 13 % of patients overall ≥75 years [25] (Table 17.1). There was improved survival in the accelerated hyperfractionated arm compared with the ODRT treatment (5-year survival 26 % versus 16 %; $p=0.04$) at the expense of increased rates of grade 3 esophagitis (27 % versus 11 %; $p<0.001$) which can be of concern in elderly patients who may be more susceptible to rapid clinical deterioration and malnutrition as a result [10]. A retrospective subgroup analysis of this trial compared the outcome of patients aged <70 years to those aged ≥70 years [25]. Severe hematological toxicities (grades 4–5: 61 % versus 84 %; $p<0.01$) and fatal toxicities (1 % versus 10 %; $p=0.01$) occurred more often among older patients, but there were no differences in the frequency of nonhematological toxicities. There was no difference in 5-year event-free survival (19 % versus 16 %; $p=0.18$), but 5-year overall survival (22 % versus 16 %; $p=0.05$) favored the younger group.

These results were echoed in the retrospective analysis of the North Central Cancer Treatment Group study comparing ODRT to split-course BDRT given concurrently with chemotherapy [26]. Two hundred and sixty-three patients with LS-SCLC were randomized including 54 (21 %) elderly patients (age >70 years old). Although elderly patients were more likely to have weight loss, poorer performance status, and increased pulmonary toxicity and to die as a result of the treatment, survival was not found to be significantly worse in older individuals.

Finally, Quon et al. examined the impact of age on the delivery, tolerance, and efficacy of thoracic RT for LS-SCLC in two Canadian randomized controlled trials (BR3 and BR6) addressing the optimization of thoracic RT in combination with chemotherapy [27]. A total of 608 patients were deemed evaluable in the two trials and of those 88 were ≥70. Age did not impact on the delivery, tolerance, or efficacy of thoracic RT although in the BR6 study elderly patients were less likely to complete thoracic RT given at a dose of 40 Gy in 15 fractions compared to their younger counterparts (nonsignificant difference).

Further studies showed that compliance to chemotherapy in the concurrent setting is the main issue in elderly patients. Rates of nonhematological toxicities (particularly radiation esophagitis and pneumonitis rates) and treatment-related deaths were not increased in the elderly according to the limited literature available [10, 27]. The two Canadian studies reported by Quon et al. [27] showed in the first study (BR3) that although there was no significant difference between elderly (>70 years of age) and younger patients in terms of toxicity, elderly patients were subject to a greater

Table 17.1 Summary of toxicities in selected trials involving LS-SCLC patients over the age of 70 treated with CTRT

Study	Full-course CTRT completed	Hematological toxicity grade 3+	Selected nonhematological toxicity grade 3+	Treatment-related deaths and cause
Yuen et al. [25]	39/50 (78 %)	Neutropenia 41/50 (82 %)[a] Thrombocytopenia 18/50 (36 %)	Esophagitis 12/50 (24 %) Pneumonitis 4/50 (8 %)	5/50 (10 %) 2 (4 %) – infection 1 (2 %) – pulmonary 1 (2 %) – coagulation 1 (2 %) – hemorrhage
Schild et al. [26]	Not reported	Neutropenia 48/54 (89 %) Thrombocytopenia 25/54 (46 %) Anemia 6/54 (11 %)	Esophagitis 3/54 (6 %) Pneumonitis 3/54 (6 %)	3/54 (6 %) Pneumonitis 3/54 (6 %)
Murray et al. [29]	49/55 (89 %)	Not reported[b]	Not reported[b]	3/55 (6 %) 2 (4 %) – pneumonitis 1 (2 %) – sepsis

[a]Grade 4+ toxicity rates – grade 3 not reported
[b]Toxicity rates not reported but authors stated rates of toxicities similar to that seen in younger patients

number of chemotherapy dose omissions. In the second study (BR6), no difference between elderly patients and their youngest counterparts with regard to treatment omissions or toxicities was reported. The findings of this study contradict those of the retrospective analysis of elderly patients in the Turrisi trial in which elderly patients were more likely to experience both chemotherapy dose omissions and higher rates of grade 4+ hematological toxicities [25].

In a study which included patients with lung cancer conducted at a tertiary cancer center and examining acceptance of treatment-related toxicity in the elderly, 244 patients were interviewed using two sets of hypothetical vignettes to examine (1) the influence of age on a patient's acceptance of cancer therapy and (2) whether older patients were as likely to trade an increased survival for maintaining quality of life [28]. The authors found that older patients (>65 years) were just as likely to accept chemotherapy regardless of disease stage and likely toxicity as their younger counterparts. However, older patients were less willing to select a more toxic treatment which might result in a reduction in quality of life (QoL) in order to gain an advantage in overall survival time.

Considering Yellen's findings and the fact that elderly patients are more likely to experience chemotherapy dose omissions/delays, a treatment strategy is to consider an abbreviated chemotherapy schedule combined with RT. In a prospective study by Murray et al. [29], 55 patients with LS-SCLC were treated with two cycles of chemotherapy (1 cycle of CAV and 1 cycle of EP) with an interval between courses of 3 weeks. CAV included cyclophosphamide 1,000 mg/m^2 intravenously (IV), doxorubicin 50 mg/m^2 IV, and vincristine 2 mg IV on day 1; the EP regimen included etoposide 100 mg/m^2 IV and cisplatin 25 mg/m^2 IV on days 22, 23, and 24. RT was commenced concurrently with EP chemotherapy, and target volume included pre-chemotherapy tumor plus a 2 cm margin and encompassing the entire mediastinum. Although median survival rates were slightly shorter compared with younger patients treated at the time (the median survival time was 54 weeks), the 2- and 5-year survival rates of 28 and 18 % correlated well with outcomes for younger patients.

Another strategy in elderly patients for whom there is a concern regarding the tolerability of concurrent CTRT is to consider sequential CTRT associated with a lower risk of radiation esophagitis and hematological toxicity [30].

Prophylactic Cranial Irradiation

Prophylactic cranial irradiation is considered standard treatment in patients with complete response on chest X-ray following systemic therapy for LS-SCLC. A meta-analysis demonstrated that PCI reduces the incidence of brain metastases (relative risk 0.46; 95 % confidence interval, 0.38–0.57; $p<0.001$) and improves overall survival from 15.3 to 20.7 % at 3 years (relative risk of death 0.84; 95 % confidence interval 0.73–0.97) [13]. Subgroup analysis showed that the reduction in risk of brain metastasis persisted in the 25 % of patients ≥65 years (relative risk 0.37, 95 % confidence interval 0.25–0.59). Although the oldest patient in the trials pooled for meta-analysis was 80 years, the median age was only 59 years, and therefore, the role of PCI in patients with LS-SCLC ≥75 years remains uncertain.

Patel et al. [31] reported a SEER data review of 7,995 patients with LS-SCLC. Of these, 670 were identified as having PCI. Greater overall and cause-specific survival was observed in patients treated with PCI. The 2- and 5-year survival rates were 23 and 11 % without PCI and 42 and 19 % with PCI, respectively. The analysis indicates a significant magnitude of benefit with PCI for both the cause-specific survival and overall survival endpoints regardless of age.

A retrospective review of patients with LS-SCLC treated at Princess Margaret Hospital from 1997 to 2007 showed that patients older than 65 years of age were significantly less likely to receive PCI than patients aged 65 years or less, 45.7 % versus 54.3 % ($p=0.01$) [32]. One explanation for this finding is that despite improved survival with PCI, the possibility of severe lethargy and long-term neurotoxicity remains one of the major concerns among oncologists particularly in vulnerable elderly patients. Long-term sequelae including memory loss, intellectual impairment, tremors, somnolence, ataxia, and cortical atrophy have been described. However, it should be noted that in the few studies where baseline neuropsychological testing was conducted, the majority of patients had evidence of impaired cognitive function prior to starting PCI [33, 34]. Furthermore, in elderly patients the evaluation of the long-term effects of PCI is confounded by the multiple comorbidities associated with age such as cerebrovascular disease and dementia.

Neuropsychological testing and QoL assessment were carried out in the international PCI study comparing two doses of radiation (25 or 36 Gy) [35]. A mild deterioration across time of communication deficit, weakness of legs, and intellectual deficit and memory was reported in both groups (all $p<0.005$). No conclusion could be made regarding the toxicity of PCI in the elderly from this study as the protocol specified an upper age limit of 70 years for the European patients resulting in the recruitment of only 5 % of patients above that age, exclusively from US centers.

More reassuringly two randomized controlled trials, employing rigorous pre- and posttreatment neuropsychologic assessment, did not demonstrate any difference in neurocognitive function related to PCI use within the first few years after treatment [36, 37]. However, patients aged >70 years were excluded from one study [36] and, in the second, the median age was 60 years [37]. Therefore, because of the expected increased incidence of neurocognitive comorbidities in this age group, it is important not only to counsel these patients when consenting for PCI but also to consider using neuropsychometric assessment tools prior to the start of treatment.

Conclusions and Future Directions

In conclusion, elderly patients should neither be undertreated nor overtreated with RT or CTRT. Selection of treatment should not be made on the basis of chronological age and should take into account performance status, stage, comorbidities, nutritional status, and patients' preference. The benefits of concurrent CTRT have to be balanced against the risks of radiation esophagitis and pneumonitis more likely to lead to hospitalization, malnutrition, and deterioration of QoL in the elderly compared to their younger counterparts. Future studies in SCLC including elderly patients are urgently needed with emphasis on toxicity, QoL, and efficacy. The use of geriatric assessments may help to define groups of patients more likely to benefit from aggressive treatments such as concurrent CTRT and may also enable more robust stratification of elderly patients in prospective studies. Furthermore, advances in RT planning and delivery, such as omitting elective nodal irradiation, 4-D conformal RT planning, intensity-modulated radiotherapy (IMRT), and image-guided radiotherapy (IGRT), are likely to widen the therapeutic window, and the resulting reduction in toxicity should make future RT more tolerable for elderly patients.

The CONVERT trial (NCT00433563) is a large international multicenter phase III randomized controlled trial comparing BDRT (45, 1.5 Gy per fraction, 3 weeks) with a dose-escalated OD regimen (66, 2 Gy per fraction, 6.5 weeks) concurrently with cisplatin/etoposide chemotherapy. There is no upper age limit for inclusion to the trial. This study uses involved field irradiation using a 3D conformal plan and will provide important information about the tolerability of CTRT in elderly patients in the era of modern RT.

References

1. Owonikoko TK, Ragin CC, Belani CP, et al. Lung cancer in elderly patients: an analysis of the surveillance, epidemiology, and end results database. J Clin Oncol. 2007;25(35):5570–7.
2. Lally BE, Geiger AM, Urbanic JJ, et al. Trends in the outcomes for patients with limited stage small cell lung cancer: an analysis of the Surveillance, Epidemiology, and End Results database. Lung Cancer. 2009;64(2):226–31.
3. Govindan R, Page N, Morgensztern D, et al. Changing epidemiology of small cell lung cancer in the United States over the last 30 years: analysis of the surveillance, epidemiologic, and end results database. J Clin Oncol. 2006;24:4539–44.
4. Bayman N, Sheikh H, Kularatne B, et al. Radiotherapy for small-cell lung cancer – where are we heading? Lung Cancer. 2009;63(3):307–14.
5. Faivre-Finn C, Lorigan P, West C, et al. Thoracic radiation therapy for limited-stage small-cell lung cancer. Unanswered questions. Clin Lung Cancer. 2005;7:23–9.
6. Van Loon J, De Ruysscher D, Wanders R, et al. Selective nodal irradiation on basis of (18)FDG-PET scans in limited disease small-cell lung cancer: a prospective study. Int J Radiat Oncol Biol Phys. 2010;77:329–36.
7. De Ruysscher D, Pijls-Johannesma M, Vansteenkiste J, et al. Systematic review and meta-analysis of randomised, controlled trials of the timing of chest radiotherapy in patients with limited-stage, small-cell lung cancer. Ann Oncol. 2006;17:543–52.
8. Fried DB, Morris DE, Poole C, et al. Systematic review evaluating the timing of thoracic radiation therapy in combined modality therapy for limited-stage small-cell lung cancer. J Clin Oncol. 2004;22:4837–45.
9. Huncharek M, McGarry R. A meta-analysis of the timing of chest irradiation in the combined modality treatment of limited-stage small cell lung cancer. Oncologist. 2004;9:665–72.

10. Turrisi 3rd AT, Kim K, Blum R, et al. Twice daily compared with once-daily thoracic radiotherapy in limited small-cell lung cancer treated concurrently with cisplatin and etoposide. N Engl J Med. 1999;340:265–71.
11. Repetto L, Balducci L. A case for geriatric oncology. Lancet Oncol. 2002;3:289–97.
12. Repetto L, Venturino A, Fratino L, et al. Geriatric oncology: a clinical approach to the older patient with cancer. Eur J Cancer. 2003;39:870–80.
13. Auperin A, Arrigada R, Pignon J-P, et al. Prophylactic cranial irradiation for patients with small cell lung cancer in complete remission. Prophylactic Cranial Irradiation Overview Collaborative Group. N Engl J Med. 1999;341:476–84.
14. Balducci L. Geriatric oncology: challenges for the new century. Eur J Cancer. 2000;36:1741–54.
15. Pignon JP, Arriagada R, Ihde DC, et al. A meta-analysis of thoracic radiotherapy for small-cell lung cancer. N Engl J Med. 1992;327:1618–24.
16. Albain KS, Crowley JJ, LeBlanc M, et al. Determinants of improved outcome in small-cell lung cancer: an analysis of the 2,580-patient Southwest Oncology Group data base. J Clin Oncol. 1990;8:1563–74.
17. Osterlind K, Andersen PK. Prognostic factors in small cell lung cancer: multivariate model based on 778 patients treated with chemotherapy with or without irradiation. Cancer Res. 1986;46:4189–94.
18. Sagman U, Maki E, Evans WK, et al. Small-cell carcinoma of the lung: derivation of a prognostic staging system. J Clin Oncol. 1991;9:1639–49.
19. Spiegelman D, Maurer LH, Ware JH, et al. Prognostic factors in small-cell carcinoma of the lung: an analysis of 1,521 patients. J Clin Oncol. 1989;7:344–54.
20. Fairchild A, Harris K, Barnes E, et al. Palliative thoracic radiotherapy for lung cancer: a systematic review. J Clin Oncol. 2008;26:4001–11.
21. Turner NJ, Muers MF, Haward RA, et al. Do elderly people with lung cancer benefit from palliative radiotherapy? Lung Cancer. 2005;49:193–202.
22. Faivre-Finn C, Lee LW, Lorigan P, et al. Thoracic radiotherapy for limited-stage small-cell lung cancer: controversies and future developments. Clin Oncol (R Coll Radiol). 2005;17:591–8.
23. Ludbrook JJ, Truong PT, MacNeil MV, et al. Do age and comorbidity impact treatment allocation and outcomes in limited stage small-cell lung cancer? A community-based population analysis. Int J Radiat Oncol Biol Phys. 2003;55:1321–30.
24. Janssen-Heijnen ML, Maas HA, Siesling S, et al. Treatment and survival of patients with small-cell lung cancer: small steps forward, but not for patients >80. Ann Oncol. 2012;23(4):954–60.
25. Yuen AR, Zou G, Turrisi AT, et al. Similar outcome of elderly patients in intergroup trial 0096: cisplatin, etoposide, and thoracic radiotherapy administered once or twice daily in limited stage small cell lung carcinoma. Cancer. 2000;89:1953–60.
26. Schild SE, Stella PJ, Brooks BJ, et al. Results of combined-modality therapy for limited-stage small cell lung carcinoma in the elderly. Cancer. 2005;103(11):2349–54.
27. Quon H, Shepherd FA, Payne DG, et al. The influence of age on the delivery, tolerance, and efficacy of thoracic irradiation in the combined modality treatment of limited stage small cell lung cancer. Int J Radiat Oncol Biol Phys. 1999;43:39–45.
28. Yellen SB, Cella DR, Leslie WT. Age and clinical decision making in oncology patients. J Natl Cancer Inst. 1994;86:1766–70.
29. Murray N, Grafton C, Shah A, et al. Abbreviated treatment for elderly, infirm, or noncompliant patients with limited-stage small-cell lung cancer. J Clin Oncol. 1998;6:3323–8.
30. Takada M, Fukuoka M, Kawahara M, et al. Phase III study of concurrent versus sequential thoracic radiotherapy in combination with cisplatin and etoposide for limited-stage small-cell lung cancer: results of the Japan Clinical Oncology Group Study 9104. J Clin Oncol. 2002;20:3054–60.
31. Patel S, Macdonald OK, Suntharalingam M. Evaluation of the use of prophylactic cranial irradiation in small cell lung cancer. Cancer. 2009;115:842–50.

32. Giuliani M, Sun A, Bezjak A, et al. Utilization of prophylactic cranial irradiation in patients with limited stage small cell lung carcinoma. Cancer. 2010;116(24):5694–9.
33. Grosshans DR, Meyers CA, Allen PK, et al. Neurocognitive function in patients with small cell lung cancer: effect of prophylactic cranial irradiation. Cancer. 2008;112(3):589–95.
34. Komaki R, Shin Dong M, Glisson BS, et al. Interdigitating versus concurrent chemotherapy and radiotherapy for limited small cell lung cancer. Int J Radiat Oncol Biol Phys. 1995;31(4):807–11.
35. Le Péchoux C, Dunant A, Senan S, et al. Standard-dose versus higher-dose prophylactic cranial irradiation (PCI) in patients with limited-stage small-cell lung cancer in complete remission after chemotherapy and thoracic radiotherapy (PCI 99–01, EORTC 22003–08004, RTOG 0212, and IFCT 99–01): a randomised clinical trial. Lancet Oncol. 2009;10(5):467–74.
36. Arriagada R, Le Chevalier T, Borie F, et al. Prophylactic cranial irradiation for patients with small-cell lung cancer in complete remission. J Natl Cancer Inst. 1995;87:183–90.
37. Gregor A, Cull A, Stephens RJ, et al. Prophylactic cranial irradiation is indicated following complete response to induction therapy in small cell lung cancer: results of a multicentre randomised trial. Eur J Cancer. 1997;33:1752–8.

Chapter 18
Chemotherapy in the Elderly: Standard Chemotherapy or Specific Regimens?

Paul Wheatley-Price and Frances A. Shepherd

Abstract Small cell lung cancer (SCLC) incidence falls with increasing age, yet 40 % of all SCLC cases occur in the 70 years and older population, and poorer survival is seen in the elderly. There is limited prospective data on chemotherapy in the elderly population, such that exists supports standard platinum based therapies that are used in younger patients, although caution should be used because of the risk of toxicity.

Keywords Small cell lung cancer chemotherapy • Lung cancer in the elderly • Chemotherapy in elderly lung cancer patients • SCLC chemotherapy • Cranial irradiation in the elderly with lung cancer

---

P. Wheatley-Price, BSc, MBChB, MRCP (UK), MD (✉)
Division of Medical Oncology,
Department of Medicine, Ottawa Hospital Cancer Centre,
Ottawa Hospital, 501 Smyth Rd.,
Ottawa, ON K1H 8L6, Canada
e-mail: pwheatleyprice@toh.on.ca

F.A. Shepherd, MD, FRCPC
Department of Medical Oncology and Hematology,
Princess Margaret Hospital,
610 University Ave., 5-104,
Toronto, ON M5G2M9, Canada

C. Gridelli, R.A. Audisio (eds.), *Management of Lung Cancer in Older People*,
DOI 10.1007/978-0-85729-793-8_18, © Springer-Verlag London 2013

The Incidence of Small Cell Lung Cancer in the Elderly

Small cell lung cancer (SCLC) represents approximately 12–15 % of all lung cancer cases, a proportion that has been falling over recent decades, likely due to the reduction in cigarette smoking rates and the routine addition of filters to cigarettes [1–3]. When looking by age, however, in an analysis of the SEER (Surveillance, Epidemiology and End Results) database, while SCLC represents about 14–16 % of all lung cancer cases in the <70 years and 70–79-year-old populations, the proportion falls to only 9–11 % of all lung cancer cases in the 80 years and older population [4]. Older data from the cancer registry of Kansas and Western Missouri support this finding, where SCLC accounted for 19–23 % of lung cancer cases in the under 70 age group, 18 % in the 70–79-year-old group, and only 13 % in the 80+ age group [5]. Further veterans data from North Carolina also demonstrate the falling incidence of SCLC in older populations [6].

This still is a significant number, however, with approximately 40 % of all SCLC cases occurring in the 70+ age group and 10 % in the 80+ age group. The same SEER analysis further reports poorer survival for the elderly SCLC population, with 5-year survival rates of 7.1, 3.9, and 2.2 % in the <70, 70–79, and 80+ age groups, respectively ($p<0.0001$) [4].

Until recently, SCLC has been staged using the Veterans Administration Lung Study Group staging system [7]. While there is some variation in the definition of limited-stage disease, it is widely accepted as being a disease that is restricted to one hemithorax, with or without lymphadenopathy that can be encompassed within an acceptable radiation field [8]. Extensive disease is therefore defined as when the cancer has progressed beyond limited stage in any manner. Approximately two-thirds of SCLC patients have extensive-stage disease at diagnosis. The limited available data suggests that this proportion does not vary across age groups [5, 9]. More recently, the International Association for the Study of Lung Cancer staging project clearly showed that tumor, node, and metastasis (TNM) staging is applicable to SCLC as well [10, 11].

The purpose of this chapter is to discuss the treatment of extensive-stage SCLC in the elderly. The topic of limited-stage disease in the elderly is discussed in Chap. 17. Where the available data come from trials investigating treatment across stage groupings, those findings are also discussed in this chapter.

Standard Therapy for Extensive-Stage SCLC

Chemotherapy is the mainstay of treatment in ES-SCLC, with radiation largely reserved for specific palliative treatments, such as treatment of superior vena cava obstruction (SVCO), painful bone metastases, or symptomatic brain metastases.

Since the introduction of chemotherapy for SCLC in the 1970s, a number of drugs have established efficacy as monotherapy, with tumor response rates of greater than 30 % in untreated patients. Active chemotherapy drugs include cisplatin, carboplatin, nitrogen mustard, ifosfamide, etoposide, doxorubicin, methotrexate, vincristine, vinorelbine, vindesine, paclitaxel, docetaxel, gemcitabine, irinotecan, and topotecan [12]. Combination chemotherapy subsequently established an advantage over single-agent therapy [13, 14], and in recent years the most frequently used chemotherapy combinations for treatment of SCLC have been CAV (cyclophosphamide, doxorubicin [Adriamycin], and vincristine) or platinum and etoposide (EP).

Platinum-containing regimens are considered slightly superior to non-platinum-containing regimens, supported by meta-analyses demonstrating a survival benefit for cisplatin-containing protocols [15, 16]. Pujol et al., in a meta-analysis of 19 trials with 4,054 evaluable patients, investigated outcomes in patients receiving platinum versus non-platinum chemotherapy [15]. This demonstrated improved response rates in those receiving cisplatin and a significant reduction in the risk of death at 1 year (HR 0.80, 95 % CI 0.69–0.93, $p = 0.002$). More recently, some centers have replaced cisplatin with carboplatin, because of its slightly lower toxicity and similar efficacy as demonstrated in one small 147-patient comparison trial in LS-SCLC [17]. The current standard chemotherapy regimen internationally is EP, for both limited- and extensive-stage disease.

Many approaches have been investigated in an attempt to improve on the outcomes seen with EP, such as different cytotoxic agents, alternating regimens, high-dose chemotherapy, or dose-dense approaches. However, to date there have been no significant advantages demonstrated [18–32].

The role of prophylactic cranial irradiation (PCI), now a standard component of the treatment of limited disease [33, 34], also has been investigated in ES disease. In a randomized trial conducted by the European Organisation for Research and Treatment of Cancer (EORTC), 286 patients with ES-SCLC, who had responded to primary chemotherapy, were randomized to PCI or observation. Treatment with PCI was associated with a significant reduction in brain metastases (16.6 % versus 41.3 %, $p < 0.001$) and a significant improvement in survival (median overall survival 6.7 versus 5.4 months; hazard ratio 0.68, 95 % confidence interval 0.52–0.88, $p = 0.003$) [35].

The overwhelming majority of patients with ES-SCLC will relapse, with a median progression-free survival (PFS) after first-line therapy in the order of 4–6 months [28]. Second-line chemotherapy treatment usually has response rates of 20 % or less, and patients resistant to first-line chemotherapy or with a short relapse-free interval are not likely to benefit [36, 37]. For those who are suitable, second-line therapy with CAV is a commonly used approach following progression after a platinum-based treatment. Topotecan, a topoisomerase I inhibitor from the same family as irinotecan, has demonstrated efficacy in the second-line setting similar to CAV [38]. More recently an oral formulation of topotecan has been studied against best supportive care in relapsed SCLC, demonstrating a significant survival benefit [39]. Amrubicin is a novel cytotoxic with combined anthracycline and topoisomerase II inhibition activity, which has now been tested in a number of SCLC settings. Two phase II studies investigated amrubicin in the second-line setting, as monotherapy or compared to topotecan, and both showed promising clinical activity [40, 41]. The subsequent phase III study, which randomized 637 patients to either amrubicin or topotecan in the second-line setting, demonstrated that treatment with amrubicin was associated with a significantly higher response rate, longer PFS, and less neutropenia, thrombocytopenia, or anemia. However, there was no significant difference in overall survival between groups [42].

Treatment of Extensive-Stage SCLC in the Elderly

In seeking guidance for chemotherapy in the elderly, data exist from different sources, including randomized trials in the elderly, subgroup analyses from randomized trials without age restrictions, retrospective institutional data, and extrapolation from data in the limited-stage setting (discussed in Chap. 17). However, the sum total from all these sources remains limited. Relevant studies are summarized in Table 18.1.

Retrospective Clinical Trial Data

Age has not been identified as a prognostic factor in a series of chemotherapy trials of ES-SCLC over a number of decades [43–46], although there are some studies that do report age as being prognostic [24, 47].

Spiegelman et al. published prognostic factors for SCLC from a series of clinical trials conducted between 1972 and 1986. Specifically in 662 patients with extensive disease, age (with a cutoff of 60 years) was not prognostic for response ($p=0.30$) or overall survival (HR 1.03, $p=0.74$) [44]. A large analysis of clinical trials from the Southwest Oncology Group (SWOG) included 2,580 patients, of whom 1,217 were enrolled to ED studies [45]. In univariate analysis, age <70 years was a positive prognostic factor in both limited and extensive diseases, but in a Cox multivariate analysis, patient age was no longer prognostic in the extensive-stage disease subgroup. Indeed, the Manchester score, a prognostic model developed to guide treatment decisions, investigated 61 possible prognostic factors in SCLC, and age was not found to be a significant factor [48]. It should be noted though that of the total cohort of 407 patients, only 163 had extensive-stage disease, and the specific age range and number of elderly patients were not reported. Artal-Cortes et al. reported a randomized study of different schedules of etoposide and cisplatin [46]. Of 411 patients, 195 had extensive disease, and there were no patients over the age of 75. While age ≥70 years was a negative prognostic factor in limited-stage disease (HR 1.86, $p=0.007$), this was not a significant factor in the extensive-stage disease cohort.

Conversely, Neill et al. published a phase III study in patients with only ES-SCLC, randomized to EP with or without paclitaxel [24]. Of 587 patients, 107 were ≥70 years of age. In this study, young patients lived significantly longer than the older patients (10.5 versus 8.6 months, $p=0.0008$). Further, in a retrospective pooled

Table 18.1 Clinical trials in elderly patients with extensive-stage small cell lung cancer

Author	Year	Age range	Treatment	Number	% ES	Response rate (%)	Overall survival (months)
Ardizzoni et al. [51]	2005	70–80	Low dose EP	28	43	39	7.2
			Standard EP	67	46	69	9.5
Gridelli et al. [52]	2011	>70	Gem/etoposide	10	100	10	9.2
			Gem/vinorelbine	30	100	37	5.3
			Gem/cisplatin	12	100	17	5.1
			Gem/carboplatin	26	100	61.5	8.5
Okamoto et al. [53]	2007	55–86[a]	EC	110	100	73	10.6
			EP	110	100	73	9.9
Quoix et al. [54]	2001	70–88	EC	38	68	60.5	7.2
Larive et al. [55]	2001	70–79	EC	34	82	59	8.5
Evans et al. [57]	1995	47–84	oEC	36	100	66	10.4
Matsui et al. [56]	1998	73–84	oEC	22	100	71	8.6
Gridelli et al. [58]	2002	65–78	Carboplatin/ vinorelbine	28	100	39	7.9
Hainsworth et al. [59]	2004	56–88[b]	Docetaxel/gem	40	100	23	4
Inoue et al. [61]	2010	70–83	Carboplatin/ amrubicin	36	58	89	18.6
Igawa et al. [60]	2010	55–82[c]	Amrubicin	27	100	70	9.3

gem gemcitabine, *EP* etoposide and cisplatin, *EC* etoposide and carboplatin, *oEC* oral etoposide and carboplatin

[a]92 % patients age ≥70 years

[b]median age 72

[c]median age 73

analysis of 1,707 patients treated in SCLC chemotherapy trials in the UK, female sex, age ≤60 years, limited-stage disease, good performance status, and normal baseline white blood cell count were all prognostic of longer survival in multivariate analysis [47]. This analysis however did not investigate the more widely accepted 70 years of age as a cutoff, and this analysis was not limited to patients with ES-SCLC.

An approach that at one time was considered attractive in the elderly was single-agent oral chemotherapy. However, two phase III trials of single-agent etoposide demonstrated this to be inferior to standard therapy [49, 50]. A phase III trial randomizing patients to oral etoposide versus alternating EP and CAV was conducted in 155 patients with ES-SCLC ranging in age from 49 to 86 years. Patients under the age of 75 years, with limited disease and ECOG performance status 0–1, were ineligible. Oral etoposide was associated with significantly *shorter* survival, but no data were reported on the efficacy in the elderly subgroup [49]. In the second study, 339 poor performance (ECOG 2–4) patients (57 % extensive stage) were randomized to oral etoposide for 10 days versus CAV or etoposide/vincristine [50]. Again, etoposide monotherapy was associated with significantly shorter survival, even though approximately one-third of the comparator cohort received a chemotherapy regimen containing neither platinum nor anthracycline. Unfortunately there was no analysis in this study by age.

Prospective Clinical Trials in the Elderly

Prospective clinical trial data in the elderly are limited; in particular very few randomized trials are available to give guidance in this area (Table 18.1). An Italian phase II study of 95 patients in the 70–80 years age range, of whom 45 % had extensive disease, randomized patients between two differing EP regimens [51]. The attenuated dose (AD) arm consisted of four cycles of cisplatin 25 mg/m^2 on days 1 and 2, and etoposide 60 mg/m^2 on days 1–3 every 3 weeks; the full dose (FD arm) was cisplatin 40 mg/m^2 on days 1 and 2, and etoposide 100 mg/m^2 on days 1–3 every 3 weeks, plus lenogastrim support. The observed response rate was significantly lower in the AD arm (39 % versus 69 %) with a shorter median overall survival (31 versus 41 weeks). Grade 3–4 hematological toxicities (10 % versus 0 %) and non-hematological toxicities (10 % versus 4 %) were more common in the FD cohort, and one death in the FD arm only was attributed to treatment toxicity.

A second Italian phase I/II study, the G-STEP program, investigated four different gemcitabine-based doublets in patients with ES-SCLC over the age of 70 years [52]. Seventy-eight eligible patients were randomized to either gemcitabine/vinorelbine, gemcitabine/etoposide, gemcitabine/carboplatin, or gemcitabine/cisplatin. Three of the doublets failed to progress beyond stage 1 in the trial design due to lack of acceptable clinical activity. Only gemcitabine/carboplatin ($n=26$) reported a response rate over 60 %, and this was the only combination that the study authors concluded may be worth further study.

The Japanese Clinical Oncology Group (JCOG) 9702 trial compared carboplatin/etoposide to cisplatin/etoposide in 220 ES-SCLC patients who either were elderly or had poor performance status [53]. Age criteria stated patients had to be ≥70 years with ECOG PS 0–2 or <70 years with PS 3. Of the 220 patients randomized, 92 % were ≥70 years. No significant differences in response rate, survival, or major toxicities were observed between the two groups, with the exception of higher rates of grade 3 or 4 thrombocytopenia in the carboplatin-receiving cohort (56 % versus 16 %, $p < 0.01$), although there were no grade 3 or 4 bleeding events in either cohort. The authors concluded that carboplatin/etoposide may be considered as an alternative to cisplatin/etoposide.

Carboplatin and etoposide also has been investigated in two small French phase II single-arm studies in the elderly. Quoix et al. reported a series of 38 patients ranging in age from 70 to 88 years, treated with carboplatin and etoposide for stage IIIb/IV small cell lung cancer [54]. The overall response rate was 60.5 % and the median overall survival was 220 days (7.2 months). Larive et al. reported the use of carboplatin and etoposide in 34 patients ≥70 years of age, of whom 28 had extensive disease [55] with similar results to Quoix et al. The overall response rate was 59 % and median overall survival 37 weeks (8.5 months).

Etoposide is also available in oral formulation and has been utilized in SCLC. Matsui et al. reported a phase II trial in 38 patients over the age of 70 years, treated with carboplatin and oral etoposide given daily for 14 days every 4 weeks [56]. Twenty-two patients had extensive-stage disease, and this group had a response rate of 71 % and median survival of 8.6 months. The regimen was well tolerated, with three reported episodes of neutropenic fever. A similar Canadian study reported the results of 47 patients who received carboplatin and oral etoposide [57]. Extensive disease was seen present in 36 patients, 33 of whom were 65 years or older. A response rate of 66 % was observed in the ED cohort, with a median survival of 45 weeks.

The combination of carboplatin and vinorelbine also has been tested in a small phase II study in the elderly [58]. Only 28 patients ≥65 years were enrolled, but three patients died while on treatment, and the overall response rate of only 39 % meant that this regimen has not been studied further.

A phase II study of weekly docetaxel and gemcitabine was investigated in 40 patients with ES-SCLC [59]. Patients had to be over 65 years, or have a performance status 2, or not be considered fit for platinum therapy in the opinion of the treating clinician. While this regimen appeared tolerable, efficacy outcomes were poor, with a partial response rate of only 27 % and a median survival of 4 months. The authors rightly concluded there was no rationale for further investigation of this combination.

Three Japanese phase II studies have investigated the use of amrubicin chemotherapy in elderly lung cancer populations [60–62]. Inoue et al. reported 36 patients over 70 years of age, treated in the first-line setting with carboplatin/amrubicin [61]. All patients were of good performance status (ECOG 0–1) and 21 patients had extensive-stage disease. The overall response rate was 89 % with a median survival of 12.8 months for the patients with extensive disease. In contrast, Igawa et al. studied amrubicin as monotherapy in patients either 75 years or older or those with a poor performance status (ECOG ≥2) [60]. In this cohort of 27 patients, the overall response rate was 70 % with a median survival in the elderly patients of 9.0 months. The third study, by Nakao et al., studied amrubicin monotherapy in previously treated lung cancer patients (SCLC and NSCLC), comparing outcomes between the young and the elderly (≥70 years) [62]. In this trial, of 51 patients in total, 31 had SCLC and 22 were ≥70 years old; response rates and toxicities did not significantly differ between age groups. Therefore, while the patient numbers are very small, it would seem that amrubicin may be a treatment option in older populations. While amrubicin is classified as an anthracycline, cardiac toxicity has not been reported in these trials, thus increasing its attractiveness as a potential agent. However, while it is approved for use in Japan, it currently is not available in North America or Europe. Finally, a small dose-escalation study investigated different dose combinations of carboplatin and irinotecan in patients with SCLC over the age of 70 years [63]. Of 18 patients enrolled, 10 had extensive disease and 9 had received prior therapy. Reported efficacy was impressive, with a response rate of 89 % and median survival of 13.3 months; however, in the context of subsequently reported negative phase III trials [27, 28], this regimen is not likely to become a standard of care.

Data from Case Series

A useful analysis, although still small patient numbers, was performed by Li et al., who reported a single institution review of SCLC cases over a 10-year period. Of a total of 126 patients, just over 50 % had ES disease, and one-third of the patients were aged 70 years or older [64]. Unsurprisingly the elderly group had more comorbidities, but the choice of chemotherapy (CAV or EP) did not significantly differ between groups. The authors reported similar response rates between the young and older groups (69 % versus 65 %, $p=0.591$) and similar median overall survival (13 versus 12 months, $p=0.263$). The elderly did experience significantly higher rates of leukopenia, neutropenia, and thrombocytopenia. The authors continued to do a further analysis using 75 as the age cutoff. Only 19/126 patients were 75+years, and in this group they still reported no significant difference in response rate or survival, but the older group was less likely to complete four cycles of therapy (24 % versus 42 %, $p=0.018$).

A smaller series of 76 patients over the age of 70 years treated between 1978 and 1983, of whom 64 % had extensive disease, was reported by Findlay et al. [65]. In this retrospective analysis, CAV was considered "intensive" treatment, while "gentle" treatment was either monotherapy or reduced dose CAV. In the ES subgroup, the authors reported a response rate of 75 % from intensive chemotherapy and 50 % from gentle therapy, with a median overall survival of 23 weeks. Grade 3 or 4 toxicities were almost exclusively seen in the intensively treated cohort, leading the authors to question whether significant toxicity should be accepted in a disease where fewer than 20 % patients survived 12 months.

An interesting case series was published by Bonn et al. reporting the use of combination vindesine/etoposide in 41 patients with ES-SCLC, described in the manuscript title as for "elderly patients or patients in reduced clinical condition" [66]. While the authors conclude that this regimen is a "practicable, equally effective, and well-tolerated alternative to standard therapies," in fact the paper describes an age range of 40–89 years with a median of 63 years, reports no age analysis, and states that 95 % of patients had an ECOG PS of 0 or 1 and that the overall response rate was 43.9 %. Therefore, it would appear that the title and conclusions did not add any meaningful information to guide treatment in the elderly with SCLC.

A series of 123 patients over the age of 70 years (including 14 over 80 years), treated between 1976 and 1988, was reported by Shepherd et al. [9]. The median survival in patients with extensive disease was 5.2 months, and 25 patients received no therapy at all (median survival 1.1 months), and a further 20 received radiation alone. The primary factors influencing longer survival were disease stage and treatment with chemotherapy ($p<0.0001$). It should be noted though that of the 77 patients who received chemotherapy, less than 50 % completed a planned six cycles of therapy, and three-quarters of all patients required two or more dose reductions.

Data from Limited-Stage SCLC

It is not necessarily appropriate to extrapolate differences in outcome by age in the setting of limited-stage disease to that of extensive-stage disease. In a condition with such an aggressive natural history, such as SCLC, it is possible that "weaker" prognostic factors may not exert any significant influence in the face of "stronger" prognostic factors (such as stage of disease). However, it is worth noting that the effect of age on outcomes in LS-SCLC is also conflicting. A review article by Pallis et al. summarizes these conflicting results [67], in which three studies of chemotherapy and radiotherapy in LS-SCLC did not demonstrate age to be a prognostic factor [68–70], and two studies did report increasing age to be associated with shorter survival [71, 72]. An analysis from the SEER database of patients treated with LS-SCLC also reported advancing age to be a negative prognostic factor (for patients over 70; $HR=1.66$, $p<0.0001$); however, the over 70 age group was also far less likely to receive radiotherapy than younger age groups ($p<0.0001$) [73]. The effect of age in limited SCLC is discussed more completely in Chap. 17.

Prophylactic Cranial Irradiation

The issue of PCI in the elderly with ES-SCLC has not been answered. Inclusion criteria for the definitive study mandated patients were between 18 and 75 years of age. The manuscript does not state the number of patients in the 70–75 age group, and no age-based analysis was reported [35]. Data from trials of in LS-SCLC have not shown any difference in the degree of benefit from PCI in different age groups. A subset analysis was performed in a meta-analysis of PCI in patients with LS-SCLC who had a complete response after chemotherapy. Approximately one-quarter of patients were 65 years old or older, and the benefits of PCI were similar in both the younger and older groups [33].

Discussion

Treatment of the elderly with SCLC is an important issue. While SCLC may represent a falling fraction of lung cancer as a whole, a significant proportion of cases occur in the elderly population, and the available data suggest that overall, their survival is shorter. While the published literature offers guidance in the treatment of extensive-stage SCLC in the elderly, there are insufficient data to provide definitive recommendations. Limitations of the available data include an inconsistent definition of the elderly, where now the more widely accepted cutoff is 70 years [74]. Another flaw is the propensity to group together the elderly patients and those with poor performance status in many trials [53, 59, 60, 66]. However, it is far from clear that these two distinct subgroups have similar outcomes, and therefore, the validity of combining them in a single study is questionable. Indeed in patients with lung cancer, comorbidities are more common in the over 70 age group, and this has been associated with slightly less aggressive therapy in small cell lung cancer [75]. A review of non-small cell lung cancer trials by the National Cancer Institute of Canada Clinical Trials Group (NCIC CTG) reported that while age did not influence overall survival, the presence of comorbidities (that were more common in the elderly) was prognostic [76].

Overall it seems clear that attempts to reduce the intensity of chemotherapy, either with reduced doses of recognized regiments or with a monotherapy approach, are likely to significantly reduce the efficacy of the treatment, even if the toxicities are reduced with such an approach. There may however be increased toxicity associated with standard therapy in the elderly. While the data are conflicting, there is reasonable evidence to suggest modestly higher rates of hematological toxicity in the 70+ population and also that the elderly are less likely to complete a course of chemotherapy and more likely to require dose reductions. Therefore, treatment should proceed with caution, to minimize toxicities in a group of patients with a very limited life expectancy.

Finally, there is extremely little data to support treatment guidelines in the over 80 age group, sometimes referred to as the “oldest old” or “extreme elderly.” The SEER database identified poorer survival in this age group [4], but while many series included a few patients over the age of 80, this subgroup was routinely not further analyzed as the numbers were so small. Furthermore, many clinical trials exclude patients over 80 years of age. Careful assessment of comorbidity and performance status is required, along with clear risk-benefit discussions with the patients in these uncommon scenarios.

In conclusion, the current standard of care in patients with ES-SCLC remains etoposide with either carboplatin or cisplatin, and while caution should be used, this should still be considered the standard of care in both the young and elderly populations.

References

1. Jemal A, Bray F, Center MM, Ferlay J, Ward E, Forman D. Global cancer statistics. CA Cancer J Clin. 2011;61(2):69–90.
2. Govindan R, Page N, Morgensztern D, et al. Changing epidemiology of small-cell lung cancer in the United States over the last 30 years: analysis of the surveillance, epidemiologic, and end results database. J Clin Oncol. 2006;24(28):4539–44.
3. Hinson Jr JA, Perry MC. Small cell lung cancer. CA Cancer J Clin. 1993;43(4):216–25.
4. Owonikoko TK, Ragin CC, Belani CP, et al. Lung cancer in elderly patients: an analysis of the surveillance, epidemiology, and end results database. J Clin Oncol. 2007;25(35):5570–7.
5. Teeter SM, Holmes FF, McFarlane MJ. Lung carcinoma in the elderly population. Influence of histology on the inverse relationship of stage to age. Cancer. 1987;60(6):1331–6.
6. DeMaria Jr LC, Cohen HJ. Characteristics of lung cancer in elderly patients. J Gerontol. 1987;42(5):540–5.
7. Zelen M. Keynote address on biostatistics and data retrieval. Cancer Chemother Rep 3. 1973; 4(2):31–42.
8. Jackman DM, Johnson BE. Small-cell lung cancer. Lancet. 2005;366(9494):1385–96.
9. Shepherd FA, Amdemichael E, Evans WK, et al. Treatment of small cell lung cancer in the elderly. J Am Geriatr Soc. 1994;42(1):64–70.
10. Shepherd FA, Crowley J, Van Houtte P, et al. The International Association for the Study of Lung Cancer lung cancer staging project: proposals regarding the clinical staging of small cell lung cancer in the forthcoming (seventh) edition of the tumor, node, metastasis classification for lung cancer. J Thorac Oncol. 2007;2(12):1067–77.
11. Vallieres E, Shepherd FA, Crowley J, et al. The IASLC Lung Cancer Staging Project: proposals regarding the relevance of TNM in the pathologic staging of small cell lung cancer in the forthcoming (seventh) edition of the TNM classification for lung cancer. J Thorac Oncol. 2009;4(9):1049–59.
12. Argiris A, Murren JR. Advances in chemotherapy for small cell lung cancer: single-agent activity of newer agents. Cancer J. 2001;7(3):228–35.
13. Alberto P, Brunner KW, Martz G, Obrecht J, Sonntag RW. Treatment of bronchogenic carcinoma with simultaneous or sequential combination chemotherapy, including methotrexate, cyclophosphamide, procarbazine and vincristine. Cancer. 1976;38(6):2208–16.
14. Lowenbraun S, Bartolucci A, Smalley RV, Lynn M, Krauss S, Durant JR. The superiority of combination chemotherapy over single agent chemotherapy in small cell lung carcinoma. Cancer. 1979;44(2):406–13.
15. Pujol JL, Carestia L, Daures JP. Is there a case for cisplatin in the treatment of small-cell lung cancer? A meta-analysis of randomized trials of a cisplatin-containing regimen versus a regimen without this alkylating agent. Br J Cancer. 2000;83(1):8–15.
16. Mascaux C, Paesmans M, Berghmans T, et al. A systematic review of the role of etoposide and cisplatin in the chemotherapy of small cell lung cancer with methodology assessment and meta-analysis. Lung Cancer. 2000;30(1):23–36.
17. Skarlos DV, Samantas E, Kosmidis P. Randomized comparison of etoposide-cisplatin vs. etoposide-carboplatin and irradiation in small-cell lung cancer. A Hellenic Co-operative Oncology Group study. Ann Oncol. 1994;5(7):601–7.
18. Evans WK, Feld R, Murray N, et al. Superiority of alternating non-cross-resistant chemotherapy in extensive small cell lung cancer. A multicenter, randomized clinical trial by the National Cancer Institute of Canada. Ann Intern Med. 1987;107(4):451–8.
19. Fukuoka M, Furuse K, Saijo N, et al. Randomized trial of cyclophosphamide, doxorubicin, and vincristine versus cisplatin and etoposide versus alternation of these regimens in small-cell lung cancer. J Natl Cancer Inst. 1991;83(12):855–61.
20. Roth BJ, Johnson DH, Einhorn LH, et al. Randomized study of cyclophosphamide, doxorubicin, and vincristine versus etoposide and cisplatin versus alternation of these two regimens in extensive small-cell lung cancer: a phase III trial of the Southeastern Cancer Study Group. J Clin Oncol. 1992;10(2):282–91.

21. Sundstrom S, Bremnes RM, Kaasa S, et al. Cisplatin and etoposide regimen is superior to cyclophosphamide, epirubicin, and vincristine regimen in small-cell lung cancer: results from a randomized phase III trial with 5 years' follow-up. J Clin Oncol. 2002;20(24):4665–72.
22. Prendiville J, Lorigan P, Hicks F, et al. Therapy for small cell lung cancer using carboplatin, ifosfamide, etoposide (without dose reduction), mid-cycle vincristine with thoracic and cranial irradiation. Eur J Cancer. 1994;30A(14):2085–90.
23. Thatcher N, Qian W, Clark PI, et al. Ifosfamide, carboplatin, and etoposide with midcycle vincristine versus standard chemotherapy in patients with small-cell lung cancer and good performance status: clinical and quality-of-life results of the British Medical Research Council multicenter randomized LU21 trial. J Clin Oncol. 2005;23(33):8371–9.
24. Niell HB, Herndon 2nd JE, Miller AA, et al. Randomized phase III intergroup trial of etoposide and cisplatin with or without paclitaxel and granulocyte colony-stimulating factor in patients with extensive-stage small-cell lung cancer: Cancer and Leukemia Group B Trial 9732. J Clin Oncol. 2005;23(16):3752–9.
25. Reck M, von Pawel J, Macha HN, et al. Randomized phase III trial of paclitaxel, etoposide, and carboplatin versus carboplatin, etoposide, and vincristine in patients with small-cell lung cancer. J Natl Cancer Inst. 2003;95(15):1118–27.
26. Noda K, Nishiwaki Y, Kawahara M, et al. Irinotecan plus cisplatin compared with etoposide plus cisplatin for extensive small-cell lung cancer. N Engl J Med. 2002;346(2):85–91.
27. Natale RB, Lara PN, Chansky K, et al. S0124: A randomized phase III trial comparing irinotecan/cisplatin (IP) with etoposide/cisplatin (EP) in patients (pts) with previously untreated extensive stage small cell lung cancer (E-SCLC). J Clin Oncol. 2008;26(20 Suppl). Abstract 7512.
28. Hanna N, Bunn Jr PA, Langer C, et al. Randomized phase III trial comparing irinotecan/cisplatin with etoposide/cisplatin in patients with previously untreated extensive-stage disease small-cell lung cancer. J Clin Oncol. 2006;24(13):2038–43.
29. Thatcher N, Girling DJ, Hopwood P, Sambrook RJ, Qian W, Stephens RJ. Improving survival without reducing quality of life in small-cell lung cancer patients by increasing the dose-intensity of chemotherapy with granulocyte colony-stimulating factor support: results of a British Medical Research Council Multicenter Randomized Trial. Medical Research Council Lung Cancer Working Party. J Clin Oncol. 2000;18(2):395–404.
30. Ardizzoni A, Tjan-Heijnen VC, Postmus PE, et al. Standard versus intensified chemotherapy with granulocyte colony-stimulating factor support in small-cell lung cancer: a prospective European Organization for Research and Treatment of Cancer-Lung Cancer Group Phase III Trial-08923. J Clin Oncol. 2002;20(19):3947–55.
31. Lorigan P, Woll PJ, O'Brien ME, Ashcroft LF, Sampson MR, Thatcher N. Randomized phase III trial of dose-dense chemotherapy supported by whole-blood hematopoietic progenitors in better-prognosis small-cell lung cancer. J Natl Cancer Inst. 2005;97(9):666–74.
32. Leyvraz S, Pampallona S, Martinelli G, et al. A threefold dose intensity treatment with ifosfamide, carboplatin, and etoposide for patients with small cell lung cancer: a randomized trial. J Natl Cancer Inst. 2008;100(8):533–41.
33. Auperin A, Arriagada R, Pignon JP, et al. Prophylactic cranial irradiation for patients with small-cell lung cancer in complete remission. Prophylactic Cranial Irradiation Overview Collaborative Group. N Engl J Med. 1999;341(7):476–84.
34. Meert AP, Paesmans M, Berghmans T, et al. Prophylactic cranial irradiation in small cell lung cancer: a systematic review of the literature with meta-analysis. BMC Cancer. 2001;1:5.
35. Slotman B, Faivre-Finn C, Kramer G, et al. Prophylactic cranial irradiation in extensive small-cell lung cancer. N Engl J Med. 2007;357(7):664–72.
36. Huisman C, Postmus PE, Giaccone G, Smit EF. Second-line chemotherapy and its evaluation in small cell lung cancer. Cancer Treat Rev. 1999;25(4):199–206.
37. Thatcher N, Faivre-Finn C, Lorigan P. Management of small-cell lung cancer. Ann Oncol. 2005;16 Suppl 2:ii235–9.
38. von Pawel J, Schiller JH, Shepherd FA, et al. Topotecan versus cyclophosphamide, doxorubicin, and vincristine for the treatment of recurrent small-cell lung cancer. J Clin Oncol. 1999; 17(2):658–67.

39. O'Brien ME, Ciuleanu TE, Tsekov H, et al. Phase III trial comparing supportive care alone with supportive care with oral topotecan in patients with relapsed small-cell lung cancer. J Clin Oncol. 2006;24(34):5441–7.
40. Ettinger DS, Jotte R, Lorigan P, et al. Phase II study of amrubicin as second-line therapy in patients with platinum-refractory small-cell lung cancer. J Clin Oncol. 2010;28(15):2598–603.
41. Jotte R, Conkling P, Reynolds C, et al. Randomized phase II trial of single-agent amrubicin or topotecan as second-line treatment in patients with small-cell lung cancer sensitive to first-line platinum-based chemotherapy. J Clin Oncol. 2011;29(3):287–93.
42. von Pawel J, Jotte R, Spigel DR, et al. Amrubicin improved response rate and progression-free survival vs. topotecan in Phase III trial. J Thorac Oncol. 2011;6(6):S274 (Abstract 2219).
43. Souhami RL, Bradbury I, Geddes DM, Spiro SG, Harper PG, Tobias JS. Prognostic significance of laboratory parameters measured at diagnosis in small cell carcinoma of the lung. Cancer Res. 1985;45(6):2878–82.
44. Spiegelman D, Maurer LH, Ware JH, et al. Prognostic factors in small-cell carcinoma of the lung: an analysis of 1,521 patients. J Clin Oncol. 1989;7(3):344–54.
45. Albain KS, Crowley JJ, LeBlanc M, Livingston RB. Determinants of improved outcome in small-cell lung cancer: an analysis of the 2,580-patient Southwest Oncology Group data base. J Clin Oncol. 1990;8(9):1563–74.
46. Artal-Cortes A, Gomez-Codina J, Gonzalez-Larriba JL, et al. Prospective randomized phase III trial of etoposide/cisplatin versus high-dose epirubicin/cisplatin in small-cell lung cancer. Clin Lung Cancer. 2004;6(3):175–83.
47. Wheatley-Price P, Ma C, Ashcroft LF, et al. The strength of female sex as a prognostic factor in small-cell lung cancer: a pooled analysis of chemotherapy trials from the Manchester Lung Group and Medical Research Council Clinical Trials Unit. Ann Oncol. 2010;21(2):232–7.
48. Cerny T, Blair V, Anderson H, Bramwell V, Thatcher N. Pretreatment prognostic factors and scoring system in 407 small-cell lung cancer patients. Int J Cancer. 1987;39(2):146–9.
49. Souhami RL, Spiro SG, Rudd RM, et al. Five-day oral etoposide treatment for advanced small-cell lung cancer: randomized comparison with intravenous chemotherapy. J Natl Cancer Inst. 1997;89(8):577–80.
50. Girling DJ. Comparison of oral etoposide and standard intravenous multidrug chemotherapy for small-cell lung cancer: a stopped multicentre randomised trial. Medical Research Council Lung Cancer Working Party. Lancet. 1996;348(9027):563–6.
51. Ardizzoni A, Favaretto A, Boni L, et al. Platinum-etoposide chemotherapy in elderly patients with small-cell lung cancer: results of a randomized multicenter phase II study assessing attenuated-dose or full-dose with lenograstim prophylaxis-a Forza Operativa Nazionale Italiana Carcinoma Polmonare and Gruppo Studio Tumori Polmonari Veneto (FONICAP-GSTPV) study. J Clin Oncol. 2005;23(3):569–75.
52. Gridelli C, Gallo C, Morabito A, et al. Phase I-II Trial of Gemcitabine-based first-line chemotherapies for small cell lung cancer in elderly patients with performance status 0-2: the G-STEP Trial. J Thorac Oncol. 2012;7(1):233–42.
53. Okamoto H, Watanabe K, Kunikane H, et al. Randomised phase III trial of carboplatin plus etoposide vs split doses of cisplatin plus etoposide in elderly or poor-risk patients with extensive disease small-cell lung cancer: JCOG 9702. Br J Cancer. 2007;97(2):162–9.
54. Quoix E, Breton JL, Daniel C, et al. Etoposide phosphate with carboplatin in the treatment of elderly patients with small-cell lung cancer: a phase II study. Ann Oncol. 2001;12(7):957–62.
55. Larive S, Bombaron P, Riou R, et al. Carboplatin-etoposide combination in small cell lung cancer patients older than 70 years: a phase II trial. Lung Cancer. 2002;35(1):1–7.
56. Matsui K, Masuda N, Fukuoka M, et al. Phase II trial of carboplatin plus oral etoposide for elderly patients with small-cell lung cancer. Br J Cancer. 1998;77(11):1961–5.
57. Evans WK, Radwi A, Tomiak E, et al. Oral etoposide and carboplatin. Effective therapy for elderly patients with small cell lung cancer. Am J Clin Oncol. 1995;18(2):149–55.
58. Gridelli C, Rossi A, Barletta E, et al. Carboplatin plus vinorelbine plus G-CSF in elderly patients with extensive-stage small-cell lung cancer: a poorly tolerated regimen. Results of a multicentre phase II study. Lung Cancer. 2002;36(3):327–32.

59. Hainsworth JD, Carrell D, Drengler RL, Scroggin Jr C, Greco FA. Weekly combination chemotherapy with docetaxel and gemcitabine as first-line treatment for elderly patients and patients with poor performance status who have extensive-stage small cell lung carcinoma: a Minnie Pearl Cancer Research Network phase II trial. Cancer. 2004;100(11):2437–41.
60. Igawa S, Ryuge S, Fukui T, et al. Amrubicin for treating elderly and poor-risk patients with small-cell lung cancer. Int J Clin Oncol. 2010;15(5):447–52.
61. Inoue A, Ishimoto O, Fukumoto S, et al. A phase II study of amrubicin combined with carboplatin for elderly patients with small-cell lung cancer: North Japan Lung Cancer Study Group Trial 0405. Ann Oncol. 2010;21(4):800–3.
62. Nakao M, Oguri T, Suzuki T, et al. Amrubicin monotherapy for elderly patients with previously treated lung cancer. Intern Med. 2010;49(17):1857–62.
63. Okamoto H, Naoki K, Narita Y, Hida N, Kunikane H, Watanabe K. A combination chemotherapy of carboplatin and irinotecan with granulocyte colony-stimulating factor (G-CSF) support in elderly patients with small cell lung cancer. Lung Cancer. 2006;53(2):197–203.
64. Li J, Chen P, Dai CH, Li XQ, Bao QL. Outcome and treatment in elderly patients with small cell lung cancer: a retrospective study. Geriatr Gerontol Int. 2009;9(2):172–82.
65. Findlay MP, Griffin AM, Raghavan D, et al. Retrospective review of chemotherapy for small cell lung cancer in the elderly: does the end justify the means? Eur J Cancer. 1991;27(12):1597–601.
66. Bonn O, Schmidt-Wolf G, Risse F, Glasmacher A, Kleinschmidt R, Schmidt-Wolf IG. Vindesine and etoposide: a practical and well-tolerated therapy for elderly patients or patients in reduced clinical condition with extensive-stage small-cell lung cancer (SCLC). Med Sci Monit. 2005;11(2):PI19–21.
67. Pallis AG, Shepherd FA, Lacombe D, Gridelli C. Treatment of small-cell lung cancer in elderly patients. Cancer. 2010;116(5):1192–200.
68. Dajczman E, Fu LY, Small D, Wolkove N, Kreisman H. Treatment of small cell lung carcinoma in the elderly. Cancer. 1996;77(10):2032–8.
69. Jara C, Gomez-Aldaravi JL, Tirado R, Meseguer VA, Alonso C, Fernandez A. Small-cell lung cancer in the elderly–is age of patient a relevant factor? Acta Oncol. 1999;38(6):781–6.
70. Siu LL, Shepherd FA, Murray N, Feld R, Pater J, Zee B. Influence of age on the treatment of limited-stage small-cell lung cancer. J Clin Oncol. 1996;14(3):821–8.
71. Nou E. Full chemotherapy in elderly patients with small cell bronchial carcinoma. Acta Oncol. 1996;35(4):399–406.
72. Ludbrook JJ, Truong PT, MacNeil MV, et al. Do age and comorbidity impact treatment allocation and outcomes in limited stage small-cell lung cancer? A community-based population analysis. Int J Radiat Oncol Biol Phys. 2003;55(5):1321–30.
73. Lally BE, Geiger AM, Urbanic JJ, et al. Trends in the outcomes for patients with limited stage small cell lung cancer: an analysis of the Surveillance, Epidemiology, and End Results database. Lung Cancer. 2009;64(2):226–31.
74. Balducci L. Geriatric oncology: challenges for the new century. Eur J Cancer. 2000;36(14):1741–54.
75. Janssen-Heijnen ML, Schipper RM, Razenberg PP, Crommelin MA, Coebergh JW. Prevalence of co-morbidity in lung cancer patients and its relationship with treatment: a population-based study. Lung Cancer. 1998;21(2):105–13.
76. Asmis TR, Ding K, Seymour L, et al. Age and comorbidity as independent prognostic factors in the treatment of non small-cell lung cancer: a review of National Cancer Institute of Canada Clinical Trials Group trials. J Clin Oncol. 2008;26(1):54–9.

Index

C. Gridelli, R.A. Audisio (eds.), *Management of Lung Cancer in Older People*,
DOI 10.1007/978-0-85729-793-8, © Springer-Verlag London 2013

MIX
Papier aus verantwortungsvollen Quellen
Paper from responsible sources
FSC® C105338

If you have any concerns about our products,
you can contact us on
ProductSafety@springernature.com

In case Publisher is established outside the EU,
the EU authorized representative is:
Springer Nature Customer Service Center GmbH
Europaplatz 3, 69115 Heidelberg, Germany

Printed by Libri Plureos GmbH
in Hamburg, Germany